Anatomy and Physiology

THEORY and PRACTICAL

for Diploma in Pharmacy Students

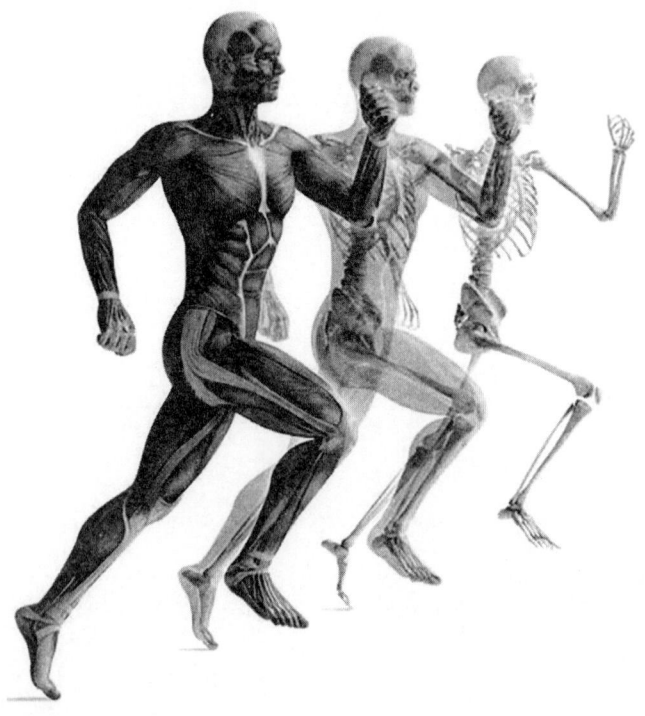

Anatomy and Physiology

THEORY and PRACTICAL

for Diploma in Pharmacy Students

Krishna Garg MBBS MS PhD FAMS FASI, Legend of Anatomy
former Professor and Head
Department of Anatomy
Lady Hardinge Medical College, New Delhi

Medha Joshi MBBS FCGP
Guest Faculty
Pt Deendayal Upadhyaya National Institute for
Persons with Physical Disabilities, New Delhi, and
Amar Jyoti Institute of Physiotherapy, Delhi

Sudipta Kundu MSc
Associate Professor and Head
Department of Physiology
Kalka Dental College
Meerut, UP

With Input from
Meenakshi Saran
Senior Dietician
Max Smart Hospital, Saket, New Delhi

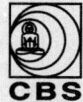

CBS

CBS Publishers & Distributors Pvt Ltd

New Delhi • Bengaluru • Chennai • Kochi • Kolkata • Mumbai
Hyderabad • Jharkhand • Nagpur • Patna • Pune • Uttarakhand

Anatomy and Physiology

THEORY and PRACTICAL

for Diploma in Pharmacy Students

ISBN: 978-93-87964-94-5

Copyright © Authors and Publisher

First Edition: 2019
Reprint: 2021

Published by Satish Kumar Jain and produced by Varun Jain for

CBS Publishers & Distributors Pvt Ltd

4819/XI Prahlad Street, 24 Ansari Road, Daryaganj, New Delhi 110 002, India.
Ph: 23289259, 23266861, 23266867   Website: www.cbspd.com
Fax: 011-23243014   e-mail: delhi@cbspd.com; cbspubs@airtelmail.in.

Corporate Office: 204 FIE, Industrial Area, Patparganj, Delhi 110 092
Ph: 4934 4934   Fax: 4934 4935   e-mail: publishing@cbspd.com; publicity@cbspd.com

- **Bengaluru:** Seema House 2975, 17th Cross, K.R. Road, Banasankari 2nd Stage, Bengaluru 560 070, Karnataka
  Ph: +91-80-26771678/79   Fax: +91-80-26771680   e-mail: bangalore@cbspd.com
- **Chennai:** 7, Subbaraya Street, Shenoy Nagar, Chennai 600 030, Tamil Nadu
  Ph: +91-44-26680620/26681266   Fax: +91-44-42032115   e-mail: chennai@cbspd.com
- **Kochi:** 42/1325, 26, Power House Road, Opp KSEB, Power House, Ernakulam 682 018, Kochi, Kerala
  Ph: +91-484-4059061-67   Fax: +91-484-4059065   e-mail: kochi@cbspd.com
- **Kolkata:** 6/B, Ground Floor, Rameswar Shaw Road, Kolkata-700 014, West Bengal
  Ph: +91-33-22891126, 22891127, 22891128   e-mail: kolkata@cbspd.com
- **Mumbai:** 83-C, Dr E Moses Road, Worli, Mumbai-400018, Maharashtra
  Ph: +91-22-24902340/41   Fax: +91-22-24902342   e-mail: mumbai@cbspd.com

Representatives

- **Hyderabad**   0-9885175004
- **Patna**   0-9334159340
- **Jharkhand**   0-9811541605
- **Pune**   0-9623451994
- **Nagpur**   0-9421945513
- **Uttarakhand**   0-9716462459

Printed at: Mudrak, Noida, UP, India

Preface

Anatomy and Physiology (Theory and Practical) for Diploma in Pharmacy Students has been designed as per the syllabus prescribed by Pharmacy Council of India (ER-2014). The best part of the book is that it contains both theoretical and practical aspects of anatomy and physiology for pharmacy course making it a "two-in-one" book.

Students these days are quite enthusiastic about taking up a career in pharmacy with the result that many of them are opting for it as a subject of their choice.

The language of the book is lucid and simple. The text has been covered in 12 chapters, providing necessary and adequate knowledge of both anatomy and physiology. At the end of each chapter "Points to Remember" are given which form the "must know" component of the concerned chapter. To evaluate the knowledge and skill acquired, examination-oriented "Multiple Choice Questions" are given with their respective answers.

The practicals on anatomy encompass the skeleton and various systems. Students have to identify the various parts and enumerate their functions. The last chapter of anatomy practical is on histology of the basic tissues. One can see the histological slides under the microscope and identify various components of the tissue. Physiology practicals include study of microscope, determination of various parameters of blood, recording of body temperature, pulse, heart rate, blood pressure and electrocardiogram. The practical component of both the subjects has been supplemented by eight coloured plates.

Diploma in pharmacy is a "stepping stone" for bachelor's and master's in pharmacy or setting up a chemist's shop. As is well known, higher studies are an unending lifelong learning.

We are grateful to Mr SK Jain, Chairman, and Mr Varun Jain, Director, CBS Publishers & Distributors, for accepting the project and encouraging us to complete it in time.

Constant and continuous support of Mr YN Arjuna, Senior Vice President (Publishing, Editorial and Publicity); Mrs Ritu Chawla, GM (Production); Mr Sanju, Graphic Designer; Mrs Sunita Rautela, DTP Operator; and Mr Mukund Kumar, Proof Reader; is deeply appreciated. Impetus provided by Mr Dignesh Vashist is also welcome.

The feedback about the book may please be sent to *dr.krishnagarg@gmail.com*

happy reading

Krishna Garg
Medha Joshi
Sudipta Kundu

Contents

PRACTICAL PART

Anatomy

Physiology

HUMAN ANATOMY AND PHYSIOLOGY FOR DIPLOMA IN PHARMACY

Theory (75 hours)

Scope of anatomy and physiology: Definition of various terms used in anatomy. Structure of cell, function of its components with special reference to mitochondria and miscrosomes.

Elementary tissues: Elementary tissues of the body, i.e. epithelial tissue, muscular tissue, connective tissue and nervous tissue.

Skeletal system: Structure and function of skeleton. Classification of joints and their function. Joint disorders.

Cardiovascular system: Composition of blood, functions of blood elements. Blood group and coagulation of blood. Brief information regarding disorders of blood. Name and functions of lymph glands. Structure and function of various parts of the heart. Arterial and venous system with special reference to the names and positions of main arteries and veins. Blood pressure and its recording. Brief information about cardiovascular disorders.

Respiratory system: Various parts of respiratory system and their functions, physiology of respiration.

Urinary system: Various parts of urinary system and their functions, structure and functions of kidney. Physiology of urine formation. Patho-physiology of renal diseases and edema.

Muscular system: Structure of skeletal muscle, physiology of muscle contraction. Names, positions, attachments and functions of various skeletal muscles. Physiology of neuromuscular junction.

Central nervous system: Various parts of central nervous system, brain and its parts, functions and reflex action. Anatomy and physiology of autonomic nervous system.

Sensory organs: Elementary knowledge of structure and functions of the organs of taste, smell, ear, eye and skin. Physiology of pain.

Digestive system: Names of various parts of digestive system and their functions, structure and functions of liver, physiology of digestion and absorption.

Endocrine system: Endocrine glands and hormones. Location of glands, their hormones and functions, pituitary, thyroid, adrenal and pancreas.

Reproductive system: Physiology and anatomy of reproductive systems.

Practicals (50 hours)

1. Study of the human skeleton
2. Study with the help of charts and models of the following system and organs—digestive system, cardiovascular system, reproductive system, respiratory system, urinary system, eye and ear
3. Microscopic examination of epithelial tissue, cardiac muscle, smooth muscle, skeletal muscle. Connective tissue and nervous tissues.
4. Examination of blood films for TLC, DLC and malarial parasite.
5. Determination of RBCs, clotting time of blood, erythrocyte sedimentation rate and haemo-globin value.
6. Recording of body temperature, pulse, heart-rate, blood pressure and ECG.

Scope of Anatomy and Physiology

Human body is unique, comprising of various organs and systems, which work both independently and interdependently according to its needs. The human body has to be studied from its normal structural and functional point of view. Once the normal structure and functions are understood, it is easy to comprehend the diseased state and necessary treatment to bring the status back to normal.

Anatomy is the science of learning the normal structure of the human. **Physiology** deals with learning and understanding the functions of the body. Thus, anatomy and physiology are the two sides of the same coin. Physiology is the enacting of various scenes in anatomy hall/theatre. The two branches of medical science are intimately related.

SUBDIVISIONS OF ANATOMY AND PHYSIOLOGY

The main subdivisions of anatomy are **gross anatomy** including neuroanatomy, **histology** or microscopic anatomy, **embryology** or developmental anatomy.

Surface anatomy is the projection of deeper structures on the skin.

Clinical anatomy emphasizes certain relations that are important to the physician/surgeon/dentist.

Radiological and imaging anatomy is the study of various components of the body by using X-ray, ultrasound, magnetic resonance imaging (MRI), etc.

PARTS OF THE BODY

The human body consists of the following parts:
1. Head, neck and brain
2. Trunk divided into upper part or thorax and lower part or abdomen (pelvis).
3. Two upper limbs
4. Two lower limbs.

Body Cavities

The organs that make up the systems of the body are contained in three cavities, i.e. cranial, thoracic and abdominopelvic cavity (Fig. 1.1).

Head is the upper most or cranial part of the body. Bone of the head is the skull (cranial cavity) which contains brain, and special sense organs like eyes, ears, nose and tongue.

Neck follows the head. Bones of neck are 1–7 cervical vertebrae. It contains big blood vessels, nerves and tubes like trachea and oesophagus.

Trunk

It is divided into:
1. An upper part or thoracic cavity.
2. A lower part or abdominopelvic cavity.

Thorax

Thorax lies below the neck. Bones in this part are 1–12 thoracic vertebrae, one sternum and 12 pair of ribs and costal cartilages. All these form the bony thoracic cavity which contains single heart, more to the left side of the body, blood vessels, right and left lungs with trachea

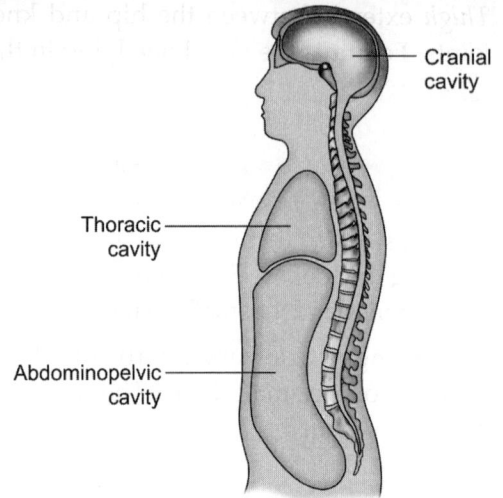

Fig. 1.1: Body cavities

and bronchi, oesophagus, nerves and lymph nodes. **Mediastinum** is the space between the lungs including the structures found there, such as heart, oesophagus and blood vessels.

Abdomen

Abdomen is present below the thorax. The thoracoabdominal diaphragm separates the two cavities. Bones here are 1 to 5 lumbar vertebrae. It contains digestive system and urinary system. It also contains spleen, suprarenal glands, blood vessels, nerves and lymph nodes. Many organs are pushed up in thoracic cavity.

Lower part of abdomen is called the **pelvis,** bounded by the two hip bones and sacrum with coccyx. The **pelvic cavity** so formed contains lower part of urinary and digestive systems. In between it contains the reproductive organs which are different in male and female.

The lowest part of abdomen is the **perineum** which contains the openings of urethra and anal canal in male and openings of urethra, vagina and anal canal in female.

Upper Limbs

They are made of the following parts:

1. *Shoulder girdle* is made of two bones, the **clavicle and scapula** and includes pectoral region in the front of chest, scapular region

in the back of chest and shoulder joint. Axilla lies between the upper aspect of thorax and the medial side of upper limb (Fig. 1.2).

2. *Arm or brachium* extends between shoulder joint and the elbow joint. Only one bone, **humerus** forms the skeleton of arm.

3. *Forearm or antebrachium* extends between the elbow and the wrist joints. Two bones, the **radius** laterally and **ulna** medially lie in this region. Radius rotates over ulna causing movements of pronation of forearm with the palm facing backwards. When the two bones are parallel to each other, the position is called supine, with the palm facing forwards.

4. Hand or carpal region extends from the wrist to the tips of the digits. Bones in this region are 8 small carpal bones, 5 metacarpals and 14 phalanges.

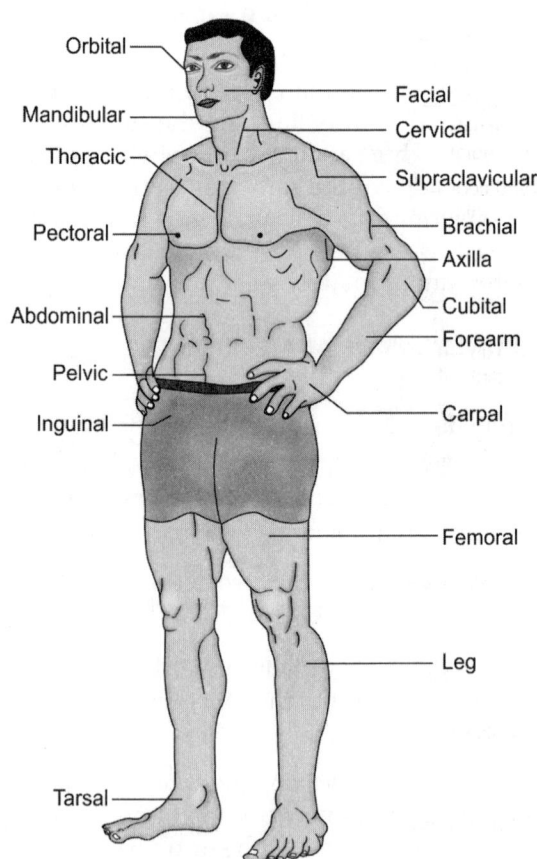

Fig. 1.2: Regions of the body

The **palm** is the region over the metacarpals and the phalanges form the skeleton of the digits.

There are five digits from lateral to medial side. These are called 1st digit or thumb, 2nd digit or index finger, 3rd digit or middle finger, 4th digit or ring finger and 5th digit or little finger (Fig. 1.3).

Lower Limbs

These are two identical limbs. Its various parts are:

1. *Pelvic girdle* comprised of two hip bones and a sacrum. Each **hip bone** is made up of three bones: (1) the ilium, (2) ischium and (3) pubis. Inguinal region in front is at the junction of abdomen and lower limb and gluteal region on the back of ilium and ischium.

2. *Thigh* extends between the hip and knee joints. **Femur** is the only bone lying in this area.

3. *Leg* extends between the knee and ankle joints. Two bones, a large **tibia** and slender **fibula** form skeleton of this region.

4. *Foot* lies distal to the ankle joint. Bones forming the foot are 7 tarsal bones, 5 metatarsal bones and 14 small phalanges.

   Phalanges are very small and form skeleton of the small digits. The digits are named from medial to lateral as 1st digit or big toe, 2nd digit or 2nd toe to 5th digit or 5th toe. The sole of the foot faces plantarwards (Fig. 1.3).

TERMINOLOGY

Anatomical Position

When a person is standing straight, with eyes looking forwards, both arms by the side of body, palms facing forwards, both feet together, the position is anatomical position. All the descriptions of viscera, vessels and nerves are done as if the body is in anatomical position (Fig. 1.4).

Supine Position

When a person is lying on his/her back, arms by the side, palms facing upwards and feet together, the position is supine position.

Prone Position

Person lying on his face, chest and abdomen, is said to be in prone position.

Lithotomy Position

Person lying on her back with legs up and feet supported with straps. In this position, the perineal region is well visualised. This position is mostly used for delivery of the baby (Fig. 1.5).

Planes

A plane passing through the centre of the body dividing it into two equal right and left halves is **median** or **midsagittal plane** (Fig. 1.6).

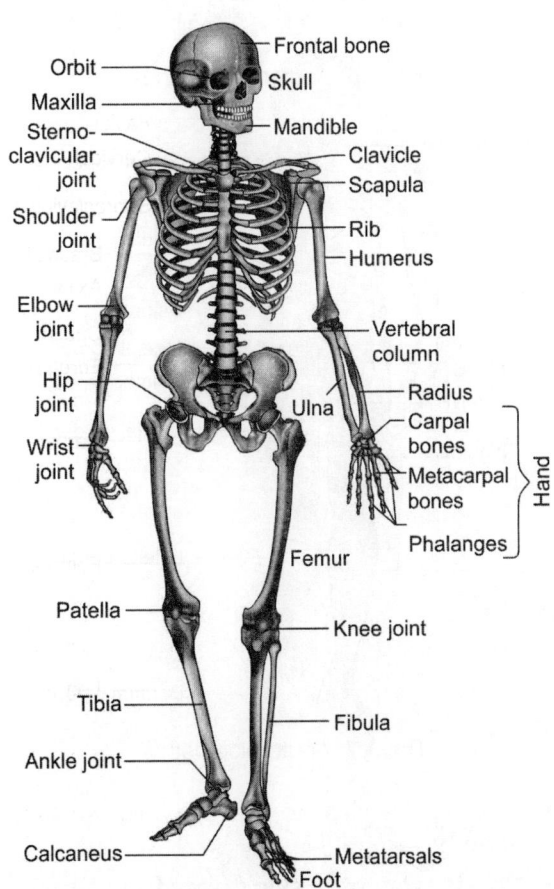

Fig.1.3: Human skeleton

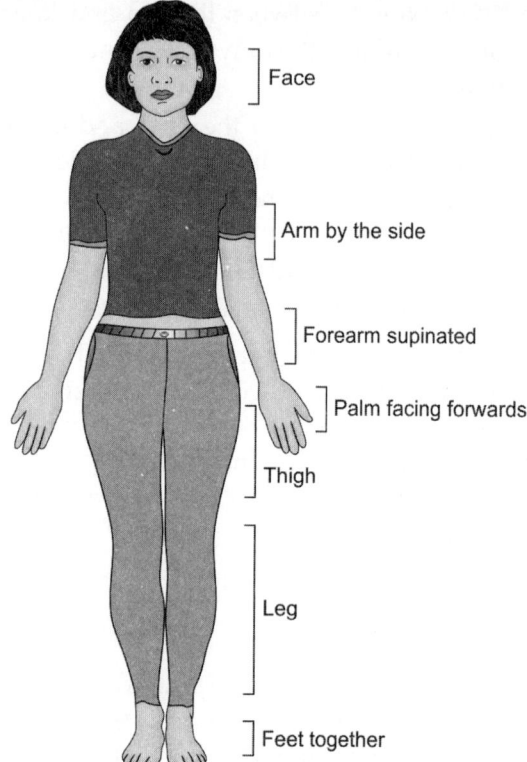

Fig. 1.4: Anatomical position

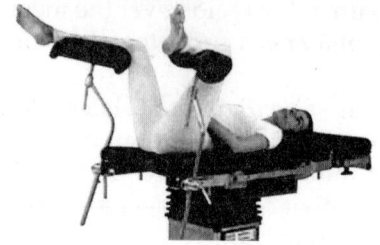

Fig. 1.5: Lithotomy position

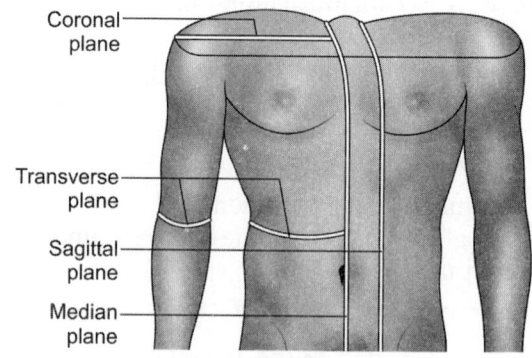

Fig. 1.6: Anatomical planes

Any plane parallel to median plane is a **sagittal plane.**

A plane at right angles to median/ mid-sagittal plane which divides the body into anterior and posterior halves is called a **coronal plane.**

A plane at right angles to both sagittal and coronal planes which divides the body into upper and lower parts is called a **transverse plane.**

Terms Used in Relation to Trunk

- *Ventral or anterior* is the front of trunk (Figs 1.7 and 1.8).
- *Dorsal or posterior* is the back of trunk.
- *Medial* is a plane close to the median plane.
- *Lateral* is plane away from the median plane.
- *Cranial/superior* is close to the head end of trunk.
- *Caudal/inferior* is close to the lower end of the trunk.

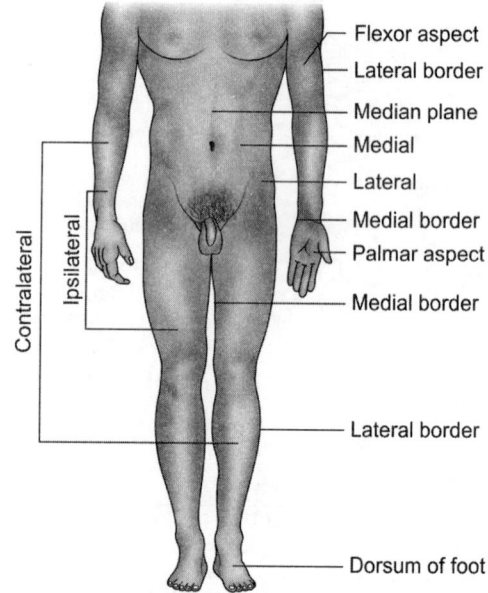

Fig. 1.7: Anatomical terms

- *Superficial* is close to skin/towards surface of body.
- *Deep* is away from skin/away from surface of body.

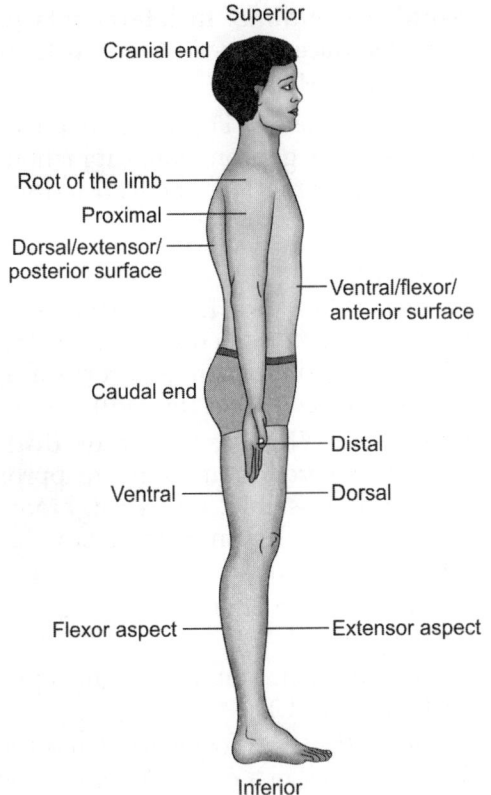

Superior
Cranial end
Root of the limb
Proximal
Dorsal/extensor/posterior surface
Ventral/flexor/anterior surface
Caudal end
Distal
Ventral
Dorsal
Flexor aspect
Extensor aspect
Inferior

Fig. 1.8: Anatomical terms

- *Ipsilateral:* On the same side of body as another structure (Fig. 1.7).
- *Contralateral:* On opposite side of body from another structure (Fig. 1.7).

Terms Used in Relation to Upper Limb

- *Ventral or anterior* is the front or flexor aspect (Fig. 1.7).
- *Dorsal or posterior* is the back aspect.
- *Medial border* lies along the little finger, medial border of forearm and arm.
- *Lateral border* follows the thumb, lateral border of forearm and arm.
- *Proximal* is close to root of limb, while **distal** is away from the root (Fig. 1.8).
- *Palmar* aspect is the front of the palm.
- *Dorsal* aspect of hand is on the back of palm.
- *Flexor* aspect is front of upper limb.
- *Extensor* aspect is back of upper limb.

Terms Used in Relation to Lower Limb

- *Ventral* aspect is the back of lower limb (Fig. 1.8).
- *Dorsal* aspect is the front of lower limb.
- *Medial border* lies along the big toe or hallux, medial border of leg and thigh (Fig. 1.7).
- *Lateral border* lies along the little toe, lateral border of leg and thigh (Fig. 1.7).
- *Flexor* aspect is back of lower limb.
- *Extensor* aspect is front of lower limb.
- *Proximal* is close to the root of limb, while **distal** is away from it.

Terms of Position of Body Movements

Movements in general at synovial joints are divided into four main categories.

1. *Gliding movement:* Relatively, flat surfaces move back-and-forth and from side-to-side with respect to one another. The angle between articulating bones does not change significantly.
2. *Angular movements:* Angle between articulating bones decreases or increases. In **flexion** there is decrease in angle between articulating bones and in **extension** there is increase in angle between articulating bones (Figs 1.9 and 1.10). **Lateral flexion** is

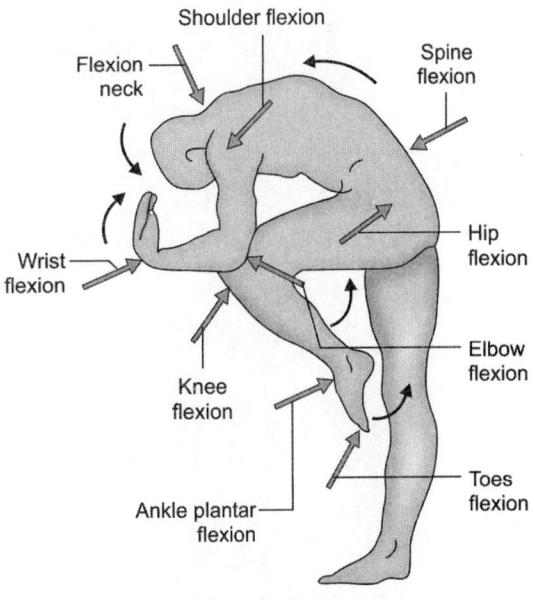

Shoulder flexion
Flexion neck
Spine flexion
Wrist flexion
Hip flexion
Knee flexion
Elbow flexion
Ankle plantar flexion
Toes flexion

Fig. 1.9: Flexion

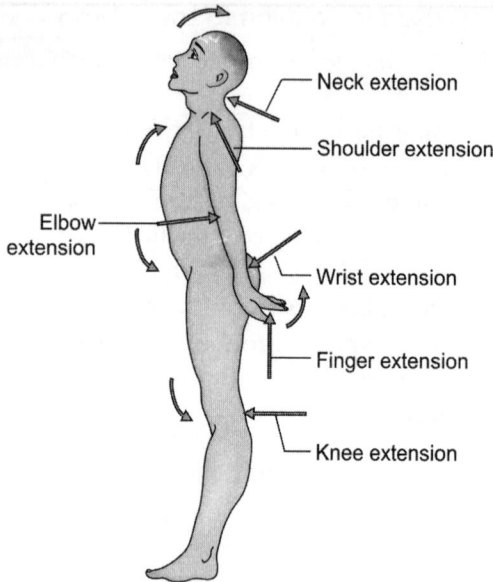

Fig. 1.10: Extension

movement of trunk sideways to the right or left at the waist. **Adduction** is movement of bone towards midline whereas **abduction** is movement of bone away from midline (Fig. 1.11)

3. *Rotation:* A bone revolves around its own longitudinal axis. In **medial rotation,** anterior surface of a bone of limb is turned toward the midline. In **lateral rotation,** anterior surface of bone of limb is turned away from midline.

4. *Special movements:* These occur only at certain joints, e.g. pronation, supination in forearm; protraction and retraction at temporomandibular joint.

In Upper Limb

1. *Flexion:* When two flexor surfaces are brought close to each other, e.g. in elbow joint when front of arm and forearm are opposed to each other (Fig. 1.9).
2. *Extension:* When extensor or dorsal surfaces are brought in as much approximation as possible, e.g. straightening the arm and forearm at the elbow joint (Figs 1.10 and 1.12).
3. *Abduction:* When limb is taken away from the body (Fig. 1.11).
4. *Adduction:* When limb is brought close to the body (Fig. 1.11).
5. *Circumduction:* It is movement of distal end of a body part in a circle. A combination of flexion, abduction, extension and

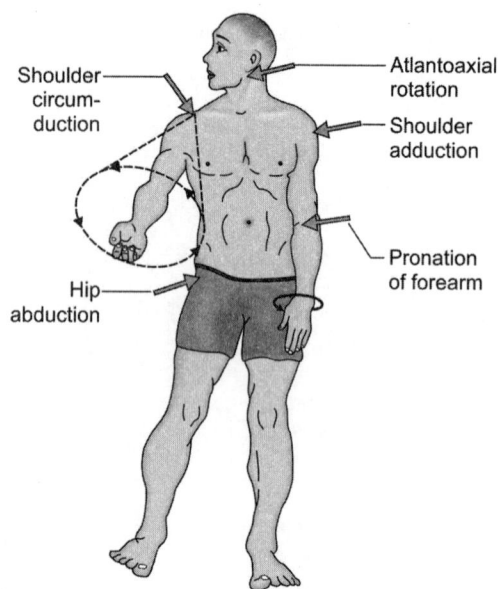

Fig. 1.11: Movements

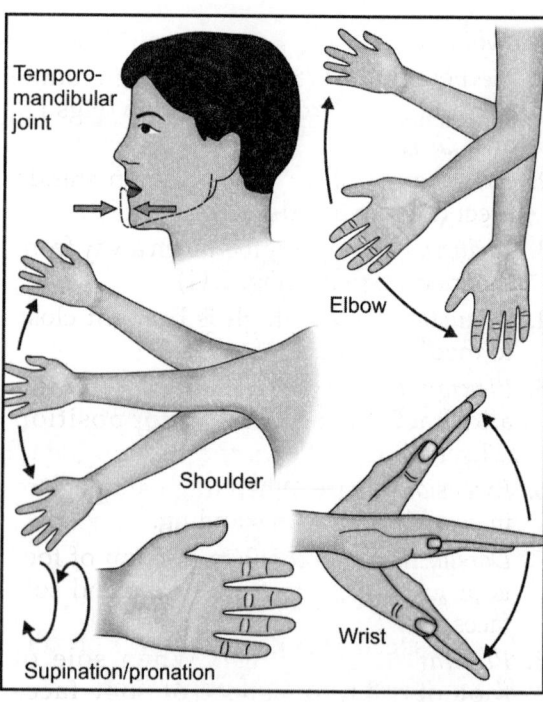

Fig. 1.12: Movements of some of the joints

adduction in a sequence is called circumduction as in bowling (Fig. 1.11).

6. *Medial rotation:* When the arm rotates medially bringing the flexed forearm across the chest.

7. *Lateral rotation:* When arm rotates laterally taking the flexed forearm away from the body.

8. *Supination:* When the palm is facing forwards or upwards, as in putting food in the mouth (Fig. 1.12).

9. *Pronation:* When the palm faces backwards or downwards, as in picking food with fingers from the plate (Fig. 1.11).

10. *Adduction of digits/fingers:* When all fingers get together (*see* Fig. 3.39A).

11. *Abduction:* When all fingers separate. The axis of movement of the fingers is the line passing through the centre of the middle finger (*see* Fig. 3.39B).

12. *Opposition of thumb:* When tip of thumb touches the tips of any of the fingers.

13. *Circumduction of thumb:* Movement of flexion, abduction, extension and adduction in sequence (Fig. 1.11).

In Lower Limb

1. *Flexion of thigh:* When front of thigh comes in contact with front of abdomen (Figs 1.9 and 1.13).

2. *Extension of thigh:* When person stands erect (Figs 1.10 and 1.13).

3. *Abduction:* When thigh is taken away from the median plane (Fig. 1.11).

4. *Adduction:* When thigh is brought close to median plane.

5. *Flexion of knee:* When back of thigh and back of leg come in opposition (Fig. 1.13).

6. *Extension of knee:* When thigh and leg are in straight line as in standing.

7. *Dorsiflexion of foot:* When dorsum of foot is brought close to front of leg and sole faces forwards.

8. *Plantar flexion of foot:* When sole of foot or plantar aspect of foot faces backwards.

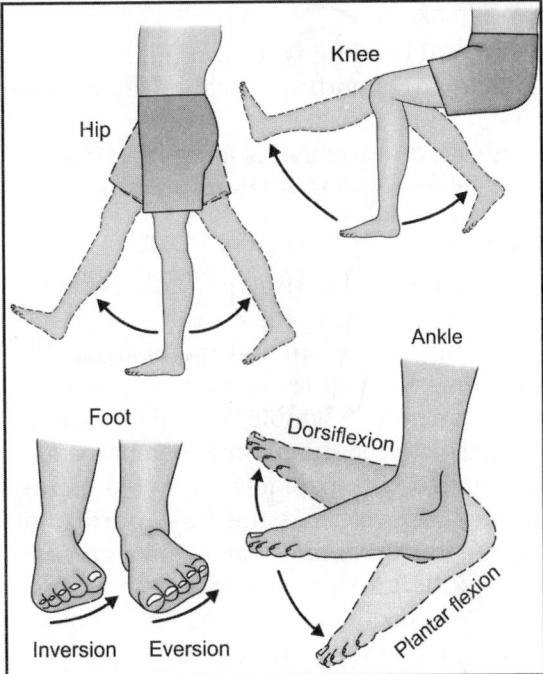

Fig. 1.13: Movements of joints of lower limb

9. *Inversion of foot:* When medial border of foot is raised from the ground (Fig. 1.13).

10. *Eversion of foot:* When lateral border of foot is raised from ground.

In the Neck

1. *Flexion:* When face comes closer to chest (Fig. 1.9).

2. *Extension:* When face is brought away from the chest (Fig. 1.10).

3. *Lateral flexion:* When ear is brought close to shoulder.

4. *Opening the mouth:* When lower jaw is lowered to open the mouth.

5. *Closure of the mouth:* When lower jaw is opposed to the upper jaw, closing the mouth.

6. *Protraction:* When lower jaw slides forwards in its socket in the temporal bone of skull (Fig. 1.12).

7. *Retraction:* When lower jaw slides backwards in its socket in the temporal bone of skull.

In the Trunk

1. Forward bending is **flexion** (Fig. 1.9).
2. Backward bending is called **extension** (Fig. 1.10).
3. Sideward movement is **lateral flexion**.
4. Sideward rotation is **lateral rotation**.

CELL: STRUCTURE AND FUNCTIONS

Cells are the smallest structural and functional units of body. Each cell consists of a plasma membrane, cytoplasm and the nucleus. The plasma membrane surrounds and contains the cytoplasm of cell. Cytoplasm is all the cellular contents between the plasma membrane and the nucleus. It consists of cytosol and organelles. Cytosol is the fluid portion of cytoplasm, containing water, ions, glucose, amino acids, fatty acids, proteins, lipids, ATP and waste products. It is the site of many chemical reactions required for a cell's existence. Organelles are specialized structures with characteristic shapes that have specific functions (Fig. 1.14).

Plasma Membrane

Also called cell membrane. It consists of two layers of lipids with some protein molecules embedded in them. The major lipids are phospholipids. The proteins in the cell membrane function as carriers, enzymes, ion channels for passage of substances and receptors. Cell membrane is semipermeable, allowing selected substances to pass through it.

Organelles

Nucleus

Every cell in the body has a nucleus surrounded by cytoplasm and a plasma membrane. The skeletal muscle fibre has several nuclei while the mature red blood cell has no nucleus. The nucleus contains the body's genetic material which directs the activities of the cell. The genetic material is present in chromosomes. Each chromosome is made up of DNA molecule. The DNA and proteins called histones inside the nucleus are coiled together to form a fine network of threads called chromatin. The chromatin becomes more tightly coiled to form chromosome. Each nucleus also has a nucleolus, a patchwork of granules rich in RNA. Nucleolus is the site of synthesis of ribosomes. The functional subunit of chromosome is called gene. Cells synthesize only the defined range of proteins appropriate to their specialized function but each cell contains the total complement of genes required to synthesize all the proteins in the body. Each human body cell has 46 chromosomes, 23 inherited from each parent.

Mitochondria

It is a sausage shaped organelle, which is the **power generating unit** of the cell. Its number in the cytoplasm is proportional to the degree of cellular activity.

It contains enzymes concerned with oxidation of glucose, amino acids and fatty acids and release the chemical energy in the form of ATP.

Lysosomes

These are large, irregular structures surrounded by a membrane. They contain digestive enzymes for breaking down larger

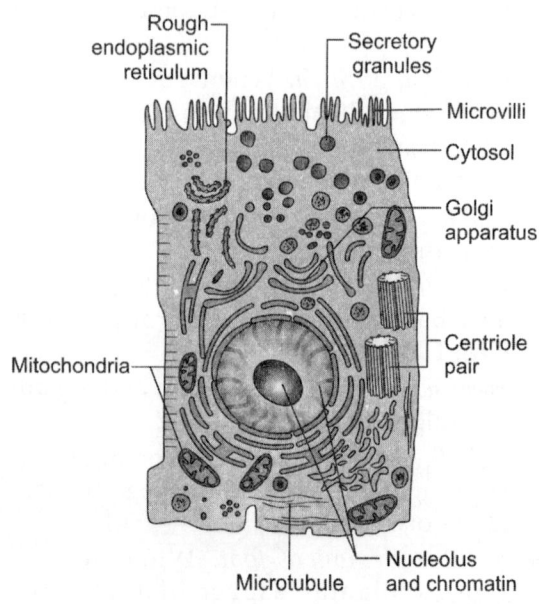

Fig. 1.14: A typical cell

molecules (of RNA, DNA, carbohydrates and proteins) inside the cell into smaller particles.

Peroxisomes

Peroxisomes are enzyme containing bodies surrounded by a membrane. These enzymes are concerned with various anabolic and catabolic reactions.

Endoplasmic Reticulum (ER)

It is a complex series of tubules in cytoplasm. The walls of tubule are made up of membrane. It is of two types: (1) smooth and (2) rough.

Smooth ER synthesises lipids and steroid hormones.

Rough ER has ribosomes attached on the surface and is the site of protein synthesis.

Ribosomes

These are tiny granules composed of RNA and proteins. They are the site of protein synthesis from amino acids.

Golgi Apparatus

It consists of stacks of closely folded flattened membranous sacs. It acts as a storehouse for the synthesized proteins which are packaged into membrane bound secretory granules.

Cytoskeleton

It is a system of fibres, made up of micro-filaments (maintain the cellular structure and provide structural support) and microtubules (permit movement of the cell and of the organelles within the cell).

Microsomes are artifacts reformed from pieces of endoplasmic reticulum when euka-ryotic cells are broken up in the laboratory. Microsomes are not present in healthy living cells.

CELL DIVISION

Cell division is the process by which cells reproduce themselves. It consists of both nuclear division and cytoplasmic division.

Cell division that results in an increase in the number of body cells is called somatic cell division and involves a nuclear division called mitosis plus cytoplasmic division. Before the mitosis, the chromosomes duplicate (replicate), so that identical chromosomes can be passed on to the next generation of cells. Mitosis results in formation of two daughter cells (Fig. 1.15).

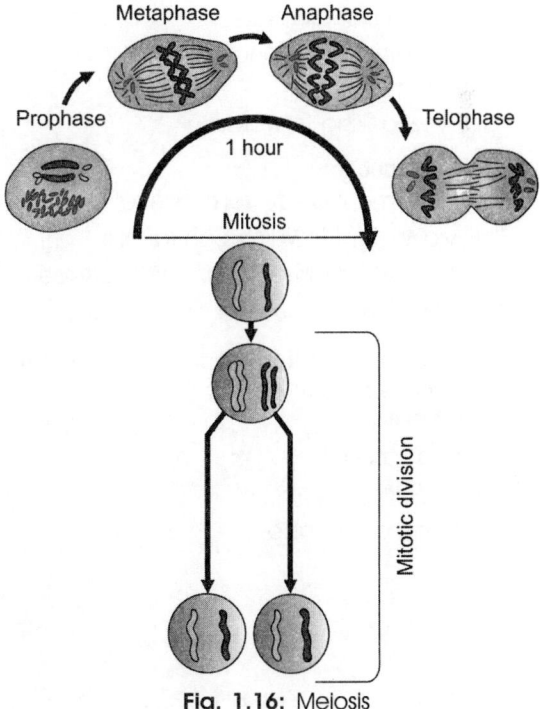

Fig. 1.16: Meiosis

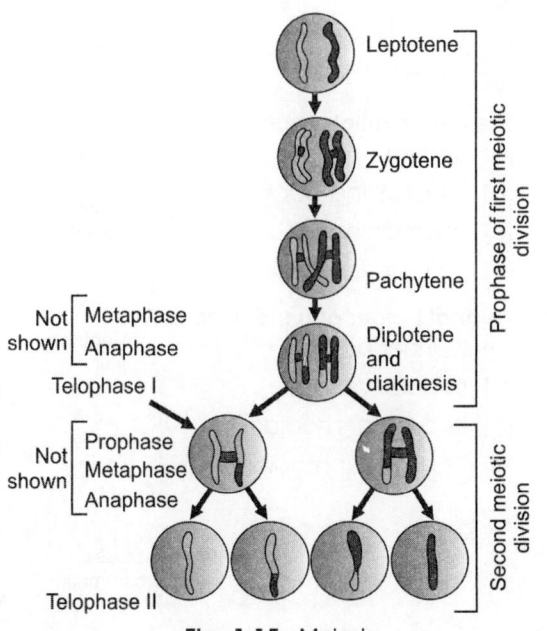

Fig. 1.15: Meiosis

Cell division that results in production of sperm and oocyte is called reproductive cell division and consists of a nuclear division called meiosis plus cytoplasmic division. Meiosis consists of a special two step division, in which the number of chromosomes in nucleus is reduced by half, followed by cytoplasmic division.

Meiotic division results in formation of four daughter cells (Fig. 1.16).

In male, all four spermatozoa are functional. In female, only one daughter cell, the ovum is functional, the remaining three are small non-functional polar bodies.

Points to Remember

1. Anatomical position is the most important position for understanding anatomy.
2. Median plane is only one plane in the trunk.
3. Pronation and supination of forearm are special movements which permit "picking up of food (pronation)" and "putting it in the mouth (supination)".
4. Big toe being in the same plane as rest of the toes is unique to human.
5. Median/midsagittal plane divides the body into right and left halves.
6. Coronal plane divides the body/any part into anterior and posterior parts.
7. Transverse/horizontal plane divides the body/part into upper and lower portions.

MCQs

1. **Anatomical position has following features except:**
   (a) Person standing erect
   (b) Forearms are pronated
   (c) Feet together
   (d) Eyes looking forwards

2. **Define abduction:**
   (a) Movement away from central axis
   (b) Movement towards central axis
   (c) Approximation of the ventral surfaces
   (d) Approximation of the dorsal surfaces

3. **What is the position of forearms in the anatomical position?**
   (a) Pronated
   (b) Supinated
   (c) Midprone
   (d) None of the above

4. **Plane at right angle to the long axis of body/body part is called:**
   (a) Sagittal
   (b) Coronal
   (c) Transverse/horizontal
   (d) Oblique

5. **The term cranial means:**
   (a) Towards the head
   (b) Towards the back
   (c) Towards the tail
   (d) Towards the front

6. **Preaxial border of upper limb is:**
   (a) Its inner border
   (b) Its outer border
   (c) Its anterior median line
   (d) Its posterior median line

Ans 1 b   2 a   3 b   4 c   5 a   6 b

Elementary Tissues

BASIC TISSUES (ELEMENTARY TISSUES)

There are four basic tissues:

1. Epithelium (epithelial tissue)
2. Connective tissue
3. Muscle (muscular tissue)
4. Neurons (nervous tissue)

Every structure/organ in the body is made up of varying combinations of these tissues.

Epithelium

Epithelial tissue form sheets of cells to cover surfaces, to line cavities and form glands.

Thus, it forms the surface lining of skin and a thin layer of cells on the outer surface of lung, stomach, intestines. It also forms an inner lining for hollow viscera like stomach, intestines.

The cells are closely packed and the intercellular substance, called **matrix**, is minimal. The cells lie on a **basement membrane** of connective tissue.

Classification of Epithelial Tissues

1. Simple epithelia if they consist of single layer of identical cells.
2. Stratified epithelia if they consist of multiple layer of cells of various shapes.

Simple epithelia are usually found on absorptive or secretory surfaces. They are of following types and are named according to shape of cells, which differ according to their functions.

1. *Squamous* (scale like) **epithelium** lines the alveoli of lungs, the blood vessels and lymphatics. This is made up of extremely thin, flattened cells closely fitted together, forming a thin and very smooth membrane. Diffusion takes place freely through this lining (Fig. 2.1).

2. *Cuboidal epithelium* lines the acini of thyroid gland, kidney tubules and small ducts of glands. It consists of cube shaped cells. It is actively involved in secretion, absorption and excretion (Fig. 2.2).

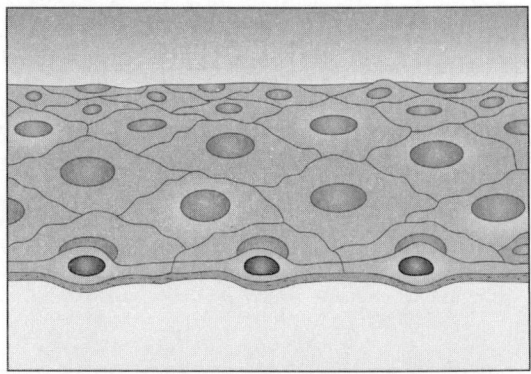

Fig. 2.1: Simple squamous epithelium

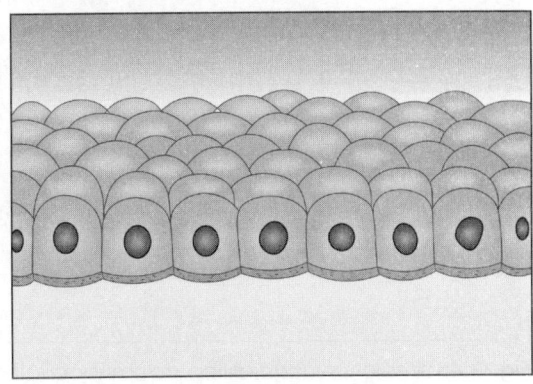

Fig. 2.2: Simple cuboidal epithelium

3. *Columnar epithelium* is made up of tall rectangular cells found in the lining of stomach and intestines. Their function is absorption of products of digestion and secretion of mucus (Fig. 2.3).

4. *Pseudostratified epithelium* is seen in trachea. The cells are of varying height giving a false appearance of layers of cells (Fig. 2.4).

5. *Ciliated epithelium* is formed by columnar cells, each of which has many **cilia** (fine, hair like processes). It is found in uterine tubes and respiratory passages. The wave like movement of cilia propels the contents of tubes (Fig. 2.5).

6. *Stratified epithelium* protects the underlying structures from mechanical wear and tear. It is of following types:

7. *Stratified squamous epithelium* is composed of multiple layers. The cells are of various shapes. In deepest layers cells are mainly columnar and as they grow towards the surface, they become flattened. It lines the oesophagus, vagina and mouth cavity in **non-keratinised** form (Fig. 2.6). **Stratified squamous keratinised** forms the epithelium of the skin, hair and nails. Here, the upper most layers of cells are converted into keratin (Fig. 2.7).

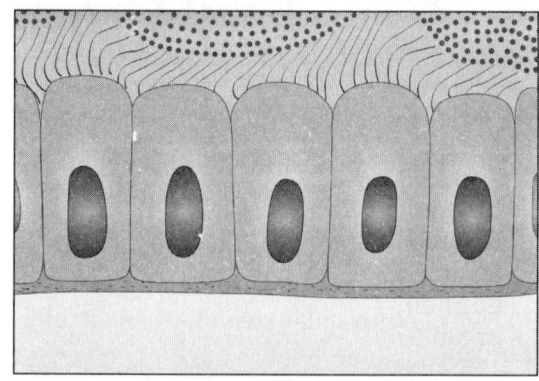

Fig. 2.5: Ciliated columnar epithelium

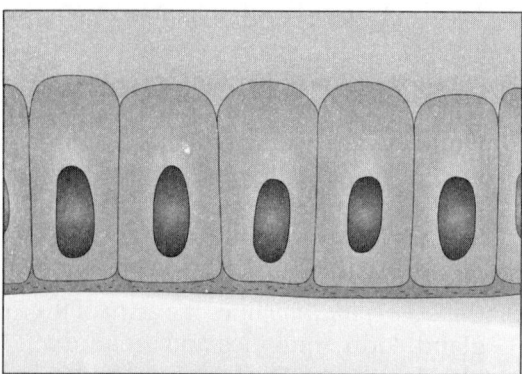

Fig. 2.3: Simple columnar epithelium

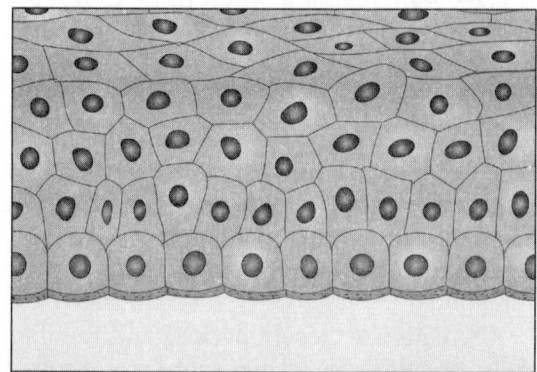

Fig. 2.6: Stratified squamous non-keratinised epithelium

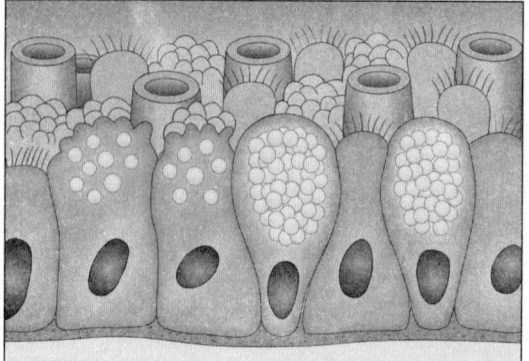

Fig. 2.4: Simple pseudostratified columnar ciliated epithelium

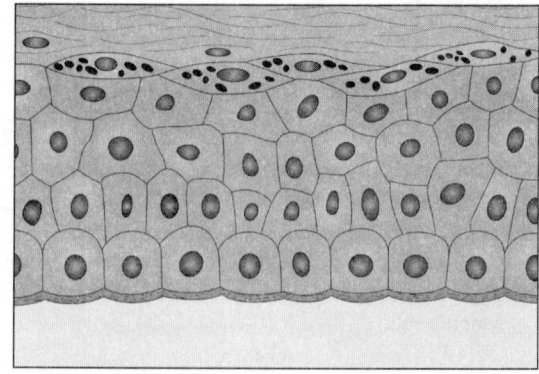

Fig. 2.7: Stratified squamous keratinised epithelium

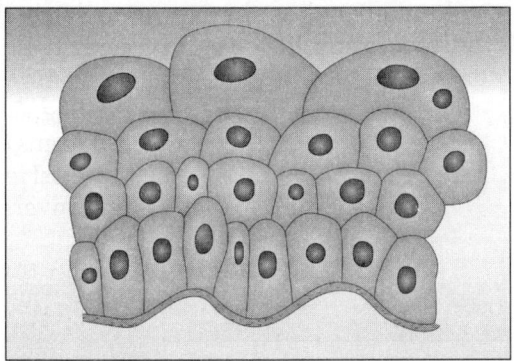

Fig. 2.8: Transitional epithelium of urinary bladder

8. *Transitional epithelium* lines the urinary bladder. The upper-most layers are not flattened but are dome shaped. The lower layers are pear shaped and columnar. This epithelium allows for distension of the organ (Fig. 2.8).

Functions of Epithelium

1. *Mechanical protection* as in case of skin, which prevents mechanical injury to the deeper tissues.
2. *Conservation of moisture:* Stratified epithelium prevents loss of water from the body.
3. *Absorption:* Single layered or simple epithelium has the property of absorption of the end products of digestion.

4. *Secretion:* Epithelial cells may become specialized to form unicellular glands, e.g. goblet cells. They may also become specialized to form multicellular glands, e.g. exocrine and endocrine glands.
5. *Excretion:* The tubular epithelium of kidney is concerned with the function of excreting the waste products of metabolism.
6. *Sensory perception:* Certain epithelial cells are greatly modified to receive sensory impulses and transmit them to the nervous system.
7. *Chemoreception:* The gustatory cells of the epithelium of the tongue are also sensory receptors, but they react to chemical substances.

Connective Tissue

It is most abundant tissue in body. It is a supporting tissue that helps to bind other tissues together. It contains not only cells but considerable amount of material around and between the cells, **the extracellular matrix.** The matrix consists of fibres and ground substance containing a variety of macromolecules.

Cells of Connective Tissue

The different types of cells of connective tissue are:

1. Fibroblasts (Fig. 2.9)

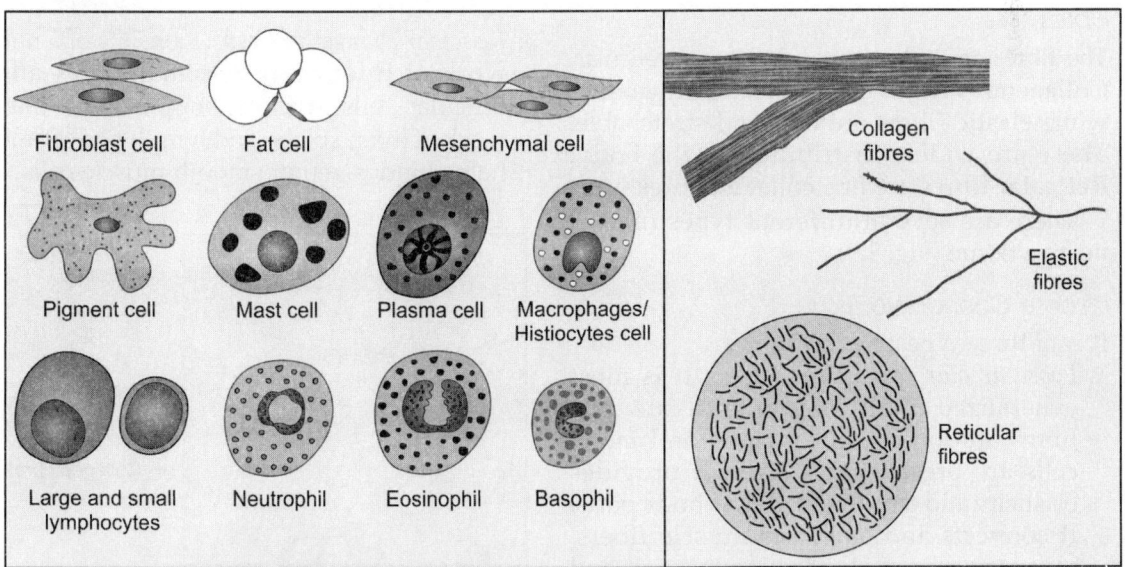

Fig. 2.9: Various types of cells and fibres of connective tissue

2. Macrophages
3. Plasma cells
4. Mast cells
5. Fat cells.

Other cells are described in Chapter 8.

The main cell type is the **fibroblast** which manufactures both the fibres and the ground substance.

Fibroblasts are large flat cells with irregular processes. They produce **collagen, elastic and reticulin fibres.** Fibroblasts are very active in wound healing (tissue repair).

The connective tissue also has **fat cells, macrophages, leukocytes and mast cells.**

Fat cells, occur singly or in groups. Fat cells are abundant in adipose tissue.

Macrophages are irregular cells with granular cytoplasm. They are important in body's defence mechanism and help the body to get rid of dead or dying cells, bacteria and other foreign bodies.

Leucocytes/white blood cells are also present in connective tissue. They secrete antibodies (by plasma cells) and play an important role in tissue defence.

Mast cells secrete heparin, histamine and other substances, which are released when cells are damaged by disease or injury.

Fibres

The **fibres** are collagenous, elastic and reticular. **Collagenous fibres** are tough and unyielding while **elastic fibres** are thin and stretchable. These are widely distributed in the body. **Reticular fibres** are fine collagen fibres.

There are several different types of connective tissue (Fig. 2.9).

I. Loose Connective Tissue

It is of three types:
1. *Loose areolar connective tissue:* It is most generalized of all connective tissue. The fibres are loosely intertwined and many cells are present (Fig. 2.10). It provides elasticity and tensile strength to body parts. It connects and supports muscle fibers, secretory cells of glands blood vessels and nerves.

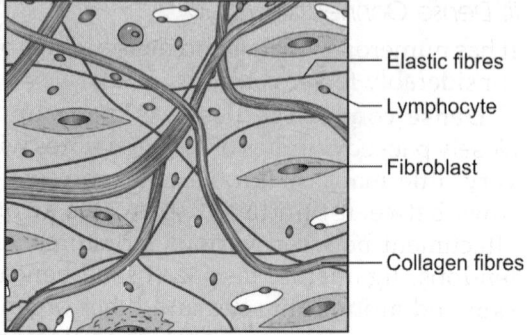

Fig. 2.10: Areolar tissue

2. *Adipose tissue:* Consists of fat cells (adipocytes). The fat cells contain fat globules in a matrix of areolar tissue. The cell is filled up with a single, large triglyceride droplet, and the cytoplasm and nucleus are pushed to the periphery of the cell (Fig. 2.11). Adipose tissue is of two types: (1) white and (2) brown. **White adipose tissue** is found supporting the kidneys and eyes, between muscle fibres and under the skin, where it acts as a thermal insulator and serves as an energy reserve. **Brown adipose tissue** is present in newborn. It has a rich blood supply. It is present in adults in only small amounts. It generates considerable heat and helps to maintain body temperature in newborn.

3. *Reticular connective tissue:* Consists of a network of interlacing reticular fibres and reticular cells. It forms supporting framework of liver, spleen and lymph nodes, and helps bind together smooth muscle cells.

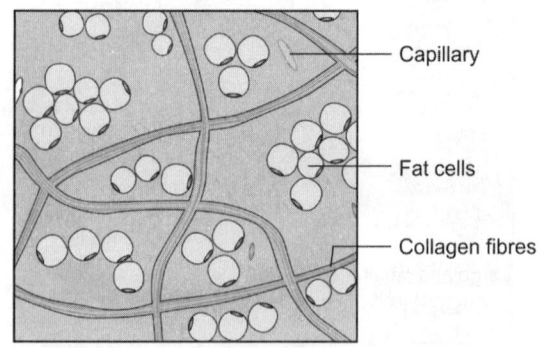

Fig. 2.11: Adipose tissue

II. Dense Connective Tissue

It has numerous, thicker and denser fibres but considerably fewer cells (Fig. 2.12).

Dense connective tissue is made up of closely packed bundles of collagen fibres with very little matrix. Fibroblasts are present in rows between bundles. It provides strong attachment between various structures, e.g. tendons, ligaments, fasciae (tissue beneath skin and around muscles and other organs), periosteum of bone, joint capsules and protective covering around various organs (kidney, liver, brain).

In **cartilage and bone,** the matrix contains many fibres. The matrix is firm in cartilage as it contains chondroitin sulphuric acid and hyaluronic acid. In bone, matrix is impregnated with calcium salts.

III. Blood

1. *Blood* is also a connective tissue where the matrix is fluid called plasma with red blood cells, white blood cells and platelets suspended in it. *Details are discussed in Chapter 4, Cardiovascular System (Blood).*

2. *Lymph* is an extracellular fluid that flows in lymphatic vessels. It is a connective tissue that consists of a clear fluid similar to blood plasma but with much less protein. *Details are discussed in Chapter 4, Cardiovascular System (Heart).*

IV. Specialised Dense Connective Tissue

1. *Cartilage:* It is a type of connective tissue where the cells, chondrocytes and fibres are embedded in a firm gel like matrix. The chondrocytes occur singly or in groups within spaces called **lacunae** in the matrix. A membrane of dense connective tissue called **perichondrium** covers the surface of most cartilage. The cartilage provides strength and elasticity. The cartilage is of three types.

- *Hyaline cartilage* is most extensively present. It covers the ends of bones, forms the costal cartilages of thorax and the cartilages of trachea and bronchi. The cells are in groups of 2 or 4 cells called the **cell-nest.** Matrix is solid and smooth with collagen fibres (Fig. 2.13).

- *Elastic cartilage,* as the name indicates contains numerous elastic fibres. The cells lie between the fibres. It is found in epiglottis, pinna of ear and auditory tube. These do not calcify (Fig. 2.14).

- *Fibrocartilage* contains high collagen fibre content. It is seen in intervertebral disc, menisci of knee joint and pubic symphysis.

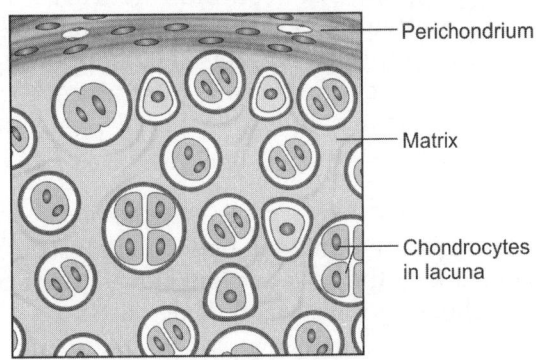

Perichondrium
Matrix
Chondrocytes in lacuna

Fig. 2.13: Hyaline cartilage: trachea

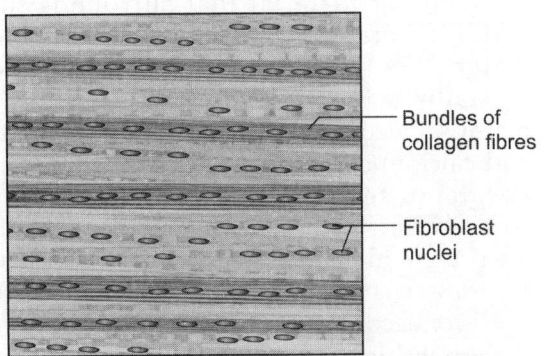

Bundles of collagen fibres

Fibroblast nuclei

Fig. 2.12: Dense connective tissue: tendon

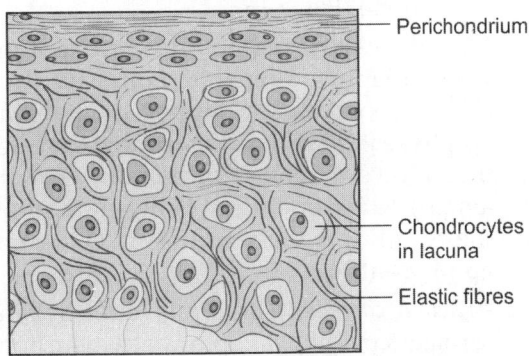

Perichondrium
Chondrocytes in lacuna
Elastic fibres

Fig. 2.14: Elastic cartilage: epiglottis

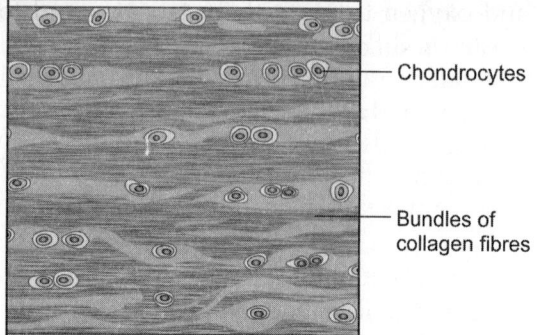

Fig. 2.15: Fibrocartilage: intervertebral disc

Fibrocartilage is devoid of perichondrium (Fig. 2.15).

Cartilage has no blood vessels and nerves. Cartilage obtains its nutrition by diffusion through the matrix. It grows by addition of cells from the perichondrium and also by the multiplication of chondrocytes.

2. *Bone:* Bone is specialized connective tissue having all the common features of connective tissue like ground substance, fibres and cells. But, this rigid supporting tissue is characterised by presence of inorganic mineral salts especially calcium and phosphate in its matrix.

Structure of Bone

The structure of a bone may be analysed by considering the parts of a long bone. A typical long bone consists of following parts:

1. *Diaphysis* is bone's **shaft,** the long, cylindrical, main portion of the bone.

2. *Epiphyses* are the distal and proximal ends of the bone (Fig. 2.16).

3. *Metaphyses* are regions in mature bone where diaphysis joins the epiphysis. In a growing bone, each metaphysis includes an **epiphyseal plate** (layer of hyaline cartilage that allows diaphysis of bone to grow in length). When bone growth in length stops, the resulting bone structure is known as **epiphyseal line.**

4. *Articular cartilage* is a thin layer of hyaline cartilage covering the epiphysis where bone forms a joint with another bone.

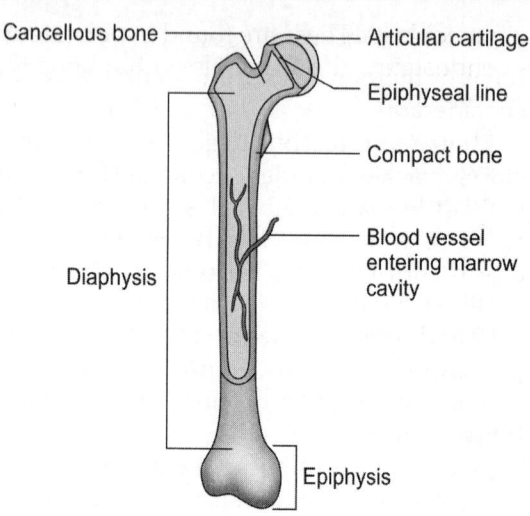

Fig. 2.16: Structure of long bone

5. *Medullary cavity/marrow cavity* is space within the diaphysis that contains fatty yellow bone marrow in adults.

6. *Periosteum* is tough sheath of dense connective tissue that surrounds the bone surface wherever it is not covered by articular cartilage. Periosteum has bone forming cells that enable bone to grow in thickness or diameter. Periosteum plays a role in healing of fractures. It also serves as an attachment point for ligaments and tendons.

7. *Endosteum* is a thin membrane lining the medullary cavity. It contains a single layer of bone forming cells and a small amount of connective tissue.

Histology of Bone Tissue

Bone tissue contains an abundant matrix of intercellular material that surrounds the widely separated cells. The matrix contains water (25%), collagen fibres (25%) and crystallised inorganic mineral salts (50%) mainly hydroxyapatite (calcium phosphate and calcium carbonate). These mineral salts are deposited in framework formed by collagen fibres of the matrix. Four types of cells are present in bone tissue:

1. *Osteogenic cells* are stem cells from which all connective tissues are formed. They are the only bone cells to undergo cells division, the resulting daughter cells develop into

osteoblasts. These are found in periosteum, endosteum and in canals within bone that contain blood vessels.

2. *Osteoblasts* are bone building cells. They synthesize and secrete collagen fibres and other organic components needed to build the matrix bone tissue. They initiate calcification. These cells surround themselves with matrix and become trapped in their secretions and become osteocytes.

3. *Osteocytes* are mature bone cells. They are main cells in bone tissue. They maintain daily metabolism of bone tissue.

4. *Osteoclasts* are large cells and are present in endosteum. They cause breakdown of bone matrix, termed **resorption,** which is part of normal development, growth, maintenance and repair of bone.

Bone tissue is classified as either compact or cancellous depending on how its matrix and cells are organised and size and distribution of spaces between its cells and matrix.

Compact Bone

Compact bone contains few spaces. It forms external layer of all bones and make up bulk of shaft of long bones. It provides protection and support and resists the stresses produced by weight and movement.

Unit of compact bone is **osteon or Haversian system.**

Blood vessels, lymphatics and nerves from periosteum penetrate the compact bone through transverse **perforating (Volkmann's) canals.** The vessels and nerves of Volkmann's canals connect with those of medullary cavity, periosteum and **central (Haversian) canals.** Central canals run longitudinally through the bone.

Around the central canals are **concentric lamellae** (rings of hard, calcified matrix). Between lamellae are small spaces called **lacunae** which contain **osteocytes.** Osteons in compact bone are aligned in same direction along lines of stress. From lacunae, **canaliculi** radiate in all directions. Canaliculi link the lacunae with each other and with Haversian canals. Canaliculi provide route for nutrients

and oxygen to reach the osteocytes and for wastes to diffuse away.

The areas between osteons contain **interstitial lamellae,** which are fragments of older osteons (Fig. 2.17).

Cancellous Bone

The cancellous bone does not contain osteons. It consists of **trabeculae,** an irregular framework of thin columns of bone. Space between trabeculae of some bones are filled with **red bone marrow.** Within each trabecula are osteocytes that lie in lacunae (Fig. 2.18). Radiating from the lacunae are canaliculi.

Cancellous/spongy bone is present in short, flat and irregular bones, epiphyses of long bones and in a narrow rim around the medullary cavity of diaphysis of long bones. Red bone marrow is present in cancellous bone of hip bones, ribs, sternum and vertebrae in an adult.

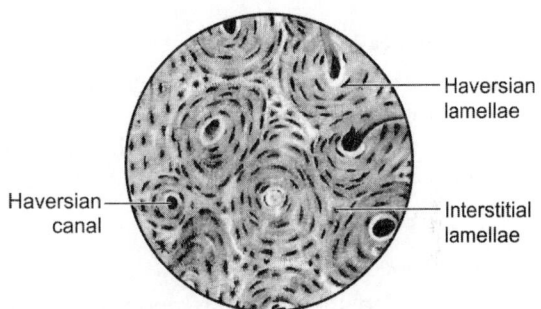

Fig. 2.17: Compact bone

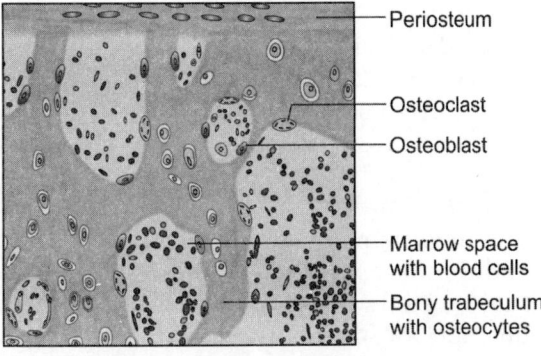

Fig. 2.18: Cancellous bone

Functions of Connective Tissue

The functions of connective tissue are manifold depending on its type.

1. *Mechanical:* It provides support for the body. Bones and cartilage are primarily concerned with providing a framework for the body. Loose connective tissue binds and connects different types of tissues, e.g. skin with muscle or muscle with bone. It also holds together different groups of the same tissue as in case of muscle fibre.

2. *Nutrition:* The ground substance or matrix of connective tissue holds large amounts of water in which electrolytes are dissolved. Thus water balance is maintained in tissues and cells are provided with nutrition.

3. *Defence:* The wandering cells of connective tissue act as defence forces of the body. They are responsible for phagocytosis and development of immunological reactions.

4. *Repair:* Fibroblasts present in the connective tissue are the agents involved in repair of tissues following injury.

Muscular Tissue

The power of contractility is especially present in the muscular tissue. Muscle cells are thin and long and are called **muscle fibres.** There are three types of muscle fibres: (1) skeletal, (2) cardiac and (3) smooth.

Skeletal Muscle

It is also called striated or striped muscle. The muscle fibre is multi-nucleated, the nuclei situated just beneath the cell membrane.

Each muscle fibre receives its branch of motor nerve fibre. So, these are under the **control of will** and are called **voluntary muscle** (Fig. 2.19). These are present in the limbs, abdominal wall, muscles of larynx, tongue.

Smooth Muscle

The myofilaments are arranged differently and do not give striated appearance. Hence these muscle fibres are called unstriated/unstriped or smooth. These are found in blood vessels and walls of hollow viscera like

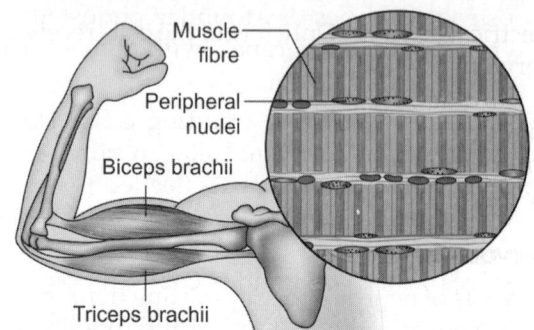

Fig. 2.19: Striated muscle (longitudinal section): tongue

stomach, intestine, urinary bladder and uterus (Fig. 2.20).

This muscle fibre is narrow spindle shaped (thickest in middle and tapering at both ends) with a **single central nucleus.** It is supplied by **autonomic nerves.** Most smooth muscle fibres do not receive nerve fibres so the impulse passes via special intercellular junctions called the **gap junctions or nexuses** to the neighbouring cells.

Cardiac Muscle

It is present only in the heart. These muscle fibres also have striations. Each fibre has only one central nucleus. The fibre is like a short cylinder with branches.

The fibres are attached to each other "end-on", where their cell membranes get folded against one another. This is called as *intercalated disc.* It helps in fast conduction of

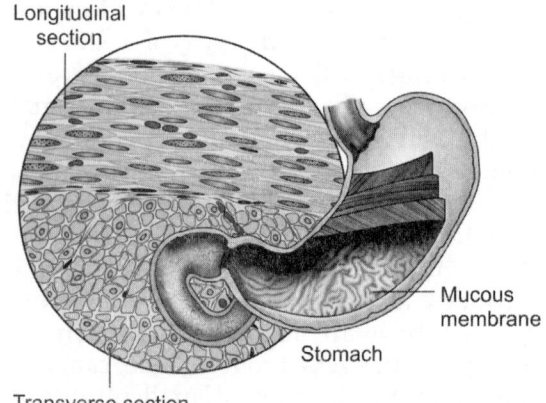

Fig. 2.20: Smooth muscle: stomach

electrical impulse. Only few of the cells receive nerve fibres (Fig. 2.21).

Cardiac muscle has inherent property of rhythmicity, i.e. regularly beating from early embryonic life till death. The rate is controlled by autonomic nerves.

Nervous Tissue

Consists of neurons, the supporting neuroglia cells. Neuron is the anatomical and functional unit of the nervous tissue.

Neuron

Neurons are the excitable cells. They initiate, receive, conduct and transmit information. It consists of a cell body containing the nucleus and its processes. The processes are **multiple dendrites and a single axon** in a multipolar

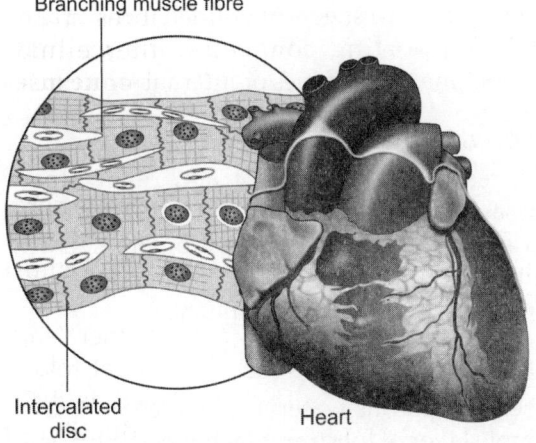

Fig. 2.21: Cardiac muscle: heart

neuron (Fig. 2.22). Cell body also contains Nissl granules, mitochondria and Golgi apparatus.

Dendrite forms the **"receptive zone"** of the neuron. Impulses reach neuron through the dendrites. Axon carries the response of the neuron to other neurons/muscle fibre/gland. It is the **"conducting zone"** of the neuron.

The axon ends by dividing into many fine processes called **axon terminals.** The membrane of the axon is called **axolemma.** Large axons and those of peripheral nerves are surrounded by a **myelin sheath.** This consists of a series of **Schwann cells** arranged along the length of the axon. Each one is wrapped abound the axon so that it is covered by a number of concentric layers of Schwann cell plasma membrane. Between layers of plasma membrane **myelin** is present. There are tiny areas of exposed axolemma between adjacent Schwann cells, called **nodes of Ranvier,** which assist in rapid transmission of nerve impulses. In **non myelinated nerve fibres,** a number of axons are embedded in Schwann cell plasma membranes.

The adjacent Schwann cells are closely associated and there is no exposed axolemma.

Grey Matter

Part of nervous tissue, containing the cell bodies of neurons with neurolgia is called grey matter. Collection of cell bodies of neuron is also called nuclei like the dentate nucleus of cerebellum. Collection of cell bodies in the

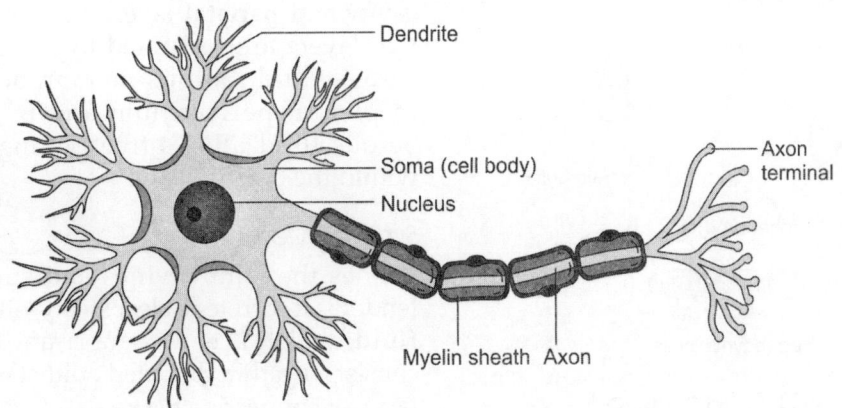

Fig. 2.22: Parts of a neuron

peripheral nervous system are called the ganglia.

White Matter

Part of nervous tissue containing only the nerve fibres is called the white matter. Such collections in brain and spinal cord are called tracts, and in peripheral nervous system are called the peripheral nerves.

Supporting Cells

The cells supporting the neurons in central nervous system are called neuroglial cells. The supporting cells in peripheral nervous system are called the Schwann cells. These lay myelin sheath for the peripheral nerves.

Neuroglia are more numerous than the neurons. These are of four types: (1) astrocytes, (2) oligodendrocytes, (3) microglia and (4) ependymal cells (Fig. 2.23).

Astrocytes are main supporting tissue of the central nervous system. They supply nourishment to the neurons and form the blood brain barrier. These are of protoplasmic and fibrous types.

Oligodendrocytes are smaller than astrocytes. They lay down myelin sheath within the central nervous system, providing insulation to the nerve impulse.

Microglia are phagocytic cells for removing the dying/dead cells.

Ependymal cells form the epithelial lining of the ventricles of brain and central canal of spinal cord. These secrete cerebrospinal fluid and assist in its circulation.

Tumours of nervous system arise only from neuroglia, not from neurons as these are too evolved to divide.

Membranes

Membranes are sheets of epithelial tissue and their supporting connective tissue that covers/lines the cavities or internal structures.

Mucous Membrane/Mucosa

It lines the alimentary tract, respiratory passages and genitourinary tract. Epithelial cells forming mucous membrane secrete **mucus,** which protects the cells from mechanical and chemical injury.

Serous Membrane/Serosa

It secretes serous watery fluid. It consists of a double layer of loose areolar connective tissue lined by simple squamous epithelium. **Visceral layer** surrounds organs within the cavity and **parietal layer** lines a cavity. The two layers are separated by a thin layer of serous fluid. Serous membrane is found in pleura, pericardium and peritoneum. Serous fluid allows free gliding of organ within the cavity.

Synovial Membrane

It lines the joint cavities and surrounding tendons. It secretes a clear sticky, oily **synovial fluid,** which acts as a lubricant to joint. It consists of a thin flattened epithelial cells on a layer of connective tissue.

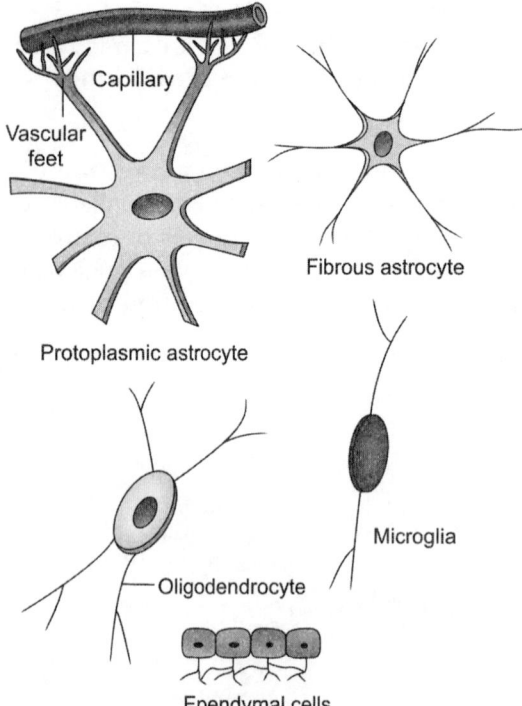

Fig. 2.23: Types of neuroglia

Glands

Glands are composed of epithelial cells which produce specialised secretion. The glands can be:

1. *Endocrine glands:* Directly discharge their secretions into blood and lymph, e.g. pituitary, thyroid, parathyroid, suprarenal.
2. *Exocrine glands:* Discharge their secretions into ducts, e.g. salivary glands.

CLINICAL ASPECTS

Tumour/new growth/neoplasm is a purposeless uncontrolled multiplication of group of cells. The tumour can be benign or malignant.

- **Benign tumours** are slow to grow, cells are differentiated. The tumour is surrounded by a capsule and does not spread.
- **Malignant tumours** are fast growing with undifferentiated cells. The tumour is not surrounded by the capsule. The critical point is that the malignant tumours can spread to any part of the body.
- **Origin of tumours:** The exact reason is unknown. Cigarette smoke, aniline dyes, X-rays, ultraviolet rays of sun and some viruses are some of the known reasons for origin of tumours. The age, diet and genetic constitution also influences the growth of tumour.

Points to Remember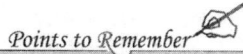

1. There are four basic tissues of the body—epithelial tissue, connective tissue, muscular tissue and nervous tissue.
2. Epithelial tissue may be simple or stratified.
3. Cartilages are of 3 types—hyaline, elastic and fibrocartilages.
4. Nervous system is made of neurons and neuroglia (the supporting tissue)

MCQs

1. **Columnar epithelium is seen in:**
   (a) lining of arteries
   (b) lining of trachea
   (c) lining of skin
   (d) lining of stomach

2. **Cells of connective tissue are all of following types *except*:**
   (a) Plasma cells
   (b) Fat cells
   (c) Fibroblast
   (d) Osteocyte

3. **Elastic cartilage is present in:**
   (a) Pinna of the ear
   (b) Compact bone
   (c) Trachea
   (d) Tendon

4. **Grey matter of brain contains:**
   (a) cell body of neuron
   (b) fibrous astrocyte
   (c) less capillaries
   (d) most of the axon

Ans! 1 d 2 d 3 a 4 a

Skeletal System and Joints

Skeletal system comprises bones and cartilages. The cartilage has been described in Chapter 2. Bones are described below:

Bone is a type of connective tissue. It consists of water (25%), organic constituents-osteoid and bone cells (25%), and inorganic constituents, mainly calcium phosphate (50%).

It is a highly vascular structure that is continuously remodelled.

FUNCTION AND CLASSIFICATION

Function

- Bones provide a framework of the body.
- Bones support and protect the various organs. The **skull** forms cavity for lodging the brain, eyes, ears, nose, tongue and pituitary. The **thoracic cavity** encloses the heart and lungs and **abdominal cavity** protects the abdominal viscera (*see* Fig. 1.3).
- Bones give attachment to muscles and tendons for the movements of the body.
- Bones form a storehouse for calcium and phosphorus.
- **Bone marrow** produces red blood cells, granular white blood cells and platelets.
- Bones articulate with each other to form joint responsible for movements.

Classification

These can be classified in following ways:

According to Position

1. *Axial skeleton*, e.g. bones of skull, thorax, vertebral column.
2. *Appendicular skeleton*, bones of upper and lower limbs.

According to Shape

1. *Long bones* are with two ends and a shaft, e.g. humerus, femur, tibia (Fig. 3.1).
2. *Short bones* are small bones, e.g. carpal and tarsal bones (Fig. 3.2).
3. *Long short bones* are small long bones, e.g. metacarpal and metatarsal bones.
4. *Flat bones* are plates of bones with spongy bone within, e.g. sternum, skull bones and scapula (Fig. 3.3).
5. *Irregular bones* are of irregular shape, e.g. vertebrae.
6. *Pneumatic bones* are with spaces containing air, e.g. frontal, maxilla, ethmoid. The air spaces are called sinuses and if infected the condition is called sinusitis (Fig. 3.4).
7. *Sesamoid bones* are present in certain tendons, e.g. patella or knee cap in front of knee present in the tendon of quadriceps femoris muscle (*see* Fig. 1.3).

According to Structure

1. *Compact or solid bone* with little spaces, e.g. shaft of long bones.
2. *Cancellous or spongy bone* with more spaces for bone marrow, e.g. ends of long bones.

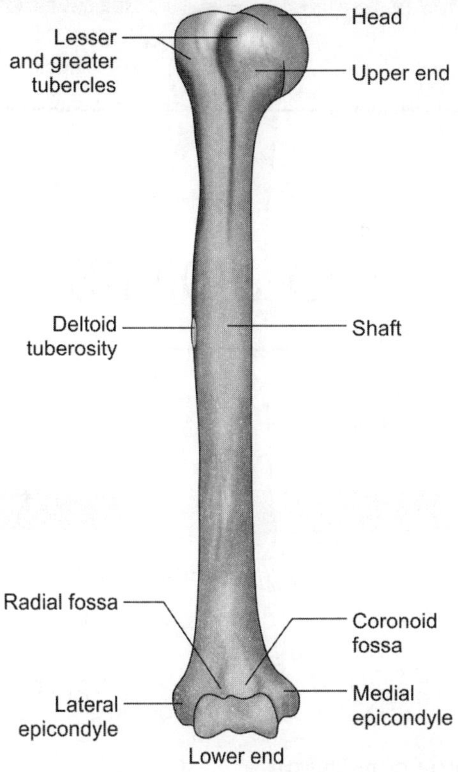

Head

Upper end

Lesser
and greater
tubercles

Deltoid
tuberosity

Shaft

Radial fossa

Coronoid
fossa

Lateral
epicondyle

Medial
epicondyle

Lower end

Fig. 3.1: Long bone

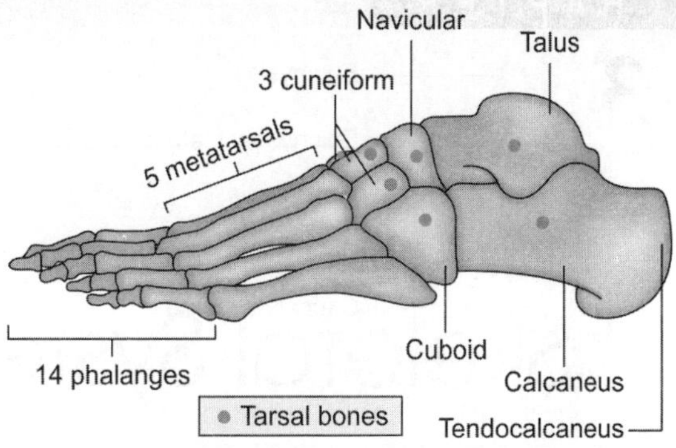

Navicular

Talus

3 cuneiform

5 metatarsals

14 phalanges

Cuboid

Calcaneus

Tendocalcaneus

• Tarsal bones

Fig. 3.2: Short bones

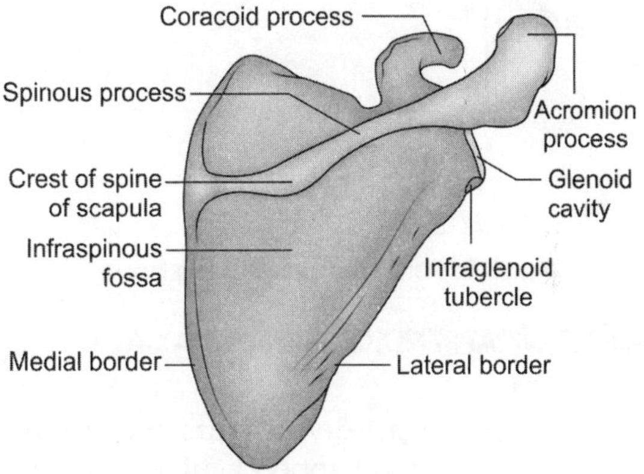

Coracoid process

Spinous process

Acromion
process

Crest of spine
of scapula

Glenoid
cavity

Infraspinous
fossa

Infraglenoid
tubercle

Medial border

Lateral border

Fig. 3.3: Flat bone

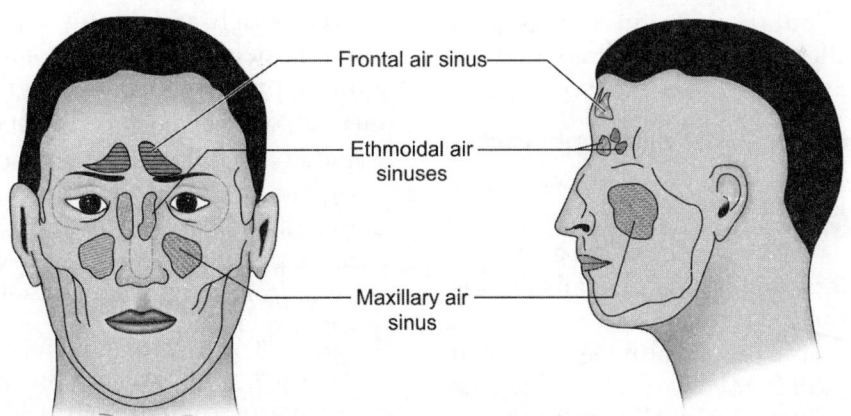

Frontal air sinus

Ethmoidal air
sinuses

Maxillary air
sinus

Fig. 3.4: Paranasal air sinuses

STRUCTURE OF BONE

A typical long bone consists of three parts:
(Fig. 3.5).

1. *Diaphysis*, the mid shaft

2. *Epiphysis*, the ends of the bone

3. *Metaphysis*, the area between diaphysis and
   epiphysis

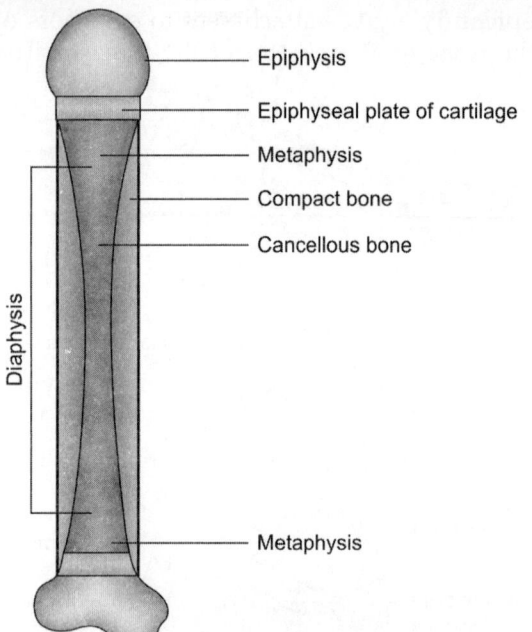

Fig. 3.5: Parts of a developing bone

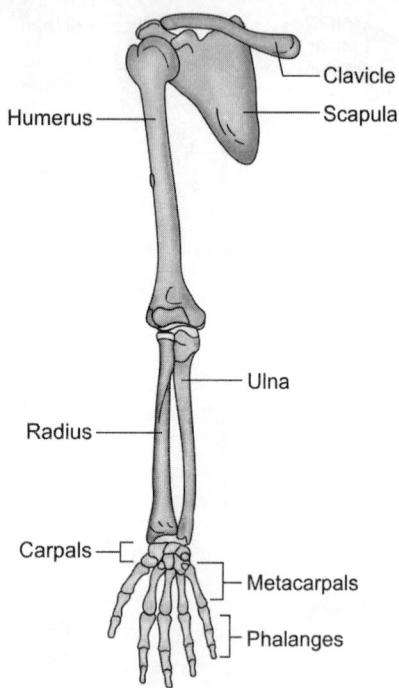

Fig. 3.6: Bones of upper limb

BONES OF APPENDICULAR AND AXIAL SKELETON

Bones of skeleton are divided into two groups: (1) axial skeleton, (2) appendicular skeleton.

Bones of Appendicular Skeleton

The appendicular skeleton consists of shoulder girdle with the upper limbs and the pelvic girdle with the lower limbs.

Bones of Shoulder Girdle and Upper Limb

- Scapula and clavicle form the shoulder girdle (Fig. 3.6).
- Humerus is the only bone of the arm.
- Radius laterally and ulna medially are the two bones of the forearm.
- Hand consists of 8 carpal bones arranged in two rows of four bones each forming the wrist. 1st to 5th metacarpals form the bones of the palm.
- 14 phalanges, 2 in the thumb and three each in index, middle, ring and little fingers.

Scapula

Scapula is a flat triangular bones lying on the posterolateral aspect of the upper back. It is suspended by various muscles (Fig. 3.3).

Scapula consists of:

1. *2 surfaces*—costal and dorsal
2. *3 angles*—superior, inferior and lateral angles. The lateral angle bears a pear shaped shallow cavity called the **glenoid cavity** which articulates with head of humerus to form the most mobile **shoulder** joint. Supraglenoid tubercle gives attachment to long head of biceps brachii muscle.
3. *3 borders*—medial, lateral and superior
4. 3 processes:
   - *The coracoid process* which gives attachment to pectoralis minor and short head of biceps brachii muscle.
   - *The spine* of scapula.
   - *Acromion process* (the lateral continuation of spine of scapula), both give attachment to deltoid muscle used for giving intramuscular injections.

Clavicle

Clavicle is long bone placed horizontally between the sternum medially and the acromion process of scapula laterally (Fig. 3.7). It is convex anteriorly in its medial

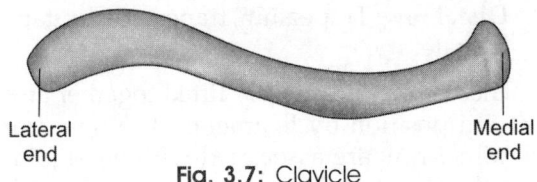

Lateral
end

Medial
end

Fig. 3.7: Clavicle

part (2/3rd) and concave in its lateral part (l/3rd).

It forms **sternoclavicular joint** medially with manubrium of sternum and **acromioclavicular joint** laterally with acromion process of the scapula.

Medially two muscles arise from it. These are pectoralis major of the pectoral region and **sternocleidomastoid** of the neck. The latter turns the chin to the opposite side.

Laterally also two muscles **trapezius and deltoid** are attached to it. Trapezius is the shrugging muscle. Deltoid is large triangular muscle from scapula and clavicle going down to the middle of the shaft of humerus in which intramuscular injections are given.

The clavicle provides the only bony link between the upper limb and the axial skeleton.

Humerus

It is the largest bone of the upper limb (Fig. 3.1). It has two ends: (1) upper and (2) lower and an intervening shaft.

Upper end comprises a rounded head forming the shoulder joint, and two tubercles giving attachments to the muscles arising from the scapula.

Shaft is long and cylindrical. On its lateral aspect in the middle region is the insertion of **deltoid** muscle. Back of the shaft gives origin to **triceps brachii** muscle which is an extensor of elbow joint. Front of the shaft gives origin to flexor of elbow joint **brachialis** muscle. Anterior to brachialis lies biceps brachii muscle, which arises from scapula.

Lower end has lateral and medial **epicondyles** on the two sides. In addition, there are **radial and coronoid fossae anteriorly** and a deep olecranon fossa on its back. **Medial epicondyle** gives attachment to flexors of the wrist and pronator of the forearm. **Lateral**

epicondyle gives attachment to extensors of the wrist and supinator of the forearm. The lower end articulates with the radius and ulna to form the elbow joint.

Radius

Radius is the lateral bone of the forearm (Fig. 3.8). It is comprised of:
• **Upper end** made of head, neck and tuberosity
• **Shaft** is the long middle part
• **Lower end** is broad with a pointed styloid process laterally.

Head articulates with lateral part of lower end of humerus forming the elbow joint. Medially it articulates with the radial notch of ulna to form **superior radioulnar joint.**

Tuberosity gives attachment to a very important flexor of elbow and supinator of forearm called the **biceps brachii** muscle.

Shaft on its concave anterior surface gives attachment to flexors of the digits while posterior surface gives attachment to extensors of the digits. Medially there is an interosseous border providing attachment to interosseous membrane between radius and ulna.

Lower end articulates with two bones of proximal row of carpus to form the wrist joint.

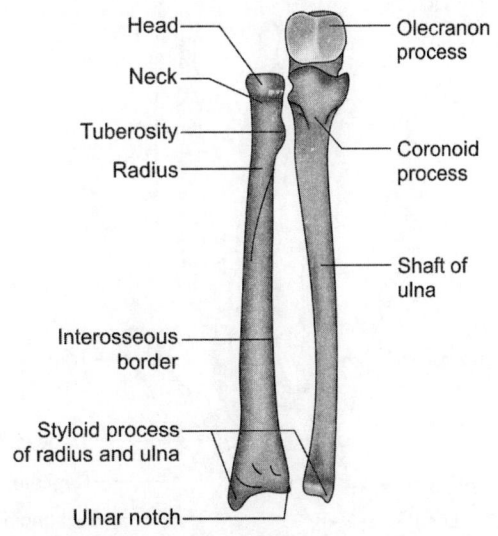

Head

Neck

Tuberosity

Radius

Interosseous
border

Styloid process
of radius and ulna

Ulnar notch

Olecranon
process

Coronoid
process

Shaft of
ulna

Fig. 3.8: Right radius and ulna (anterior view)

Medially there is a notch which articulates with head of ulna to form the **inferior radio-ulnar joint.**

Ulna

Ulna is the thin medial bone of the forearm and is longer than the radius.

Upper end has a **coronoid process** and a large beak like **olecranon process.** Brachialis is inserted into the coronoid process. Triceps brachii gets inserted into the olecranon process.

Shaft is thin.

Lower end consists of a rounded head and a medially placed styloid process.

Ulna forms superior radioulnar joint and an inferior or distal radioulnar joint with the radius.

Anterior surface of shaft gives origin to flexors of the digits, while posterior surface gives origin to extensors of the digits.

Olecranon process fits into olecranon fossa of humerus during full extension of elbow, while coronoid process fits into coronoid fossa of humerus during full flexion of elbow joint.

Hand

The wrist is formed of 8 carpal bones arranged in two rows of 4 each. From outside inwards they are (Fig 3.9):

1. **Proximal row:** Scaphoid, lunate, triquetral, pisiform.

2. **Distal row:** Trapezium, trapezoid, capitate, hamate.

These bones are closely fitted together and held in position by ligaments. The bones of proximal row are associated with wrist joint and those of the distal row form joints with the metacarpal bones.

The lateral bone of the distal row is called trapezium. It articulates with the base of 1st metacarpal to form the important 1st carpometacarpal joint which permits movement of opposition with the fingers.

The skeleton of palm is formed of 1st, 2nd, 3rd, 4th and 5th metacarpal bones. 1st metacarpal is the shortest and stoutest and lies at right angles to the other 4 bones, allowing the movements of opposition.

There are 14 phalanges for the 5 digits. 2 for the thumb and three each, i.e. proximal, middle and distal for 2nd to 5th digits.

Bones of the Pelvic Girdle and Lower Limb

1. *Hip bone* and sacrum forms the pelvic girdle. Hip bone is made of three components, i.e. ilium, ischium and pubis (Fig. 3.10).

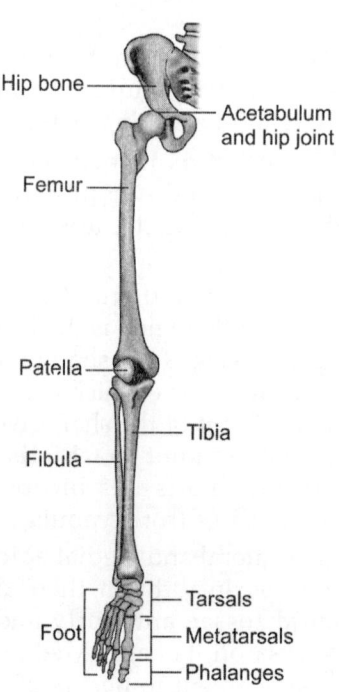

Fig. 3.10: Bones of lower limb

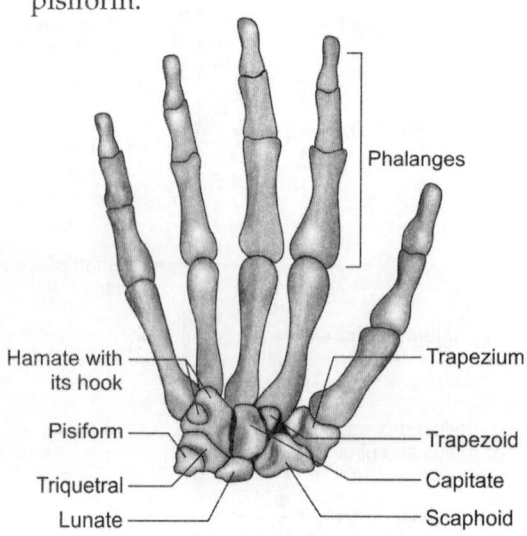

Fig. 3.9: Bones of the right hand

2. *Femur*, the longest bone of the body is present in the thigh.
3. *Stout tibia* medially and delicate fibula laterally form the skeleton of the leg.
4. *Foot* comprises 7 tarsal bones, 5 metatarsal bones and 14 phalanges (Figs 3.2 and 3.10).

Hip Bone

It is a large irregular bone comprised of 3 bones fused together—**ilium** situated above and laterally; **ischium** on the posterior aspect with a tuberosity on which one sits; and a **pubis** which lies anteroinferiorly (Fig. 3.11). The two pubic bones articulate with each other to form the **pubic symphysis**, a joint presents in the midline in the lowest part of the abdomen.

On the lateral aspect of the hip bone is a deep fossa the **acetabulum**, which articulates with the head of femur to form the **hip joint**. All the three parts of hip bone join together at acetabulum.

Ilium forms the large flat bone lying below the waist. Its posterior part articulates with the lateral surface of sacrum to form the strong **sacroiliac joint** which transmits the weight of the body to the ground via the lower limbs.

Muscles of gluteal region arise from the lateral or gluteal surface of ilium. The intramuscular injections are given in the gluteus medius muscle on the lateral side.

Ischium forms the lower and posterior part of the hip bone. Its tuberosity gives attachment to muscles of back of thigh and a part of this bone is used for sitting.

Pubis provides attachment to muscles of medial side of thigh.

Between the ischium and the pubis anteriorly is a large **obturator foramen** covered with a membrane providing attachment to the muscles.

Femur

It is the longest and strongest bone of the body. It is comprised of an upper end, a long shaft and a large lower end (Fig. 3.12).

Upper end contains a rounded head which articulates with acetabulum to form the mobile **hip joint.** In addition, there are two projections of bones, i.e. the greater and lesser trochanters which give attachment to muscles.

Shaft is long with a convex anterior surface. It gives attachment to parts of large muscle of front of thigh called the **quadriceps femoris** muscle. It also gives insertion to adductor muscles of thigh at its back.

Lower end is broad and bears two large condyles, the medial and lateral condyles. These take part in formation of a complex joint, **the knee joint.**

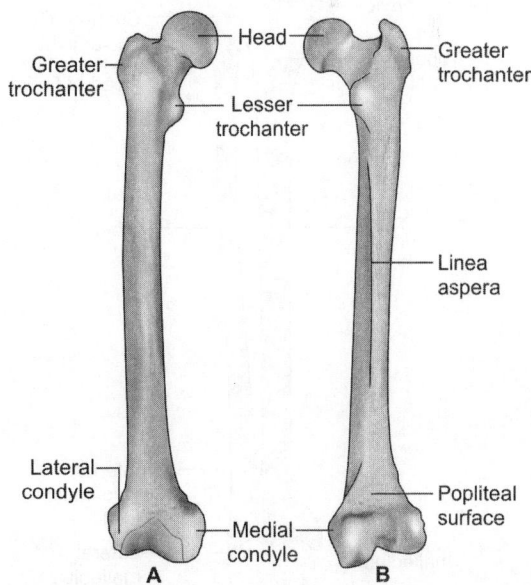

Fig. 3.12: Right femur (A) anterior view, (B) posterior view

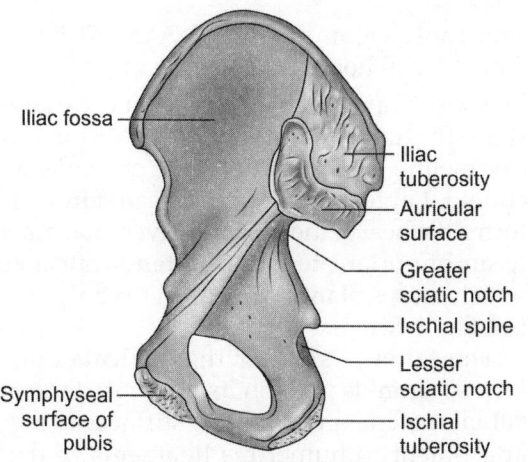

Fig. 3.11: Right hip bone (lateral view)

Patella

It is also known as **knee cap** (Fig. 3.10). It is a triangular sesamoid bone in the tendon of quadriceps femoris muscle (*see* Fig 1.2). All the four parts of the strong quadriceps muscle are inserted into the patella. From the apex of patella, the **ligamentum patellae** starts which gets attached to the tibial tuberosity. The whole muscle is the chief extensor of the knee joint. Rectus femoris part of the muscle is called "Kicking muscle".

Tibia

It is the strong bone of the leg, present on the medial side (Fig. 3.13). It comprises an upper end, shaft and a lower end.

Upper end consists of two concave **condyles** which form the important knee joint and a tibial tuberosity giving attachment to the **ligamentum patellae,** tendon of **quadriceps femoris** muscle of the thigh.

Shaft is long and cylindrical. Its medial surface is subcutaneous and can be felt through the skin. Lateral surface gives attachment to **tibialis anterior** muscle. The lateral border gives attachment to the **interosseous membrane** presents between tibia and fibula.

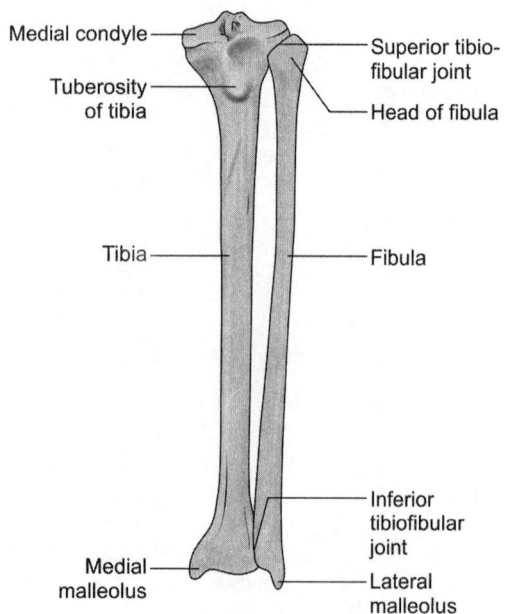

Medial condyle
Tuberosity of tibia
Superior tibio-fibular joint
Head of fibula
Tibia
Fibula
Inferior tibiofibular joint
Medial malleolus
Lateral malleolus

Fig. 3.13: Left tibia and fibula (anterior view)

Lower end is hollowed to articulate with talus forming the ankle joint. On its medial side is a prominent downward projection, the **medial malleolus,** which can be easily seen and felt through the skin (Fig. 3.13). On the front and back of lower end, various tendons crossing across the ankle joint can be seen and felt.

Fibula

It is a long slender lateral bone of the leg. It does not articulate with femur and so does not participate in the formation of knee joint. This bone gives attachment to number of muscles and helps in the formation of the ankle joint.

It consists of an upper end, long shaft and a lower end which is characterised by the presence of a subcutaneous projection, called the **lateral malleolus** (Fig. 3.13).

Upper end articulates with a facet on the posterolateral aspect of tibia to form the **superior tibiofibular joint.**

The medial surface of lower end of shaft of fibula similarly articulates with lateral surface of tibia to form the **inferior tibiofibular joint**.

In the middle part, it articulates with shaft of tibia through the interosseous membrane. The shaft gives attachment to dorsiflexor muscles of ankle joint on its anterior surface; to the plantar flexor muscles on its posterior surface. In addition, the evertor muscles arise from its lateral surface.

Lower end articulates with talus to form the ankle joint.

The Foot

The foot is comprised of 7 tarsal bones, 5 metatarsal bones and 14 phalanges.

Tarsal bones are seven in number and are larger than the carpal bones. Tarsal bones are calcaneum, talus, cuneiform (3), navicular and cuboid. Largest bone is the **calcaneum** which forms the heel of the foot and gives attachment to an important tendon the **tendocalcaneus** which causes **plantar flexion** at the ankle joint (*see* Fig. 1.13).

The **talus** is smaller than calcaneum. It forms the ankle joint on its upper surface and subtalar joint on its lower surface. It gives attachment to numerous ligaments of these joints, but has no muscle attachment.

Out of the other tarsal bones, **navicular** gives attachment to tibialis posterior. **Medial cuneiform** provides insertion for tibialis anterior and peroneus longus muscles. **Cuboid, middle cuneiform and lateral cuneiform** are other tarsal bones. The groove on the plantar aspect of cuboid gives passage to the tendon of peroneus longus muscle.

Metatarsal bones are five in number and are numbered from medial to lateral side as 1st, 2nd, 3rd, 4th and 5th bones. These are long short bones. The first metatarsal is the thickest and strongest bone and helps in transmission of weight to the ground.

The **phalanges** are very small bones, numbering 14 in number. The big toe or hallux or 1st toe has 2 phalanges, proximal and distal. The 2nd to 5th toes have 3 phalanges each, the proximal, middle and distal. These are small bones especially in the 5th digit.

Arches of Foot

Bones of the foot have a bridge like arrangement and are supported by muscles and ligaments, so that a series of three arches are formed both longitudinally and transversely. These arches help to provide ideal distribution of body weight in standing and moving, act as a spring to propel the body forwards, and protect the nerves and vessels on plantar aspect.

Medial longitudinal arch is higher and more mobile. It is formed by calcaneum, talus, three cuneiforms and first three metatarsals.

Lateral longitudinal arch is lower and less mobile. It is formed by calcaneum, cuboid, 4th and 5th metatarsals.

Transverse arch is formed by metatarsal bones and is half arch (hemidome) and becomes complete arch only when both the feet are kept together.

Bones of the Axial Skeleton

These are the bones lying in the centre of the body forming its axis. These are:
1. **Skull** including the mandible and six ossicles of ears, three on each side
2. **Hyoid bone**
3. **Sternum**
4. **12 pairs of ribs** are also considered here
5. **Vertebral column.**

Skull

This bone forms the cranial most part of the axial skeleton. It is composed of 28 bones. Out of these 8 bones form the cap and base of skull, 14 form the bones of the face and six are ossicles of the middle ear. Some are paired and others are unpaired. These are shown in Table 3.1.

Cap or vault surrounds the brain and covers it and on the base the brain rests. These bones are joined together by joints **sutures,** which are immovable. These bones also have numerous opening/perforations through which nerves, blood vessels pass.

Single frontal bone forms the bone of the forehead. It articulates with two parietal bones, ethmoid bone and two nasal bones (Fig. 3.14). The joint between frontal and two parietal bones is the **coronal suture,** part of frontal lobe of brain lies behind it. It also forms roof of the orbital cavity. This bone also contains two air filled cavities or sinuses.

Parietal bones are paired bones. These form the top of the skull or the cap. The two are joined to each other with a suture called the **sagittal suture.** Further these are joined with frontal bone at the **coronal suture.** Inferiorly each parietal bone articulates with temporal process of squamous temporal at **squamous**

Table 3.1		
	Paired	*Unpaired*
Skull cap and base (8)	Parietal Temporal	Frontal Occipital Sphenoid Ethmoid
Ossicles (6)	Malleus, incus, stapes	
Face (14)	Zygomatic Maxilla Nasal Inferior nasal concha Lacrimal Palatine	Vomer Mandible

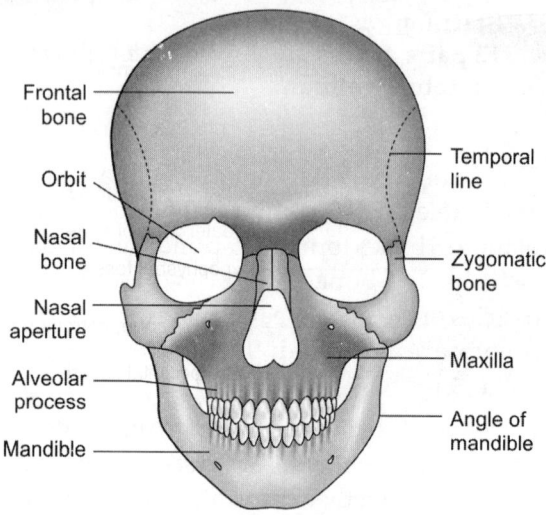

Fig. 3.14: Skull from the front

Occipital bone is a single bone forming the back of the skull cap. It also forms part of the base of the skull. It contains occipital lobe of cerebrum and cerebellum. It contains the largest foramen of the skull, the **foramen magnum** through which medulla oblongata continues as the spinal cord.

Occipital bone also has two articular condyles and forms the joint with the atlas, the first bone of vertebral column.

Sphenoid is also a single bone resembling a butterfly, forming the base of skull. The **hypophysis cerebri** or pituitary gland is situated in the sphenoid bone (Fig. 3.16). There is a big **superior orbital fissure** through which the contents of the orbit are connected to the parts of the brain lying in relation to this bone. This bone also contains an air sinus called the **sphenoidal air sinus** which drains into the lateral wall of the nasal cavity.

Ethmoid is a single very light bone forming the anterior part of base of skull. It lies between the medial wall of orbit and the nasal cavity. It also lodges 3 sets of **ethmoidal air cells** which all open into the nasal cavity. These form part of the paranasal sinuses (Fig. 3.4). It also forms part of the nasal septum and roof of nasal cavity (by cribriform plate).

Zygomatic bones are a pair of bones forming the cheek bones. Each bone articulates with temporal and maxilla bones.

suture and posteriorly with occipital bone at the **lambdoid suture.** Deep to this bone lies part of frontal and parietal lobes of the brain.

Temporal bones are paired bones situated above the pinna or external ear. In this bone is lodged the middle and internal ear. A process of this bone, the mastoid process projects behind the ear. The temporal lobe of brain is lodged deep to this bone. Zygomatic process of temporal bone articulates with temporal process of zygomatic bone to form the zygomatic arch. Temporal bone also articulates with mandible at **temporomandibular joint** (Fig. 3.15).

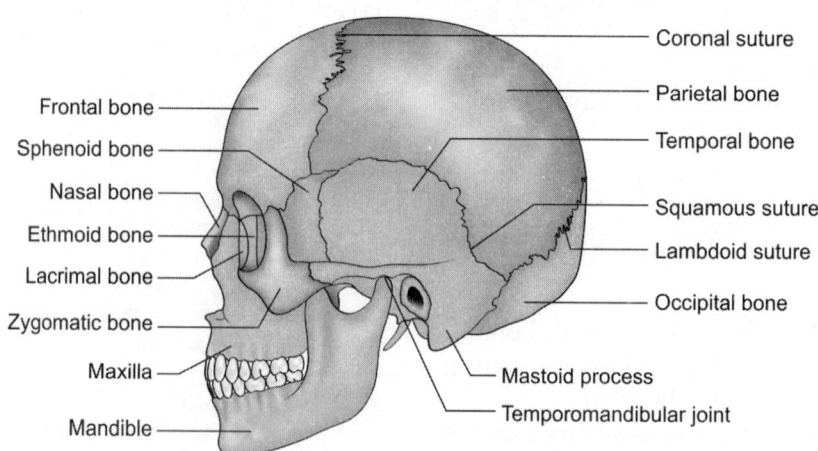

Fig. 3.15: Skull (from the side)

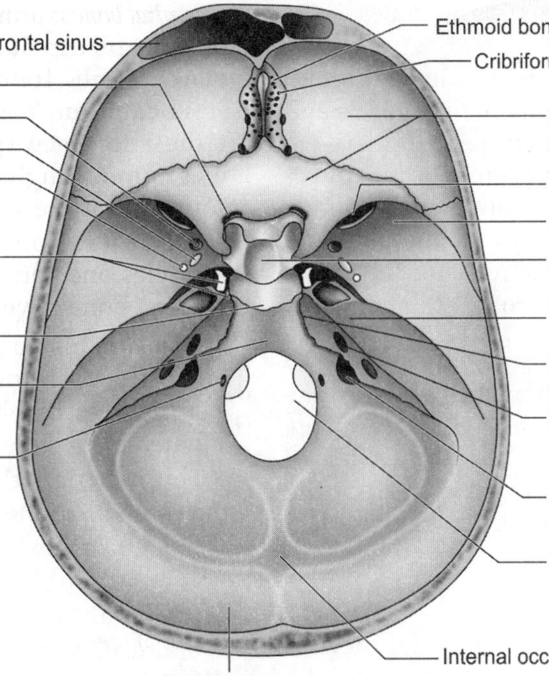

Frontal sinus

Ethmoid bone

Cribriform plate of ethmoid

Optic canal

Foramen rotundum

Foramen ovale

Foramen spinosum

Frontal bone, lesser wing of sphenoid bone

Superior orbital fissure

Greater wing of sphenoid bone

Hypophyseal fossa

Foramen lacerum and apex of petrous temporal

Dorsum sellae

Clivus

Temporal bone, petrous part

Petro-occipital fissure

Internal acoustic meatus

Hypoglossal canal

Jugular foramen

Foramen magnum

Internal occipital protuberance

Occipital bone

Fig. 3.16: Cranial fossae

Maxilla or upper jaw is a pair of bones forming a large part of the face. Each bone contains 8 **upper teeth.** It also contains a large air space called **maxillary air sinus** which drains into the nasal cavity (Fig. 3.4). Since the same nerve supplies the air sinus and upper teeth, the pain of sinusitis may be referred to teeth and vice versa. One of its process, palatal process from the large anterior part of the hard palate.

Nasal bones are a pair of small bones forming the upper part of the external nose. External nose has only the nasal bone, rest are all cartilages.

Inferior nasal concha is a pair of separate bones lying in the lateral wall of nasal cavity. Below and above this concha are a number of openings.

Lacrimal bones are a pair of delicate bones lying behind each nasal bone. This bone forms part of the medial wall of the orbit.

Palatine bones are also a pair of L-shaped bones. Horizontal parts unite and form the posterior part of the hard palate and perpendicular parts

project upwards to form part of the lateral walls of the nasal cavity.

Vomer is a single bone forming part of the nasal septum.

Mandible is a single strong bone of the face. It lodges 16 teeth, 8 each on right and left sides of the jaw (Fig. 3.17). Each half of mandible consists of 2 parts: (1) **body** with **alveolar ridge** containing the lower teeth and (2) **ramus**

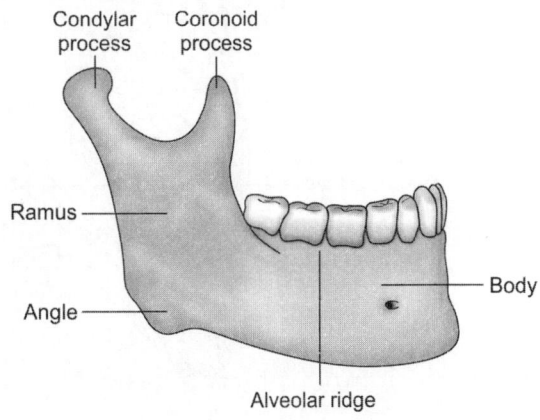

Condylar process   Coronoid process

Ramus

Angle

Body

Alveolar ridge

Fig. 3.17: Right mandible (lateral view)

which projects upwards at right angles to the posterior end of body.

At upper end ramus divides into **coronoid process** that gives attachment to a muscle and **condylar process** which articulates with temporal bone to form mobile **temporomandibular joint.** The point where ramus joins the body is the **angle** of the jaw. The inferior alveolar nerve supplying the lower teeth is related to this bone.

Hyoid Bone

It is a small single bone present between the mandible above and the thyroid cartilage (Adam's apple) below. Many muscles of pharynx, mouth, tongue, front of neck are attached to it. It does not articulate with any other bone.

Sternum

It is a single flat bone lying in the median region of anterior wall of the thoracic cavity. Its upper broad end is called manubrium sterni, middle long part is the body of sternum and lowest small part is the xiphoid process (Fig. 3.18).

Manubrium articulates on each side with the medial end of the clavicle forming the **sternoclavicular joint.** On each side the body of sternum articulates with 1st to 7th pairs of costal cartilages, continuation of the respective ribs. In between the costal cartilages and ribs are the **intercostal spaces** occupied by three layers of muscles.

Ribs

There are 12 pairs of ribs, extending from the vertebrae posteriorly, then forming the lateral wall of the thoracic cavity continue as the costal cartilage which mostly articulate directly or indirectly with the sternum (Fig. 3.18).

The ribs are classified into 3 sets:

1. *True or vertebrosternal ribs:* These extend from the thoracic vertebrae behind to the sternum in front through the costal cartilages. 1st to 7th ribs belong to this type.

2. *False or vertebrochondral ribs:* These extend from the lower thoracic vertebrae to the costal cartilages. 8th, 9th, 10th ribs belong to this variety.

3. *Floating or vertebral ribs:* These ribs have free lateral ends and are not attached to sternum at all. 11th and 12th ribs belong to this variety.

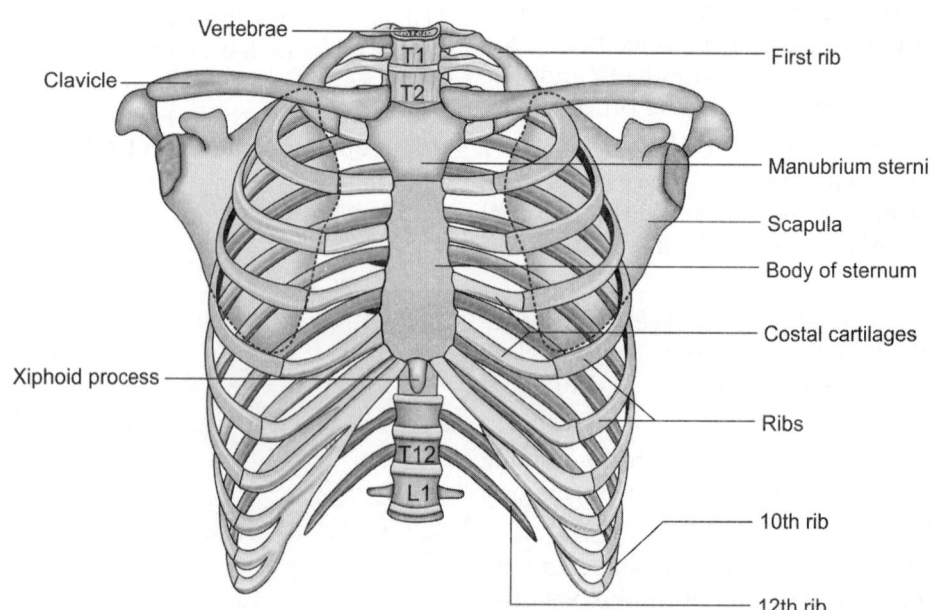

Fig. 3.18: Skeleton of thorax (front)

The ribs of both sides, vertebrae behind and sternum in front form a **thoracic cavity** which lodges the heart and a pair of lungs. Besides this, the cavity also lodges part of liver and stomach.

Along the lower border of the ribs is a **costal groove** which encloses the intercostal vein, artery and nerve (VAN) in order from above downwards (*see* Fig. 7.14).

Vertebral Column

It is a long column formed of irregular bones, the **vertebrae,** forming the central axis of the body. Lying in between the vertebral bodies is a fibrocartilaginous **intervertebral disc** (Fig. 3.19).

The 33 vertebrae are of 4 types according to the regions. These are 7 cervical, 12 thoracic, 5 lumbar, 5 sacral, 4 coccygeal.

Typical vertebra is comprised of a **body** placed anteriorly and **2 pedicles** placed postero-laterally (Fig. 3.20). From the pedicles **transverse processes,** extend laterally, and **laminae** extend medially which fuse to form the **spine.** Between the laminae and the body is a **vertebral canal** which lodges the very important **spinal cord.**

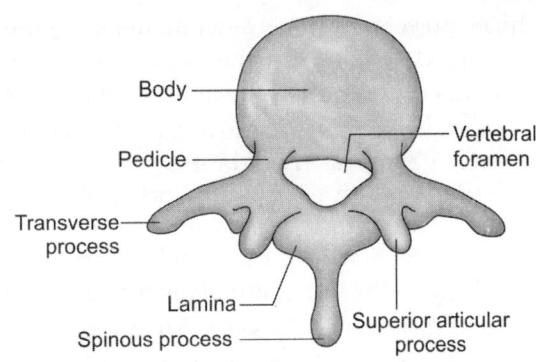

Fig. 3.20: A lumbar vertebra showing the features of a typical vertebra (viewed from above)

All the vertebrae articulate with each other to form continuous vertebral canal. This vertebral canal encloses the spinal cord and all 3 meninges till lower border of first lumbar vertebra in the adult, while the lower part contains the various nerve roots and meninges. Dura mater and arachnoid mater end at second sacral vertebra, while pia mater enclosing filum terminale ends at the coccyx.

Features of Various Types of Vertebrae

1. *Cervical vertebrae:* Typical vertebra contains a foramen in the transverse process. 1st and 2nd are atypical. **1st vertebra** is called **atlas** and **2nd vertebra** is called the **axis** (Fig. 3.21). The atlas is simply a ring of bone with two short transverse processes. Axis vertebra has an upward projecting **odontoid process** which articulates with the anterior arch of atlas vertebra. These special

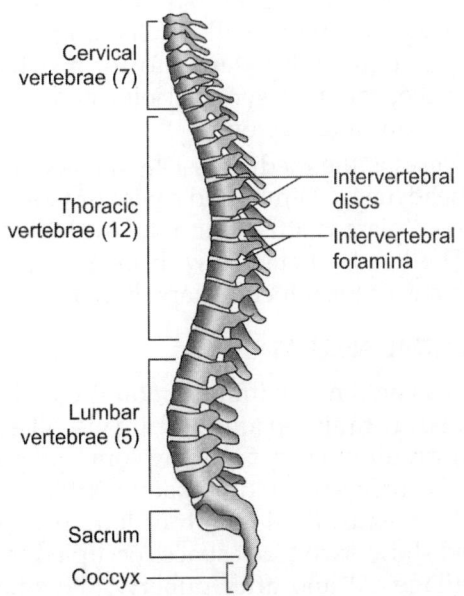

Fig. 3.19: Vertebral column

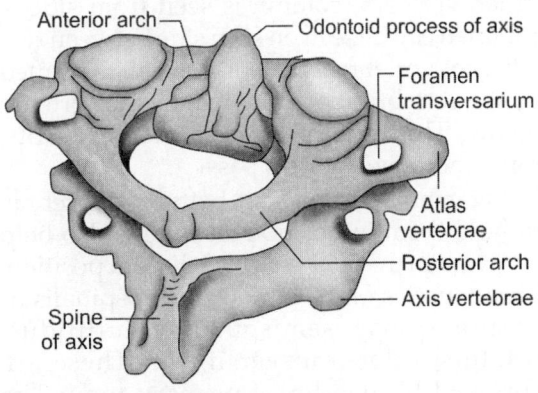

Fig. 3.21: Articulation between atlas and axis vertebrae

vertebrae permit the movements of flexion and extension with the skull and movements of rotation at the atlantoaxial joints.

2. *Thoracic vertebrae:* These are 12 in number; each vertebra articulates with at least 2 ribs, one on each side. 2nd to 9th ribs articulate with two adjacent vertebrae on each side. Bodies of the vertebrae are small to begin with, but gradually increase in size.

3. *Lumbar vertebrae:* These are 5 in number and are very big in size. The transverse processes are small.

4. *Sacral vertebrae:* These are also 5 in number but all fuse with each other to form a single piece of bone, the **sacrum,** which forms the posterior boundary of the pelvic cavity. On each side, the sacrum articulates with ilium to form sacroiliac joint. Its upper part articulates with 5th lumbar vertebra and lower part articulates with coccyx.

5. *Coccygeal vertebrae:* These are 4 very small vertebrae, which have fused to form **coccyx.** These are non-functional in human beings, but represent the bones of tail of the lower animals.

The bodies of adjacent vertebrae are separated by **intervertebral discs.** These are thinnest in cervical region and become progressively thicker towards the lumbar region. These have a shock absorbing function and also contribute to the flexibility of the vertebral column. Each disc consists of an outer fibrous ring called **annulus fibrosus** and inner soft, highly elastic **nucleus pulposus.** When vertebral column is seen from side, a **foramen** can be seen on each side between two adjacent vertebrae. Half of the wall is formed by the vertebra above and half by the vertebra below. Through these spinal nerves, roots, rami and blood vessels pass.

Ligaments are present between vertebrae to hold them in position and these also help to maintain the intervertebral discs in position. True muscles of the back are sacrospinalis or erector spinae, semispinalis, multifidus, rotators, inter-transversii, etc. These are supplied by the dorsal primary rami. The movement permitted in the vertebral column include **flexion** (forward bending), **extension** (backward bending), **lateral flexion** (bending to the side) and **rotation.**

Functions: Besides protecting the spinal cord the vertebral column supports the skull. It also forms the axis of trunk, giving attachment to muscles of shoulder girdle and upper limbs, ribs and pelvic girdle and lower limbs.

Curvatures: When viewed from side, the vertebral column shows four slight bends called **normal curves.** Relative to the front of body, **cervical and lumbar** curve are **convex** (bulging out), whereas **thoracic and sacral** curves are concave (cupping in). Thoracic and sacral curvatures are primary curvatures, while cervical and lumbar curvatures are secondary curvatures.

Ossicles of Middle Ear

Ossicles of the middle ear are three very small bones in the middle ear. These are malleus, incus and stapes.

1. *Malleus* is the lateral bone comprising of head, neck and handle. Head articulates with incus to form saddle variety of synovial joint known as incudomalleolar joint. The handle is embedded in the tympanic membrane.

2. *Incus* is the middle ossicle, consisting of a body and a long and short process. Head articulates with malleus. Its long process articulates with stapes to form ball and socket variety of synovial joint, and is called incudostapedial joint.

3. *Stapes* is the medial ossicle. It consists of a head, neck, 2 limbs and a base or foot plate. Foot plate is attached to the oval window. The head articulates with long process of incus of form incudostapedial joint.

CLINICAL ASPECTS

Bones contain maximum amount of calcium and so are radio-opaque and are visualised by plain radiographs. Growing long bone of a child contains non radio-opaque cartilage near both its ends. Radiograph of long bone of a child shows two black spaces occupied by the cartilage. At and after puberty, the ends of the bone fuse with the shaft. These black spaces should not be mistaken for fractures.

Radiographs or X-rays show the site and type of fracture and also show the progress of its healing and finally its union. Fractures can be:

- *Simple:* The broken ends do not protrude through the skin.
- *Compound:* The broken ends protrude through the skin to the external environment.

Plastering the site of fracture including the joint proximal and distal to it prevents the mobility of fractured ends and promotes healing of the fracture.

Achondroplasia

Achondroplasia is a genetic disease. The epiphyseal cartilage of long bones grows abnormally. The person is short in height with normal sized skull and trunk.

Osteogenesis Imperfecta

There is congenital defect of osteoblasts, resulting in failure of ossification. The bones are brittle and fracture easily.

Osteomyelitis

Osteomyelitis is infection of ends of long bones, mostly seen in children. Infection reaches via blood (usually) or through skin in compound fracture. It is usually caused by *Staphylococcus aureus*. It usually heals completely with antibiotics if diagnosed in the early stages.

Fracture of the Bone

Fracture of skull or vertebra acquires importance because of injury to the underlying brain or spinal cord.

Vitamin D Deficiency

Rickets is due to lack of vitamin D in children. Vitamin D helps in the absorption and proper use of calcium and phosphate for the development of bones and teeth. In rickets, the bones do not ossify properly and there is accumulation of osteoid. If lack of vitamin D occurs in adults, the condition is called **osteomalacia.**

Osteoporosis

Osteoporosis usually occurs after 45 years of age and is more common in females. The bony tissue is reduced, making them more vulnerable to fractures. Osteoporosis leads to bone pain, compression of vertebrae and fractures. It is more common in women after menopause because estrogen production declines (estrogen and testosterone stimulate osteoblast activity and synthesis of bone matrix). Calcium intake must be supplemented after 45 years to prevent osteoporosis. Low dose of estrogen, alendronate (inhibits bone resorption by osteoclasts) are also useful. Weight-bearing exercises and adequate calcium intake in early age are beneficial for prevention of osteoporosis.

Neoplasms

Primary malignant tumour or neoplasm of bone is most commonly osteosarcoma while the most common benign primary tumour is osteochondroma. Secondary tumours or metastases reach the bones from primary tumour of prostate, lung and breast.

Spina Bifida

It is a congenital defect of vertebral column in which the laminae fail to unite in the midline. In severe cases, the membranes around the spinal cord or spinal cord itself protrude through the opening producing paralysis and loss of urinary bladder control.

Scoliosis, Kyphosis and Lordosis

1. **Scoliosis** is lateral bending of vertebral column.
2. **Kyphosis** is an exaggeration of the thoracic curve of the vertebral column.
3. **Lordosis** is an exaggeration of the lumbar curve of the vertebral column.

Flat Foot and Pes Cavus

1. **Flat foot** is decrease in the height of the medial longitudinal arch of foot.
2. **Pes cavus** is abnormally increased medial longitudinal arch of foot.

JOINTS

DEFINITION

The area of articulation of two or more bones or cartilage is called a joint. The joint allows growth of bones in length, gives stability to the bones and allows free movement in some joints. Joints form cavities like cranial, thoracic and abdominal cavities. Movements of joints of thoracic cavity help in respiration.

TYPES OF JOINTS

There are various types of joints. These are:

I. *Fibrous joints* where union of two bones is by fibrous tissue, e.g. sutures of skull, gomphosis (between teeth and maxilla/mandible). These allow no movement (Figs 3.22 and 3.23).

II. *Cartilaginous joints* where binding tissue between the bones is a pad of cartilage. These allow very slight movement. These are of two varieties:

- *Primary cartilaginous joint*, e.g. between the diaphysis and epiphysis of a long bone (Fig. 3.24). Such a joint allows growth in length of the bone.

- *Secondary cartilaginous joint*, e.g. pubic symphysis, intervertebral joints where fibrocartilaginous disc is present between the bones (Fig. 3.25). These give strength to the joint.

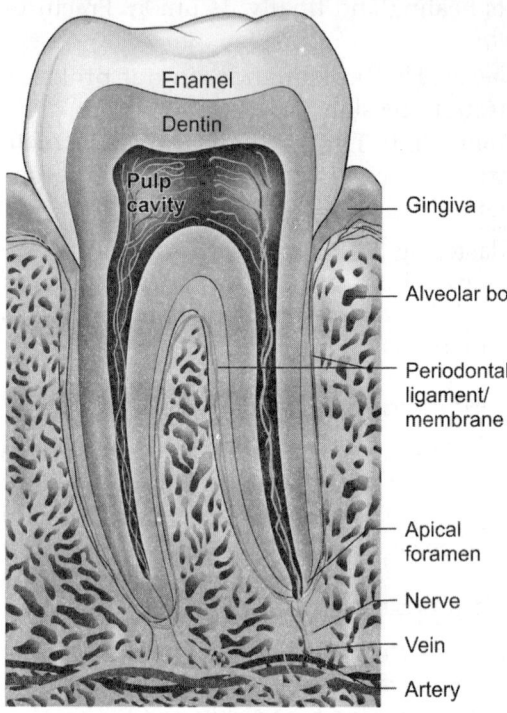

Fig. 3.23: Gomphosis

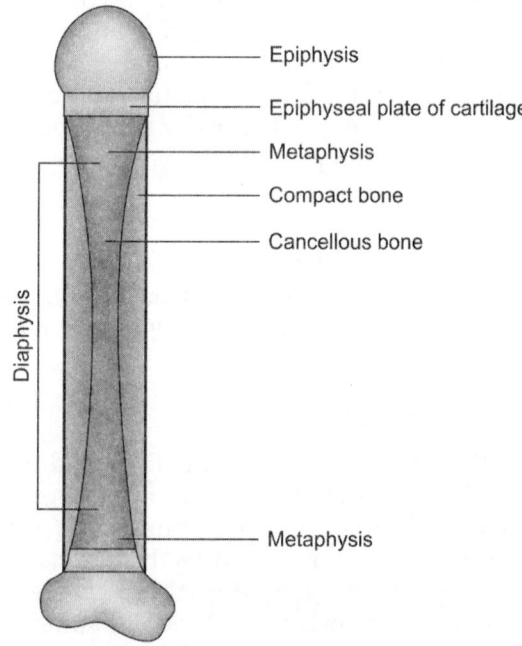

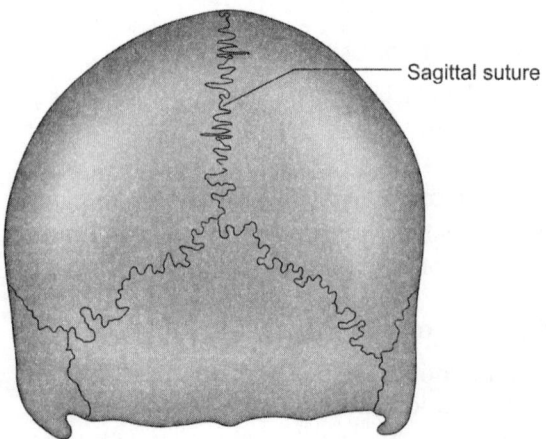

Fig. 3.22: Skull viewed from behind

Fig. 3.24: Primary cartilaginous joint

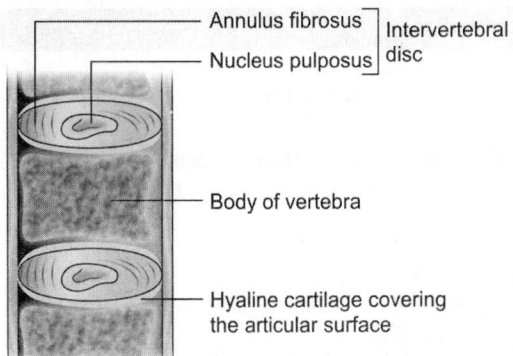

Fig. 3.25: Secondary cartilaginous joint

III. *Synovial joints* where the ends of the bones are enclosed within the **capsule** of the joint. The capsule is lined by a thin layer called the **synovial membrane** which secretes a lubricating **synovial fluid** (Fig. 3.26). The parts of the bones which are in contact are covered by hyaline cartilage. It provides a smooth articular surface. Ligament, muscles and tendons provide additional stability at most joints. These joints allow movement between the bones. These are of following varieties according to the range of movement possible.

1. *Multiaxial joint:* Which allows movement in many axes, e.g. shoulder and hip joint (ball and socket variety) and between trapezium and base of 1st metacarpal (saddle variety). These permit flexion, extension, abduction, adduction, medial and lateral rotation and circumduction (Figs 3.27A and B).

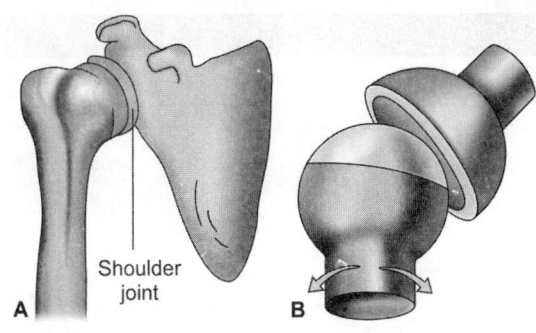

Figs 3.27A and B: Multiaxial ball and socket joint

2. *Biaxial joint:* Which allows movements in two axes, e.g. flexion, extension and abduction, adduction movements, e.g. wrist joint (Figs 3.28A and B), atlanto-occipital joint.

3. *Uniaxial joint:* Which allows movement in one axis only, e.g. flexion, extension, e.g. elbow joint (Figs 3.29A and B); rotation of atlas around the dens of axis vertebra (Fig. 3.21). Even rotation of radius over

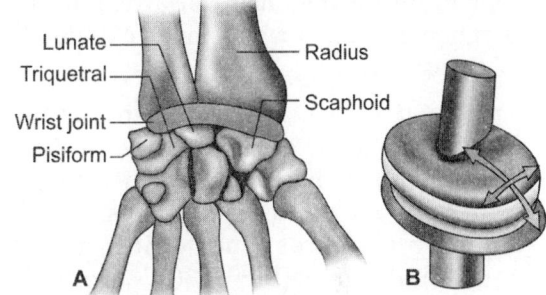

Figs 3.28A and B: Biaxial joint/wrist joint

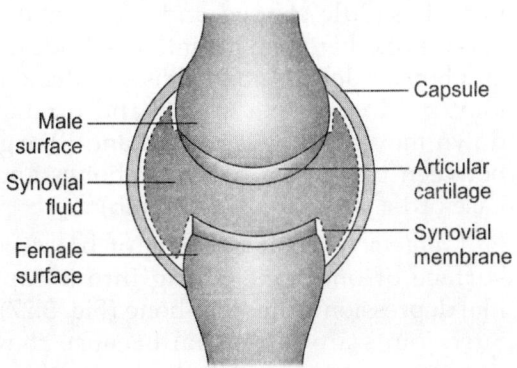

Fig. 3.26: Synovial joint

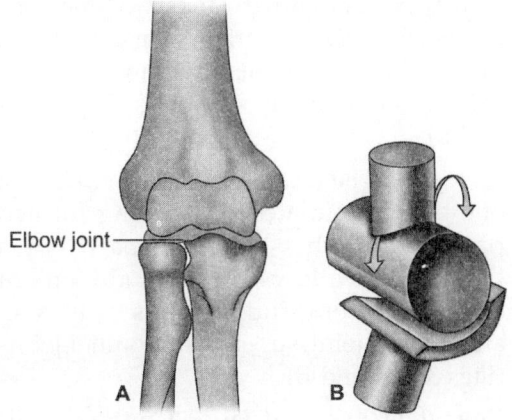

Figs 3.29A and B: Uniaxial hinge joint

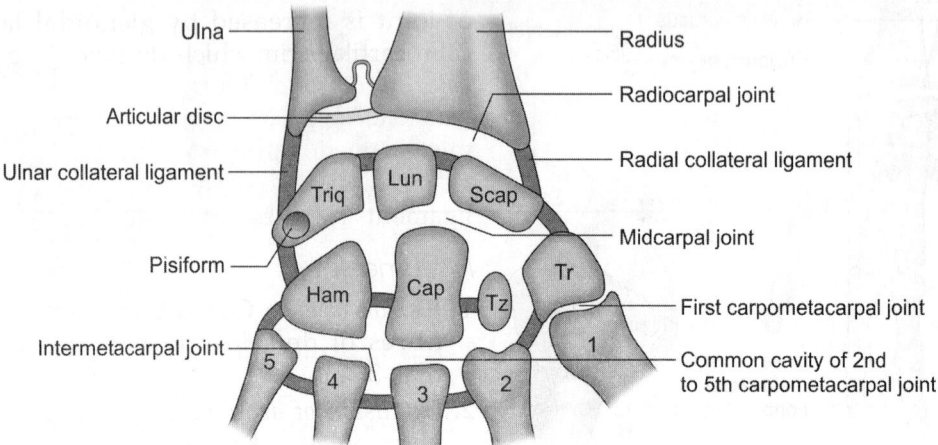

Fig. 3.30: Planar joint

ulna, e.g. supination, pronation of the forearm occurs at the uniaxial radioulnar joints (Fig. 3.30).

4. *Plane or gliding joint:* Allows gliding movements only, e.g. midcarpal joint (Fig. 3.30).

Depending on the shape of articulating parts of bones, the synovial joints are divided into 7 types:

1. *Planar joint:* Articular surfaces are flat or slightly curved. They permit side to side and back-and-forth gliding movements, e.g. joint between articular processes of adjoining vertebrae, 2nd to 5th carpometacarpal joints (Fig. 3.30), acromioclavicular joint, midcarpal (between carpal bones) joints.

2. *Hinge joint:* The convex surface of one bone fits into the concave surface of another bone. These allow movement around a single axis, e.g. ankle and elbow joints (Figs 3.29A and B).

3. *Pivot joint:* The round or pointed surface of one bone articulates with a ring formed partly by another bone and partly by a ligament. It allows rotation movement around its longitudinal axis only, e.g. atlantoaxial joint, superior radioulnar joints (Figs 3.31A and B).

4. *Condyloid/Ellipsoid joint:* Convex oval-shaped projection of one bone fits into

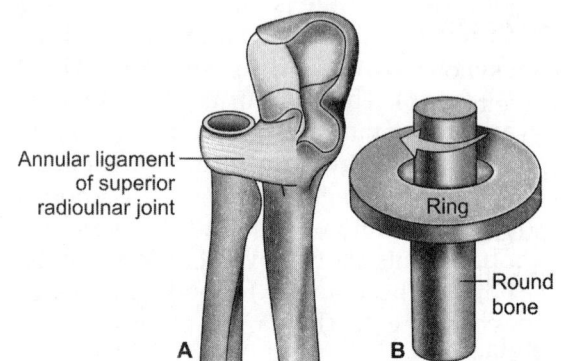

Figs 3.31A and B: Pivot joint

oval-shaped depression of another bone. It permits movement in two axes, e.g. wrist joint (Fig. 3.28), metacarpophalangeal joints for 2nd to 5th digits, knee joint, temporomandibular joint.

5. *Saddle joint:* The articular surface of one bone is saddle shaped and the articular surface of other bone fits into the "saddle" as a horse rider would sit. It is a multiaxial joint producing side to side and up and down movements (Figs 3.32A and B), e.g. between trapezium of carpal bones and base of 1st metacarpal (of thumb).

6. *Ball and socket joint* consists of ball-like surface of one bone fitting into a cup-like depression of another bone (Fig. 3.27). Such joints are multiaxial because they permit movement in all the three directions, e.g. shoulder joint and hip joint.

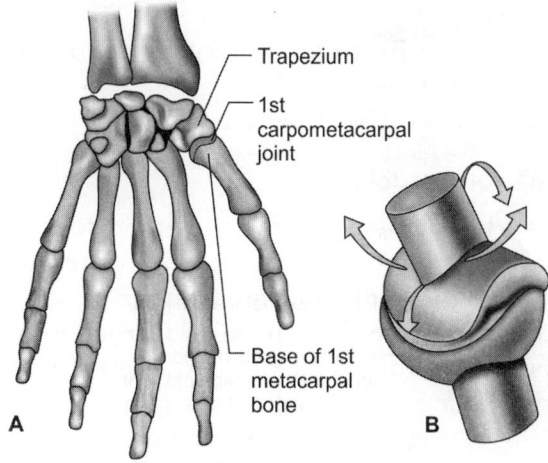

Figs 3.32A and B: Saddle joint

MAJOR SYNOVIAL JOINTS OF THE BODY

Major synovial joints of the body are shoulder joint, elbow joint, wrist joint, hip joint, knee joint, ankle joint, subtalar joint and temporomandibular joint.

Shoulder Joint

This ball and socket type of joint is formed by head of humerus and glenoid cavity of scapula. It has a wide range of movement because of the laxity of capsule inferiorly (Fig. 3.33). It is an **unstable joint.** The stability of joint is increased by glenoidal labrum (fibrocartilage rim which deepens the glenoid cavity), rotator cuff formed by short muscles, coracoacromial arch formed by coracoacromial ligament, acromion and coracoid process.

The joint is also supported by extracapsular ligaments but these are weak.

Movements

1. *Flexion of arm:* Coracobrachialis, anterior fibres of deltoid and pectoralis major (Fig. 3.34).
2. *Extension of arm:* Teres major, posterior fibres of deltoid and latissimus dorsi.
3. *Abduction:* Supraspinatus, deltoid, serratus anterior and trapezius (Fig. 3.35).
4. *Adduction:* Subscapularis, teres major and latissimus dorsi.
5. *Medial rotation:* Pectoralis major, teres major, latissimus dorsi, subscapularis and anterior fibres of deltoid.
6. *Lateral rotation:* Infraspinatus, teres minor and posterior fibres of deltoid.

Elbow Joint

It is a hinge type of joint formed by lower end of humerus, trochlear notch of ulna and head of radius (Fig. 3.36). It is strengthened by medial and lateral collateral ligament.

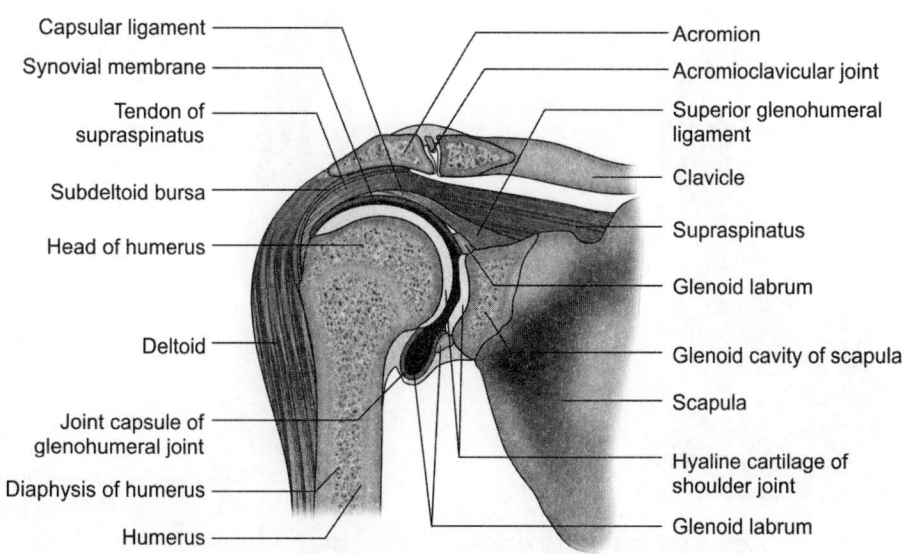

Fig. 3.33: Shoulder joint (section viewed from front)

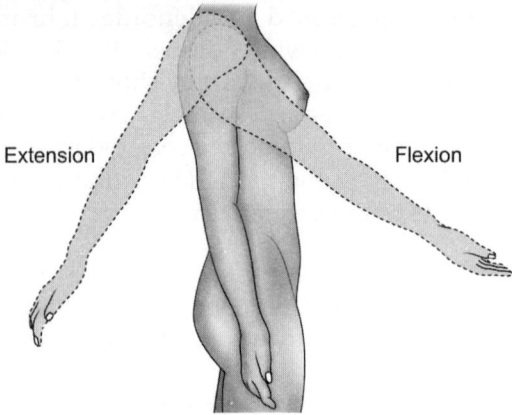

Fig. 3.34: Flexion and extension of arm

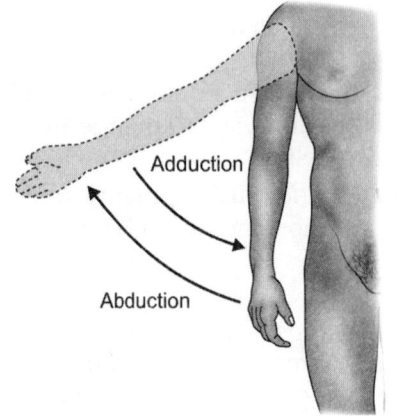

Fig. 3.35: Abduction and adduction of arm

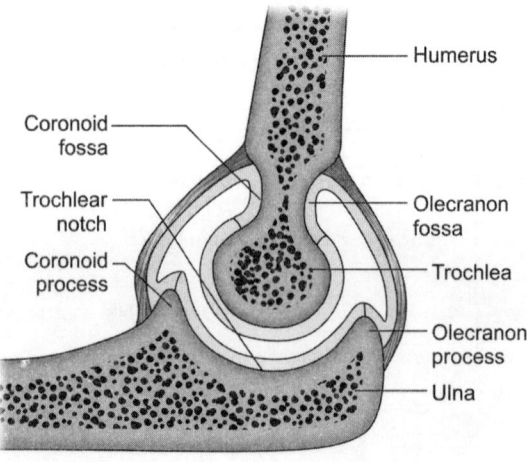

Fig. 3.36: Elbow joint (section viewed from the side in partial flexion)

Movements

1. *Flexion:* Brachialis, biceps brachii and brachioradialis.
2. *Extension:* Triceps brachii.

Radioulnar Joints

Proximal radioulnar joint is pivot joint formed between circumference of head of radius rotating in radial notch of ulna (Fig. 3.31). **Middle radioulnar joint** is fibrous joint between radius and ulna by interosseous membrane. **Distal radioulnar joint** is pivot joint between head of ulna and distal and of radius (Fig. 3.37).

Movements

1. **Supination:** Supinator and biceps brachii.
2. **Pronation:** Pronator teres and pronator quadratus (Figs 3.38A and B).

Wrist Joint

It is an ellipsoid joint between distal end of radius and proximal ends of scaphoid, lunate

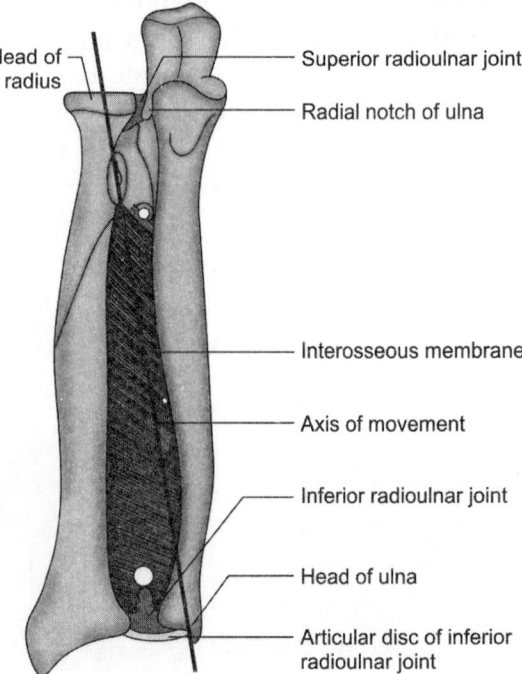

Fig. 3.37: Radioulnar joints

and triquetral bones (Fig. 3.28). Wrist joint is supported by medial, lateral, anterior and posterior ligaments.

Movements

1. *Flexion:* Flexor carpi radialis and flexor carpi ulnaris (*see* Fig. 7.5).
2. *Extension:* Extensor carpi radialis longus and brevis, and extensor carpi ulnaris (*see* Fig. 1.12).
3. *Adduction:* Flexor and extensor carpi ulnaris.
4. *Abduction:* Flexor carpi radialis and extensor carpi radialis longus and brevis.

Joints of Hand

There are synovial joints between carpal and metacarpal bones, between metacarpals and proximal phalanges and between phalanges. The movements at these joints are produced by the muscles of the forearm which have tendons extending into the hand. Movements at the first carpometacarpal joint are flexion, extension, abduction, adduction, opposition and circumduction (Fig. 3.32). Movements of the fingers are flexion, extension, abduction and adduction (Figs 3.39A and B).

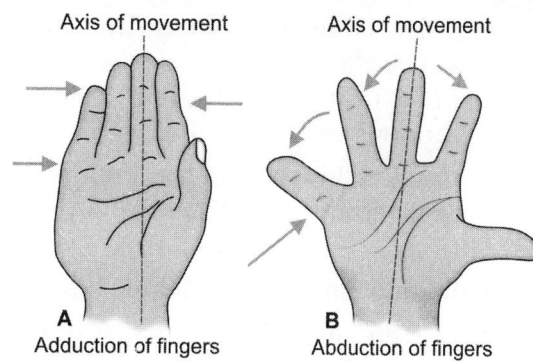

Figs 3.39A and B: Adduction and abduction of fingers

Hip Joint

It is a ball and socket joint between head of femur and cup-shaped acetabulum of hip bone (Fig. 3.40). Its stability is increased by acetabular labrum (ring of fibrocartilage attached to rim of acetabulum deepens the cavity) and strong ligaments around the hip.

Movements

1. *Flexion:* Psoas, iliacus, rectus femoris and sartorius.

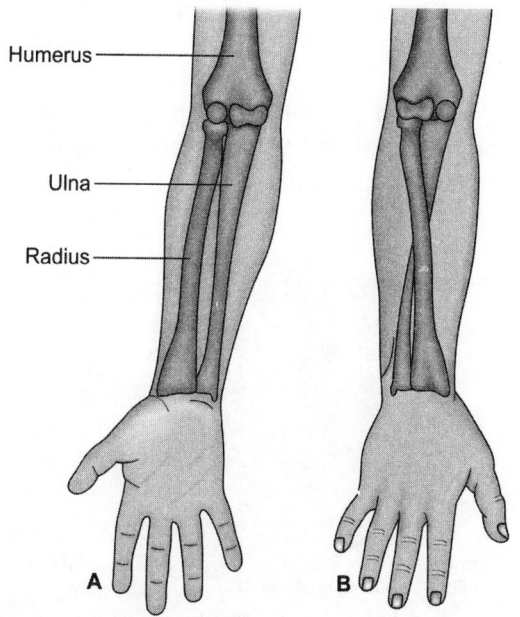

Figs 3.38A and B: Supination and pronation of forearm

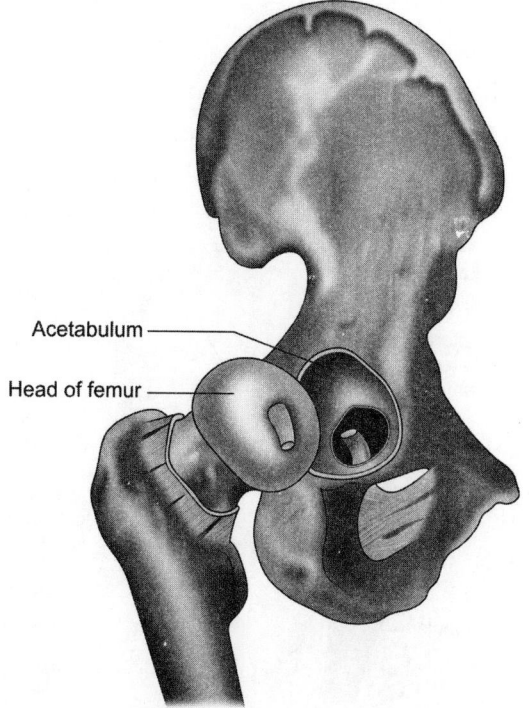

Fig. 3.40: Hip joint (section)

2. *Extension:* Gluteus maximus and hamstrings (*see* Fig. 7.25).

3. *Abduction:* Gluteus medius and minimus, and sartorius.

4. *Adduction:* Adductor longus, brevis and magnus, pectineus and gracilis.

5. *Medial rotation:* Anterior fibres of gluteus medius and minimus, and adductors.

6. *Lateral rotation:* Piriformis, obturator internus and externus, and quadratus femoris.

Knee Joint

It is a hinge joint between condyles of femur, condyles of tibia and posterior surface of patella. It is the largest joint (Fig. 3.41).

The knee joint is stabilised by tendon of quadriceps femoris muscle anteriorly, cruciate ligaments and medial and lateral collateral ligaments. **Menisci** (semilunar cartilages) are wedge shaped incomplete discs of fibrocartilage lying on top of articular surface of tibia. They also help to stabilise the joint.

Movements

1. *Flexion:* Gastrocnemius and hamstrings.

2. *Extension:* Quadriceps femoris (*see* Fig. 1.13).

Ankle Joint

It is a hinge joint formed by distal end of tibia including medial malleolus, distal end of fibula including lateral malleolus and body of talus. It is strengthened by ligaments on all the four sides (Fig. 3.42).

Movements

1. *Dorsiflexion:* Tibialis anterior, extensor digitorum longus, extensor hallucis longus and peroneus tertius.

2. *Plantar flexion:* Gastrocnemius and soleus (*see* Fig. 1.13).

Subtalar Joint

It is formed between inferior surface of body of talus and posterior facet on upper surface of calcaneum.

Movement of inversion and eversion occur between joints formed by tarsal bones (*see* Fig. 1.13).

Temporomandibular Joint

It is a condylar joint between temporal bone above and head of mandible below. It is supported by ligaments and is divided into two compartments by articular disc (Fig. 3.43).

Movements

1. *Protraction* (forward movement of mandible): Medial and lateral pterygoids of both sides acting together.

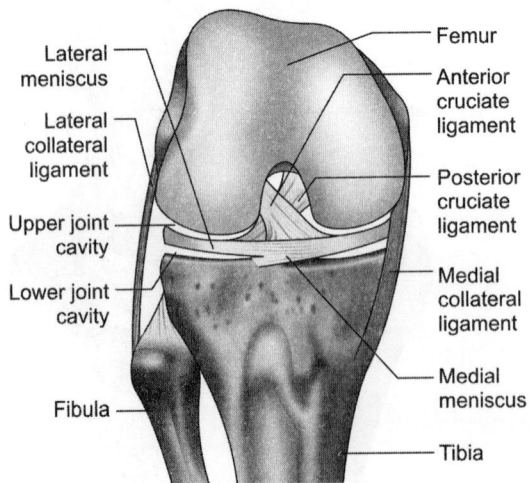

Fig. 3.41: Knee joint (section viewed from front)

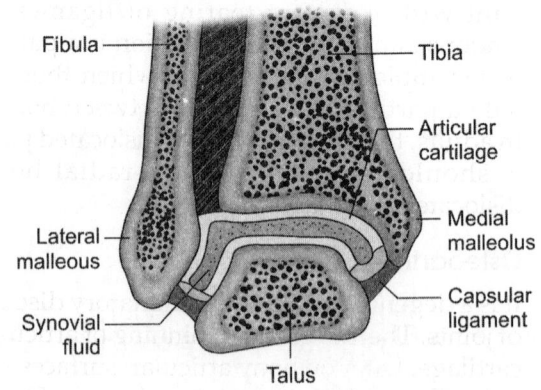

Fig. 3.42: Ankle joint (section viewed from front)

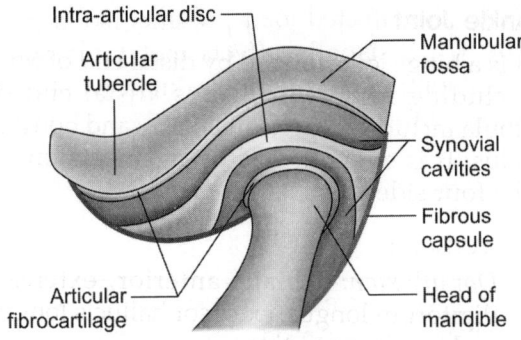

Fig. 3.43: Temporomandibular joint

2. *Retraction* (backward movement of mandible): Posterior fibres of temporalis (*see* Fig. 1.12).
3. *Elevation* (closure of mouth): Masseter, temporalis and medial pterygoid.
4. *Depression* (opening of mouth): Lateral pterygoid, digastric and mylohyoid.
5. *Side to side movement:* Lateral and medial pterygoid of one side acting alternately with the other.

CLINICAL ASPECTS

Sprain and Strain

Sprain results from forcible movement of joint that tears its ligaments. It may also damage the surrounding blood vessels; tendons, muscles or nerves. Strain results from partial tearing of the ligament.

Dislocation and Subluxation

Dislocation is displacement of a bone from a joint with resultant tearing of ligaments, tendons and capsule. Subluxation is a partial or incomplete dislocation, in which there is only a partial loss of contact between bones. In adults, the most commonly dislocated joint is shoulder and in children radial head dislocates most commonly.

Osteoarthritis

It is a degenerative non-inflammatory disease of joints. There is gradual thinning of articular cartilage. Later on bony articular surfaces are also affected and their shape changes. There is outgrowth of bone at articular margins at edges forming osteophytes. Patient usually presents with pain and restricted movement of affected joint. Usually, it is due to ageing and affects the large weight bearing joints, e.g. knees, hips and spine.

Rheumatoid Arthritis

It is a chronic inflammatory autoimmune disease. There is primarily involvement of synovial membrane but heart, blood vessels and skin are also affected. It is more common in females and mainly affects 30–55 years age group. There is formation of autoantibodies. Antigen antibody complexes (rheumatoid factor) form and are found in blood. Usually, the smaller joints of hand and feet are affected, i.e. metacarpophalangeal and proximal interphalangeal joints. It usually occurs bilaterally. There is hyperplasia and hypertrophy of synovial membrane with effusion into joint. There is erosion of articular cartilage and growth of granulation tissue (pannus) which erodes the bone.

Patient presents with pain, deformity of affected joints, loss of function, muscle wasting.

Ankylosing Spondylitis

It is an autoimmune inflammatory arthritis but the rheumatoid factor is absent. It usually affects the sacroiliac joints, spine and bigger joints, e.g. hip, shoulder. The sacroiliac and vertebral joints become progressively ossified. It is commoner in males and affects 20–40 years age group.

Acute Septic Arthritis

The joints can be affected by the bacterial infection. It usually spreads by blood. It is more common in children. Most commonly knee joint is affected. Usually, it is caused by *Staphylococcus aureus*. The patient presents with high grade fever, loss of movement of affected joint, effusion into the joint and local temperature is raised.

Gout

It is an inflammatory disorder caused by deposition of sodium urate crystals in joints and tendons. It is commoner in males. It occurs in persons with raised blood uric acid due to either over production or defective excretion by kidneys. Uric acid is a waste product of the breakdown of nucleic acids, i.e. DNA and RNA. The affected joint presents like septic arthritis. It usually affects metatarsophalangeal joint of big toe, ankle, knee, wrist and elbow joints.

Points to Remember

1. Inorganic calcium salt as clacium hydroxy-apatite [$Ca_{10}(PO_4)_6(OH)_2$] is present in the bone.
2. Periosteum does not cover the sesamoid bones and the 3 bony ossicles of middle ear.
3. Bone fractures are seen more often in persons without adequate protein, calcium and vitamin D.
4. Intramembranous ossification is quicker one step process compared to intracartilaginous, two step process.
5. Joints are classified as fibrous, cartilaginous and synovial types.
6. Joints are vital for locomotion.
7. The secondary cartilaginous joints are in midline of the body.
8. Joints in the laryngeal cartilages help us in speech.

MCQs

1. **What percentage of calcium of the body is stored in the bones?**
   (a) 90%   (b) 80%
   (c) 97%   (d) 75%

2. **Length of the bone increases by multiplication of cells at:**
   (a) Periosteum
   (b) Epiphysis
   (c) Epiphyseal plate
   (d) Diaphysis

3. **Which of the following joints contains an intra-articular disc?**
   (a) Ankle joint

   (b) Sternoclavicular joint
   (c) Elbow joint
   (d) Shoulder joint

4. **All the statements about synovial membrane are correct *except*:**
   (a) It is avascular
   (b) It is modification of deep fascia
   (c) It scretes synovial fluid
   (d) If damaged, it regenerates

5. **Condylar joints are:**
   (a) Uniaxial   (b) Biaxial
   (c) Multiaxial   (d) Symphysis

Ans   1 c   2 c   3 b   4 a   5 b

Cardiovascular System

BLOOD

FUNCTIONS OF BLOOD

Blood is a connective tissue. It helps in communication between cells of different parts of the body and external environment. Its functions are as follows:

1. It transports digested food from gastro-intestinal tract to tissues and organs.

2. It provides clotting factors to prevent loss of blood in case of injury.

3. It provides buffers to maintain the blood pH and acid–base balance.

4. It distributes hormones released by endocrine glands to various target organs.

5. It distributes heat to various parts of the body.

6. Blood maintains the internal environment within limits.

7. **Red blood cells** carry oxygen and carbon dioxide from blood to tissues and back.

   White blood cells protect our bodies from viruses, bacteria and provide immunity by forming antibodies.

   Platelets are essential for clotting mechanism. Lack of iron causes anaemia.

   Blood makes up 7% of body weight, e.g. it is about 5.6 litres in 70 kg man and is slightly less in females. Blood is always moving within blood vessels. Its continuous flow gives constant environment for the cells of the body.

COMPOSITION OF BLOOD

Blood consists of a cellular part and a liquid part. The latter is called the plasma and constitutes 55% of blood volume. The volume occupied by the cells is packed cell volume and is 45% in normal blood. Plasma contains the following:

1. *Proteins:* Albumin, globulin, fibrinogen, clotting factors.

2. *Minerals:* Calcium, phosphorus, iron, copper and magnesium.

3. *Electrolytes:* Sodium, potassium, chloride and bicarbonate.

4. *Nutrients:* Glucose, amino acids, fatty acids, glycerol and vitamins.

5. *Waste products:* Urea, uric acid, creatinine.

6. *Gases:* Oxygen, carbon dioxide, nitrogen.

7. *Hormones:* Thyroxine, cortisone, etc.

8. *Enzymes:* Certain clotting factors.

   The details of composition are as follows:

Plasma Proteins

The plasma proteins make up about 7% of plasma and are contained within the blood. The plasma proteins exert the osmotic pressure of blood which keeps plasma fluid within the circulation. If level of plasma proteins falls due to any reason, the osmotic pressure of plasma is reduced and fluid exudes out of the capillaries into the tissues causing **oedema** or swelling of soft tissues especially of the dependent parts, i.e. around ankles.

Albumins: These are formed in the liver and are responsible for maintenance of normal osmotic pressure.

Globulins: These are mainly formed in the liver. The globulins function as:

1. Antibodies, i.e. immunoglobulins, which play an important role in immunity.
2. Transporting agents of some hormones, e.g. thyroglobulin carries the hormone thyroxine.

Clotting factors: These are required for coagulation of blood. Plasma minus the clotting factors is **serum. Fibrinogen** is a very important clotting factor and is synthesized by the liver.

Mineral Salts

These are involved in cell formation, muscular contraction, nerve impulse transmission, and maintenance of pH of blood. The pH of blood is maintained between 7.35 and 7.45 by the various chemical activities involving buffer systems (Fig. 4.1).

Nutrients

Food is digested in the digestive system. The products of absorption are glucose, amino acids, fatty acids, glycerol and vitamins. All these along with mineral salts are required to provide heat and energy for the body besides repair, replacement and synthesis of various cells of the body tissues.

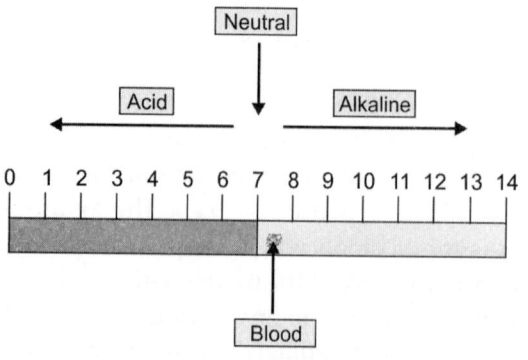

Fig. 4.1: pH scale

Waste Products

Urea, uric acid, creatinine are the waste products of protein metabolism. These reach the kidney via blood for excretion. Carbon dioxide released from all the cells reaches lungs via blood for expulsion during expiratory phase of respiration.

Hormones

These are produced by various endocrine glands and use blood as a vehicle to be transported to the target organs.

Gases

Oxygen, carbon dioxide and nitrogen are transported via the plasma.

Oxygen is carried in combination with haemoglobin and carbon dioxide is carried as bicarbonate ions in solution form in the plasma. Nitrogen also enters the body but its concentration is same in inspired air and expired air. It has no physiological function.

TYPES OF BLOOD CELLS

There are three types of blood cells:

1. Erythrocytes or red blood cells (RBC).
2. Leukocytes or white blood cells (WBC). These are granulocytes and agranulocytes.
3. Thrombocytes or platelets.

All the blood cells arise from "pluripotent stem cells" and pass through different developmental stages.

Each type of blood cell follow separate lines of development.

The blood cells are formed in red bone marrow and the process is called **haemopoiesis.**

Red Blood Cells (RBCs)

The RBCs are circular biconcave discs. These have no nucleus and are 7 µm in diameter. Certain terms about RBCs are used in clinical practice. These are:

Packed cell volume: Volume of RBCs in 1 litre or 1 mm^3 of whole blood. Normal packed cell volume is 40–50/mm^3.

RBC count: Number of RBC per litre or per mm^3 of blood.

Haemoglobin: Amount of haemoglobin present in whole blood and is measured as grams per 100 mL of blood. This is a very important measurement as it indicates the oxygen carrying capacity of blood, If haemoglobin (Hb) is less than the normal value, the condition is called **anaemia.** Normal haemoglobin in males is 13–18 g% and in females is 11.5–16.5 g%.

Mean cell volume: Average volume of cells and is measured in femtoliters (fl = 10^{-15} litre).

Mean cell haemoglobin: Average amount of haemoglobin in each cell and is measured in picograms (pg = 10^{-12} g).

Mean cell haemoglobin concentration: Amount of haemoglobin in 100 ml of red cells.

Fate of Red Blood Cells

After about 120 days, reticuloendothelial cells cause haemolysis of 'aged' RBC. The fate of RBC is shown in Fig. 4.2.

RBCs are formed in the red bone marrow. Before puberty red bone marrow is present in the medullary cavities of all long bones, marrow spaces of flat bones and ends of long bones. After puberty due to decreased need for production of RBC most of the red bone marrow is replaced by fat and is known as yellow bone marrow. However, red bone marrow persists at the ends of long bones and in flat bones like sternum and iliac crest. It is also present in the irregular bones.

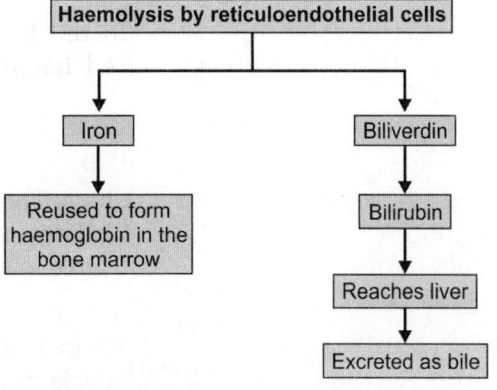

Fig. 4.2: Fate of RBC

The RBCs develop from the pluripotent stem cell to proerythroblast, erythroblast, reticulocyte to mature RBC during a period of 7 days. The cell develops, matures and also acquires haemoglobin within the cell.

During the maturation of RBCs, the size of cell decreases and loses its nucleus as well. For this process, vitamin B$_{12}$ and folic acid are necessary. Life of RBCs is about 120 days.

Haemoglobin is acquired during development of RBC. It is formed by union of a protein called **globin** and an iron containing substance known as **haem.** The haemoglobin is synthesised in the developing RBC.

Haemoglobin combines with oxygen to form oxyhaemoglobin which gives the typical bright red color to the arterial blood. Oxyhaemoglobin carries oxygen to the various cells of body. Each haemoglobin (Hb) molecule has four atoms of iron. Each atom can carry one molecule of oxygen. Therefore, one Hb molecule can carry up to 4 molecules of oxygen.

Haemoglobin also carries some amount of carbon dioxide from the tissues to the lungs to be expelled out. Rest of the carbon dioxide is carried as bicarbonate ions in solution form in the plasma.

Control of RBC formation: Normally, the rate of production and rate of destruction of RBCs is balanced. The stimulus for more production is lack of oxygen supply to the cells of the body. This may occur either because of excessive loss (menstruation) or destruction of RBCs or when oxygen tension is low as at high altitudes (Fig. 4.3).

Graveyard for RBCs: Spleen is the chief graveyard for RBCs after their lifespan is over.

Blood Groups

The blood groups are genetically controlled (Table 4.1). The major grouping is into ABO system, i.e. A, B, AB and O. This depends on two allelic genes. These genes are responsible for the potential to form the antigens known as agglutinogen A and agglutinogen B on the surface of RBC. The same genes control formation of agglutinins α and β in the blood

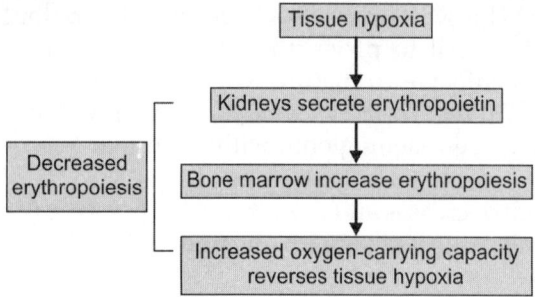

Fig. 4.3: Control of erythropoiesis: a negative feed-back mechanism

serum. Agglutinin α is responsible for agglutination of those RBCs which carry agglutinogen A and vice versa. But the arrangement is such if A agglutinogen is present, α agglutinin is absent, instead β agglutinin is present in serum. Similarly if β agglutinogen is present, then α agglutinin is present in serum. So, the serum does not agglutinate its own RBCs.

Before transfusion of blood it is imperative to see blood group named according to agglutinogen, i.e. A or B or AB or O in both the patients and the donor blood (Table 4.1).

Rhesus System

This system is also under the control of genes. This system produces either Rh +ve individuals with antigens and no antibody (85%).

Rh –ve individuals are with neither antigen nor antibody (15%). These individuals can produce antibody if RBCs carrying antigens reach in such a circulation.

If mother is Rh –ve and father is Rh +ve, Rh +ve fetus is being nurtured, and a few Rh antigen carrying RBCs escape from fetus into maternal bloodstream and are enough to stimulate her to produce antibodies which can come back to the fetus. These antibodies may be less in first pregnancy but can be in great amount in next pregnancy to be able to severely harm the fetus.

Human lymphocytic antigen (HLA) complex is a group of genes which have been identified on chromosome six. These play a major part in the identification of immune responses and foreign cells.

White Blood Cells (WBCs)

The WBCs are large cells, with nuclei, granules and no haemoglobin. Hence these are called white blood cells. There are two types of white blood cells:

1. **Granulocytes** or polymorphonuclear leukocytes: Depending upon the colour of granules, these are further classified as:
   a. Neutrophils (Fig. 4.4)
   b. Eosinophils (Fig. 4.5)
   c. Basophils.
2. **Agranulocytes:** These cells do not contain any granules and are of two types:
   a. Monocytes (Fig. 4.6)
   b. Lymphocytes, which are:
      i.   "T" lymphocytes
      ii. "B" lymphocytes

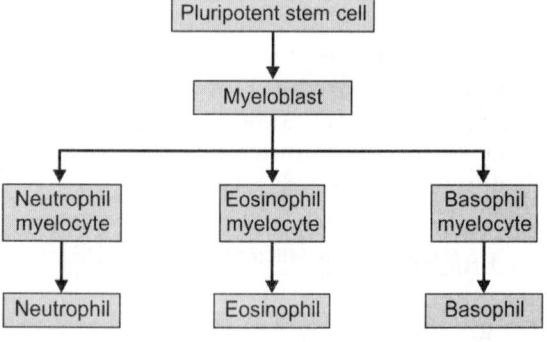

Fig. 4.4: Stages of formation of granulocytes

Table 4.1: Blood groups

Blood group	Agglutinogen	Agglutinin	Can receive blood
A	A	β	A and O
B	B	α	B and O
AB	A and B	–	AB, A, B and O
O	–	α, β	O only

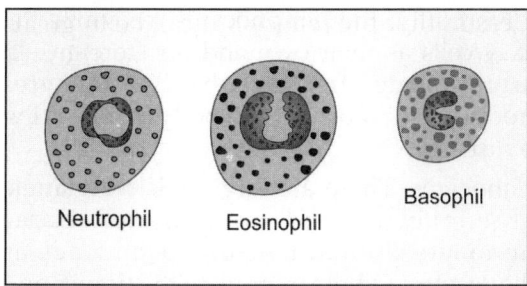

Fig. 4.5: Granulocytes (granular leukocytes)

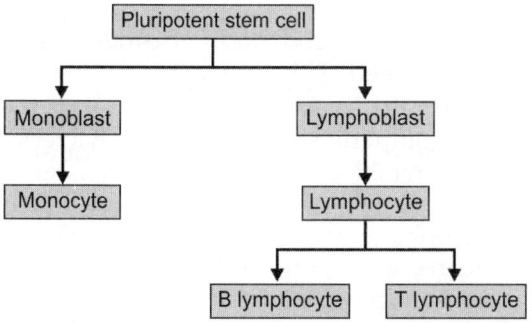

Fig. 4.6: Stages of formation of agranulocytes

Granulocytes

These cells develop from pluripotent stem cell the myeloblast which matures into three types of myelocytes (Fig. 4.4). The nuclei of granular series of cells is multilobed and their granules take up specific stains and the cells are named accordingly (Fig. 4.5).

Neutrophils: These cells form line of defence for the body. These protect the body against infecting bacteria. The bacteria enter the body to infect a particular tissue. The damaging cells produce **chemotaxins**. These **chemotaxins** attract the neutrophils to the site of infection, where these reach by amoeboid movements through the capillary wall. At the site of infection, WBCs engulf the bacteria, kill them by the enzymes contained in the granules and then phagocyte the dead bacteria.

The neutrophils are increased in:
- Any inflammatory reaction.
- Leukaemia (blood cancer).
- Bacterial infections.

Eosinophils: These cells are especially adapted to fight and kill the worms/parasites/allergic conditions. The eosinophils are found to be high in allergic conditions like asthma, allergic rhinitis, and in various skin allergies.

Basophils: These cells contain large blue granules. Their granules contain heparin which is an anticoagulant and histamine which is an inflammatory agent.

The contents of granules of basophils are released in response to an allergen, helping to fight out and remove the allergen thus protecting the body.

The mast cell is similar to basophil. It releases the contents of its granules as soon as allergen binds to the cell membrane in an attempt to destroy the allergen.

Agranulocytes

The agranulocytes contain a large nucleus and as the name indicates, no granules. These make up 25–50% of WBCs. The agranulocytes are of two types:

1. Lymphocytes (Fig. 4.7).
2. Monocytes.

Lymphocytes: These are small cells with relatively single large nucleus (Fig. 4.6). These are present in large numbers in lymph nodes, lymph nodules and spleen. These cells originate in bone marrow and reach thymus or lymph nodes. In these tissues the lymphocytes get "activated", after which these are usually able to deal effectively with the foreign proteins or antigens. There are two types of lymphocytes.

- *'T' lymphocytes:* These lymphocytes are processed in the thymus gland situated between the sternum bone and the heart. The hormone **thymosin,** produced by thymus causes the programming and maturation of lymphocytes, so that one set of "T" lymphocytes recognize one type of antigen only. These leave thymus gland to circulate in blood. The "T" cells provide **cell mediated immunity.**

The antigen (abnormal body cell, cancer cell) on coming into contact with 'T' lymphocytes stimulate the proliferation of these cells. The specialized 'T' cells are as follows:

a. **Cytotoxic 'T' cells:** These 'T' cells attach themselves to the target cells carrying antigens. Then these 'T' cells release strong toxins, thereby destroying infected cells/cancer cells.

b. **Memory 'T' cells:** These cells remember the antigen and act fast in any future attack by same antigen.

c. **Helper 'T' cells:** These cells are important as these help the 'T' cells by producing cytokines, i.e. interferons and interleukins. These helper 'T' cells help B lymphocytes in producing antibodies.

- *'B' lymphocytes:* The 'B' lymphocytes are programmed and processed in the bone marrow. These cells produce antibodies which destroy the antigen. The B lymphocytes also are very specifically matured, so that one set of 'B' cells respond to only one type of antigen. So 'B' lymphocytes produce antibody mediated immunity or **humoral immunity.**

Humoral Immunity or Antibody Mediated Immunity

'B' lymphocytes are mostly in lymph nodes, lymph nodules and in spleen. Once 'B' cells recognize the antigen, the 'B' cells start to enlarge and multiply, to produce the following two types of cells.

a. *Plasma cells:* These are modified 'B' lymphocytes. The specific plasma cells produce antibodies against a specific antigen, which was initially bound to 'B' lymphocyte.

b. *Memory 'B' cells:* The specific plasma cells remain in the body, with an imprint of the antigen. If the same antigen enters again even after years, these 'B' cells get activated and fight out with the antigen.

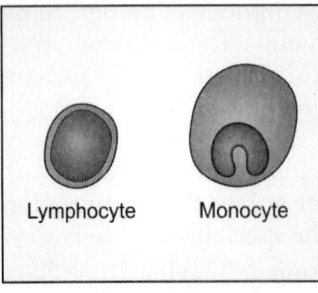

Fig. 4.7: Agranulocytes

Normally, the lymphocytes recognize the body cells as their own and not 'foreign'. In autoimmune diseases the lymphocytes produce antibodies against body cells, leading to disease.

Monocytes: These are large cells with single large nucleus and no granules. Some monocytes remain in blood and act as phagocytes. Others migrate to the tissues and mature as macrophages. Monocytes and macrophages produce interleukin I which acts as under:

a. Increases the production of programmed and activated 'T' lymphocytes.

b. Acts on the hypothalamus, and raises the body temperature especially in bacterial infections. Macrophages act a little later in inflammatory responses. After 24 hours, macrophages collect at the inflamed site, leading to chronic inflammation. The macrophages live longer than neutrophils. The macrophages phagocytose dying or dead tissues, bacteria or antigens.

Macrophages act hand in hand with monocytes of blood and with lymphocytes.

Reticuloendothelial system: This system comprises monocyte-macrophage cells. Macrophages are not only present in blood. These are also found in various tissues such as microglia in brain to phagocytose the dying or dead brain cells, Kupffer's cells in liver, macrophages in alveolar wall, reticular cells in spleen and lymph nodes.

The reticuloendothelial system helps in providing immunity to the body.

Thrombocytes or Platelets

The platelets are 2–4 micron discs which are non-nucleated. These develop from megakaryocytes in bone marrow (Fig. 4.8). The chief function of platelets is to "stop bleeding" and "promote clotting" of blood. This is possible due to number of substances present in these tiny blood cells.

The normal platelet count is 200,000–350,000/mm^3. The life span of platelets is 8–11 days. These produce a substance called **thrombopoietin.** The stages of **haemostasis**

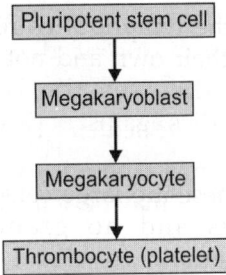

Fig. 4.8: Stages of formation of thrombocytes (platelets)

(stoppage of bleeding) following damage to blood vessel wall are as follows:

1. **Vasoconstriction:** At the site of bleeding, the damaged blood vessels get narrowed, due to serotonin released by platelets present at the site of damaged blood vessel. The narrowing of blood vessels reduce the blood flow at the site.

2. **Formation of platelet plug:** The platelets adhere to each other and clump at the site of bleeding. The release of adenosine diphosphate (ADP) attracts more platelets and these huge number of platelets form a **'platelet plug'** which acts as a temporary seal at the site of blood vessel wall damage.

3. **Blood clotting or coagulation:** Plasma protein prothrombin is converted into thrombin by the **prothrombin activator.** Thrombin converts fibrinogen into fibrin. Fibrin are thread-like pieces, which forms a mesh and hold the blood cells in between them.

   Prothrombin activator can be formed by either intrinsic or extrinsic pathway. After some time clot shrinks and serum is squeezed out.

4. **Breakdown of the clot (fibrinolysis):** The clot is broken down and healing of wall of injured blood vessel starts. As the clot is slowly removed, the healing process gets started and blood vessel gets new look.

Control of Coagulation

The coagulation is controlled by smoothness of normal blood vessel lining, presence of natural anticoagulants, e.g. heparin which inactivates clotting factors and presence of a special thrombin receptor on the cells lining blood vessels which inactivates thrombin on binding.

CLINICAL ASPECTS

Anaemia

Anaemia is a condition where the haemoglobin level is lower than nornal. It may be due to:

- Enhanced RBC loss as in hemolytic anaemias and in normocytic anaemias.
- Decreased RBC manufacture: This occurs mostly due to iron deficiency or megaloblastic anaemias due to deficiency of vitamin B_{12} and/or folic acid.

Haemolytic Anaemias

When RBCs are destroyed earlier than their life span of 120 days. These may be:

1. *Congenital haemolytic anaemia:* This is a genetic disease where Hb is abnormal and RBC are friable. This is of following types:
   - *Sickle cell anaemia:* The Hb molecule is abnormal and RBC get sickle shaped. Life span of such RBCs is less.
   - *Thalassaemia:* The protein globin synthesis is less than normal, resulting in decreased Hb synthesis. These RBC are also more friable.

2. *Acquired haemolytic anaemias:* The reasons are: *Malaria*
   - Chemicals like lead, arsenic compounds in environment.
   - Drugs like sulphonamides, primaquine taken for long periods.
   - X-rays, radioactive isotopes.

Normocytic Anaemias

The number of RBCs is less than normal. It is usually due to chronic diseases or after haemorrhage.

Decreased RBC Manufacture

1. *Iron deficiency anaemia:* This is most prevalent type of anaemia in India and is due to lack of iron in food (usually), malabsorption or increased loss of blood. Every one must eat food items containing

iron. The anaemia is responsible for breathlessness on exertion, palpitations and tachycardia. Daily requirements of iron is 1–3 mg. Children and women require more iron than male adults. Iron deficiency anaemia is microcytic (cells smaller than normal) and hypochromic (cells paler than normal).

2. *Megaloblastic anaemia:* This type of anaemia occurs in deficiency of folic acid and/or vitamin B$_{12}$. Abnormally large RBCs (megaloblasts) are found in blood.

3. *Hypoplastic anaemia:* This occurs due to depression of bone marrow. It may be due to hepatitis, ionising radiation and cytotoxic drugs.

Polycythaemia

When the number of RBCs is more than normal, the condition is known as polycythaemia. There is increased viscosity of blood which may lead to clotting within the blood vessels (intravascular clotting).

Leukopenia

When total WBC count is less than 4,000 mm^3, the condition is called leukopenia.

Neutropenia: When the neutrophils are abnormally less, the condition is called neutropenia. It may be due to leukaemia, bacterial infections, cytotoxic drugs—sulphonamides and some antibiotics. Neutropenia leads to acute and severe infections as the line of defence becomes very weak.

Leukocytosis

When the WBCs are abnormally more the condition is called leukocytosis. If WBCs are more than 11,000 mm^3, the condition is leukocytosis. It may occur as a protective response to a variety of diseases, especially infections.

Leukaemia

When there is uncontrolled production of premature or mature WBCs the condition is called leukaemia. Its reasons may be genetic, chemicals like cytotoxic drugs, ionising radiations.

Leukaemias may be acute or chronic

a. **Acute leukaemia:** There is overproduction of 'blast' cells. It may be acute myeloblastic or lymphoblastic leukaemia,

b. **Chronic leukaemia:** Here the overproduced cells are in the 'myelocyte' stage. This may also be chronic granulocytic or lymphocytic leukaemia.

Due to proliferation of WBC precursors in bone marrow there is decreased formation of other blood cells in bone marrow causing anaemia, leukopenia and thrombocytopenia.

Thrombocytopenia

This is the condition when platelet count is abnormally low to a level below 150,000/mm^3. This may be due to decreased production of platelets or enhanced destruction of platelets. A very common reason of thrombocytopenia is "dengue" fever, caused by a virus and transmitted by Aedes mosquito. Spontaneous bleeding from capillaries occur when platelet count falls below 30,000/mm^3.

Deficiency of Vitamin K

Vitamin K is required for synthesis of clotting factors II, VII, IX and X by liver. Deficiency of vitamin K leads to bleeding disorders. It may be due to deficiency of vitamin K in the diet or decreased absorption of vitamin K in the intestines.

Haemophilia

This is a sex-linked bleeding disorder. The female is the carrier and male is the sufferer. It mother is carrier and father is normal, the possibilities are—normal girl, normal boy, carrier girl and haemophilic boy.

The sufferer has bleeding episodes with very mild trauma.

LYMPHATIC SYSTEM AND ITS FUNCTIONS

Functions

- Lymphatic system produces, stores and recirculates lymphocytes. Lymphocytes are concerned with the immune responses
- Storehouse of macrophages.
- Drainage of surplus tissue fluid with macromolecules into the blood stream.
- Transport of absorbed fat from intestines into the blood stream.

Lymphoid tissue is concerned with antigen-antibody reactions. Thus they are related to allergic mechanisms. These are also related to Acquired Immunodeficiency Syndrome (AIDS). The virus of AIDS prevents proliferation of some 'T' cells, so the body's immune system fails. Lymphoid tissue is involved in lymphoid leukaemia where the lymphocytes are produced in great numbers.

Various **lymphoid organs** are lymph nodes, tonsils, spleen and thymus. Aggregations of lymphocytes are present in the gastrointestinal tract. Most of the tissues contain lymphatics except brain, spinal cord, eye and ear.

Lymphatics start as blind tubes in the tissue fluid. These drain as afferent lymphatics into the adjacent lymph node. The lymph filters through the node. The vessel leaving the node is the efferent lymphatic.

Thymus

Thymus lies in front of upper part of thorax, in front of heart and big blood vessels. It is 15 gm at birth and grows up to puberty when it regresses and is replaced by fatty tissue. It forms 'T' lymphocytes that migrate to be located in the lymphoid tissues (Fig. 4.9).

Relations:
- **Anterior:** Sternum and upper four costal cartilages
- **Posterior:** Arch of aorta and its branches
- **Superior:** Structures in the root of the neck
- **Inferior:** Heart enclosed in pericardium
- **Lateral:** Lung enclosed in pleura on each side.

Tonsils

Tonsils are collection of lymphoid tissue at oropharyngeal junction. These are palatine tonsils, seen through the open mouth. The pharyngeal tonsils are on the posterior wall of the nasopharynx. Lymphoid follicles are also present in the tongue and are called lingual tonsils. Palatine tonsils are covered with stratified squamous epithelium. Rest of the structure is same as lymph node.

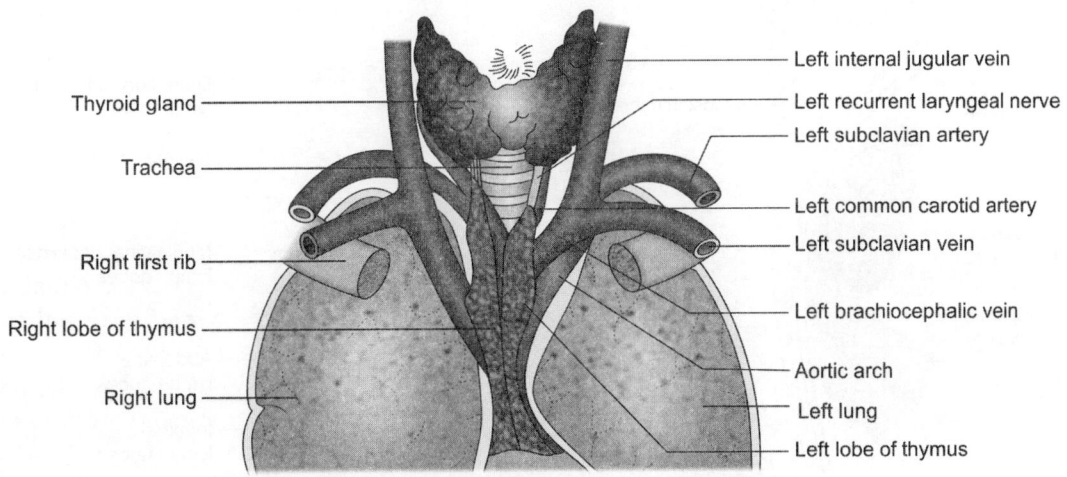

Thyroid gland — Trachea — Right first rib — Right lobe of thymus — Right lung — Left internal jugular vein — Left recurrent laryngeal nerve — Left subclavian artery — Left common carotid artery — Left subclavian vein — Left brachiocephalic vein — Aortic arch — Left lung — Left lobe of thymus

Fig. 4.9: Thymus

Waldeyer's Ring

At the oropharyngeal isthmus, there are several collection of lymphoid tissue that form the Waldeyer's lymphatic ring. It is made up of pharyngeal tonsil above, right and left palatine tonsil, right and left tubal tonsil and lingual tonsil below (Fig. 4.10).

Spleen

Spleen lies in upper left part of abdomen besides the left kidney under the left costal margin (Fig. 4.11). It is palpable when grossly enlarged. It also contains many lymphoid follicles with an arteriole running through them.

Spleen is concerned with
  i. Production of blood cells in fetal life.
  ii. Immunity (because it contains B and T lymphocytes)
  iii. Storage of blood
  iv. Phagocytosis for removal of abnormal and old erythrocytes, leukocytes and platelets.

Lymph Nodes

Lymph nodes are bean shaped structures grouped together in neck, axilla, and inguinal region, where these are palpable if enlarged. These are also present in thorax, abdomen and pelvis (Fig. 4.12).

Lymph node consists of **lymphoid follicles** within the connective tissue. In the centre of follicle is a **germinal centre** which produces new lymphocytes. Bacteria are destroyed by macrophages in the lymph node. Cancer cells mostly spread through lymphatics.

Intestines

In the mucous membrane of ileum of small intestine the lymphocytes are aggregated. These are known as Peyer's patches.

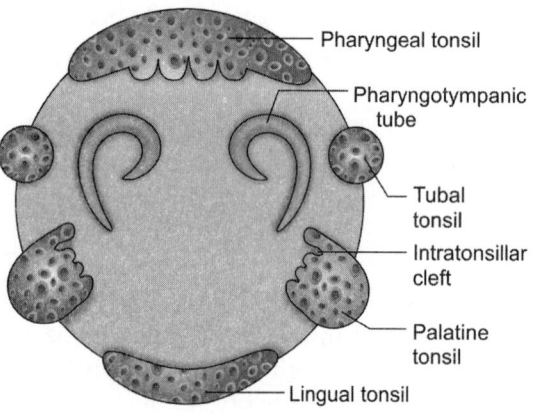

Fig. 4.10: Components of Waldeyer's ring

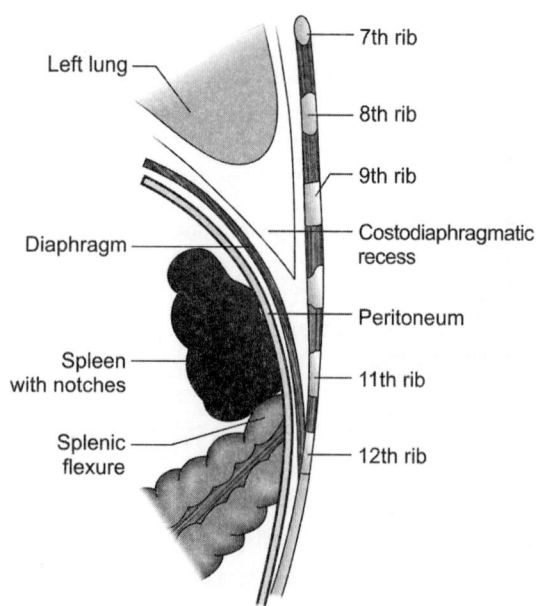

Fig. 4.11: Spleen

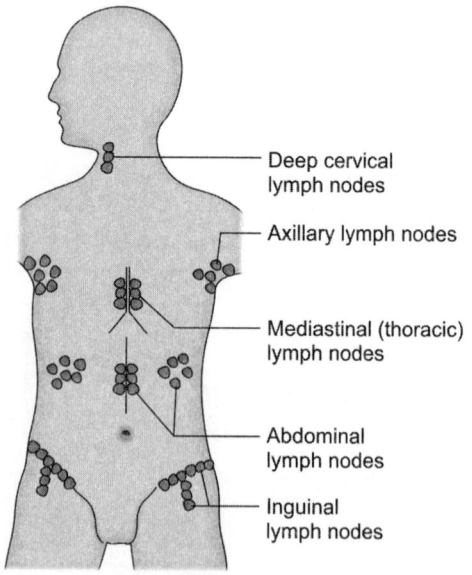

Fig. 4.12: Various groups of lymph nodes

Lymph and Lymphatic Vessels

Lymph is a surplus tissue fluid which enters the lymph capillaries. These capillaries join to form the lymphatic vessels. Lymphatic vessels are thin walled tubes with valves to permit one-way flow. They connect various lymph nodes. These drain lymph from most of the tissues and transport lymph and lymphocytes from nodes and other lymphoid tissue into blood circulation. These vessels have hardly any smooth muscle fibre. So, lymph flow depends upon pressure from surrounding structures.

The largest lymphatic duct in the body is thoracic duct (Fig. 4.13). It begins in upper abdomen, runs up in front of vertebral column to the left side of root of neck where it drains at the junction of left subclavian and left internal jugular veins. Thoracic duct drains lymph from both the lower limbs, abdomen, left side of thorax, left upper limb and left side of head and neck.

Lymph from right upper limb, right side of thorax and right side of head and neck drains into a shorter right lymphatic duct. This duct drains at the junction of right subclavian and right internal jugular vein.

CLINICAL ASPECTS

Lymphatic System

The lymph nodes guard the body against the infections. Sometimes, these guards can also be affected by acute or chronic infections.

1. *Acute infections* by various types of bacterial give rise to pain and raised body temperature.

2. *Chronic infections* are mostly due to tuberculosis, requiring proper and complete treatment by antitubercular drugs. This treatment usually lasts for 6–8 months and must be completely undertaken. In our country tuberculosis is extremely common.

3. *Tumours* of the lymph nodes are called **lymphomas.**

4. *Tonsil:* Tonsil guards the oropharynx against the antigens. Tonsil itself may be the site of acute infection. The condition is called **'acute tonsillitis'** and needs proper treatment. Tonsils if chronically inflamed

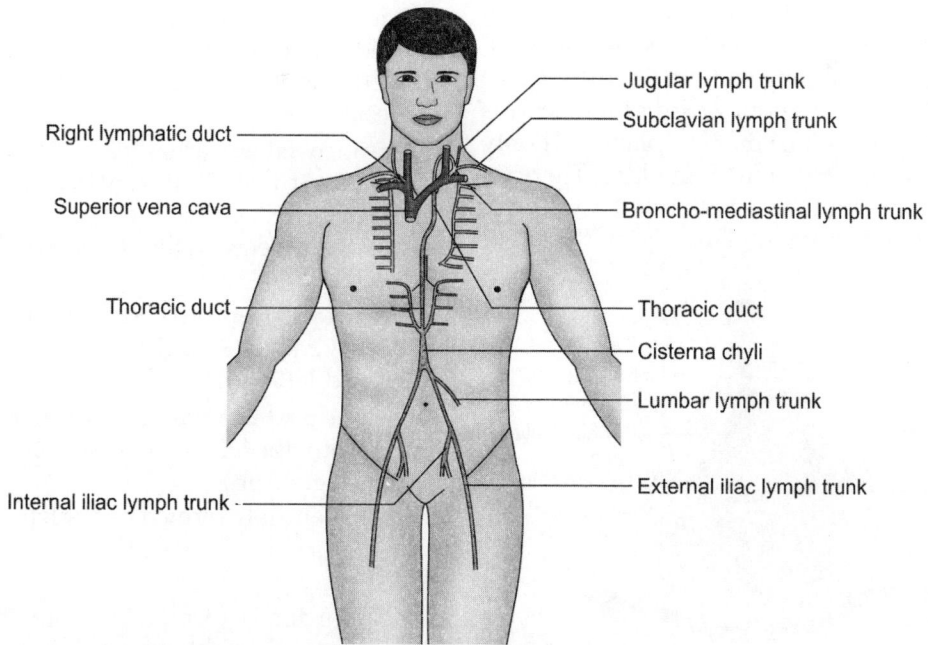

Fig. 4.13: Lymphatic system

Right lymphatic duct

Superior vena cava

Thoracic duct

Internal iliac lymph trunk

Jugular lymph trunk

Subclavian lymph trunk

Broncho-mediastinal lymph trunk

Thoracic duct

Cisterna chyli

Lumbar lymph trunk

External iliac lymph trunk

may need removal. The procedure is called **'tonsillectomy'.**

5. *Spleen:* Spleen usually gets enlarged in malaria, haemolytic anaemia and chronic myeloid leukaemia. The spleen enlarges obliquely downwards towards the right iliac fossa.

Spleen may rupture due to injury and cause excessive bleeding. In such cases, spleen has to be removed. Lymph nodes, red bone marrow and liver take over the functions of spleen.

6. *Thymus:* This gland produces 'T' lymphocytes necessary for immunity of the body. In myasthenia gravis, there is usually increase in size of the thymus.

7. *Lymph vessels:* The lymph vessels carry the lymph from distal parts of body into the main veins. These also carry the absorbed fat molecules. Lymph vessels carry the cancerous cells from its site of origin to distant areas and are responsible for the metastases of the cancer.

HEART

Heart is situated in the thoracic cavity, which protects it. In addition to the bones and cartilages forming the thoracic cage, the heart is also safe-guarded by the fibrous and serous pericardium.

Pericardium is made up of two sacs. The outer sac consists of fibrous tissue (Fig. 4.14) and the inner is a continuous double layer of serous membrane. There is a potential space between the two layers with a thin film of serous fluid between them. The pericardial fluid helps to make the contraction of heart smooth and frictionless. The inner layer of serous pericardium is known as **epicardium**.

Heart is a pumping station, almost the size of the hand's fist. About 2/3rd of the heart is situated to the left of median plane and only 1/3rd is to the right of median plane. The apex beat is palpable in the left 5th intercostal space 9 cm from the median plane.

Relations

• **Anterior:** Sternum, costal cartilages and ribs
• **Posterior:** Oesophagus, aorta and thoracic vertebrae
• **Lateral:** Lungs enclosed in pleural sac.

External Features

Heart is comprised of three surfaces, the anterior or sternocostal, inferior or diaphragmatic and posterior or base.

It has four **borders.** These are upper, right, inferior and left.

It is made up of two thin walled atria situated above and two thick walled ventricles situated below. The left ventricular wall is the thickest.

Sternocostal surface is formed by the right atrium, 2/3rd of right ventricle and 1/3rd of left ventricle. Only a little part of left atrium, the auricle projects on the sternocostal surface (Fig. 4.15A).

The diaphragmatic surface is formed by both ventricles, right ventricle forming 1/3rd and left ventricle forming 2/3rd part.

Base or posterior surface is formed by the atria, mostly the left atrium and a part of right atrium (Fig. 4.15B).

Apex is entirely formed by the left ventricle.

Borders

Upper border is formed by both the atria. Right border by right atrium. Inferior border by right ventricle. Left border by left ventricle.

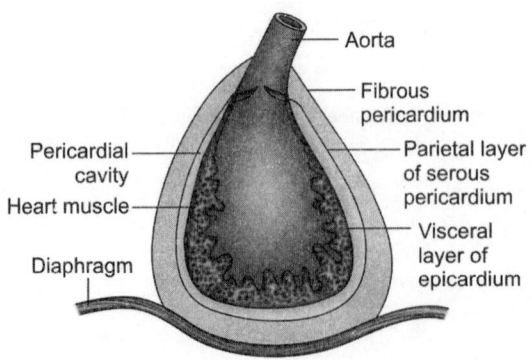

Fig. 4.14: Heart within pericardium

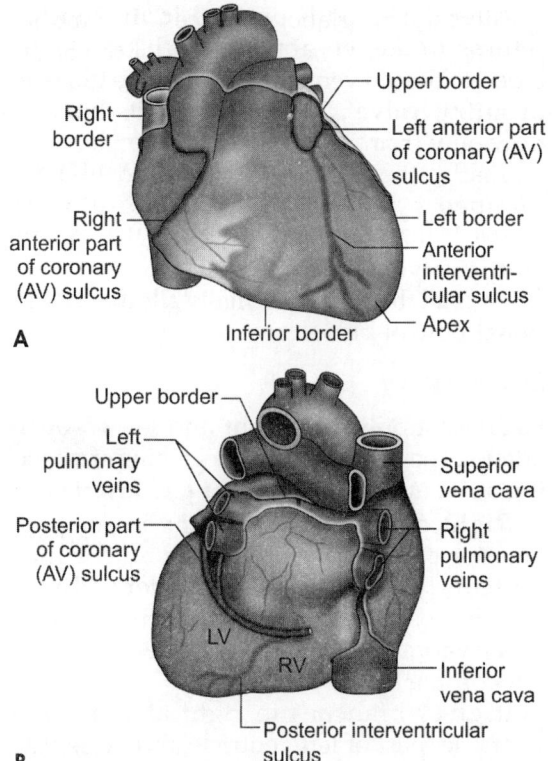

A

B

Figs 4.15A and B: Gross features: (A) sternocostal surface and (B) base of heart *(For colour Fig. see Plate 1)*

Heart also shows a circular groove in between atria and ventricles. The groove is called atrioventricular groove (AV groove).

Separating the two ventricles are the interventricular grooves sulci (IV grooves). The anterior interventricular groove lies anteriorly and posterior interventricular groove lies on the diaphragmatic surface of heart.

Chambers of the Heart

There are 4 chambers, right and left atria and right and left ventricles.

Right Atrium

It forms the right border, upper border, part of base and part of sternocostal surface of the heart. It consists of a smooth portion and a rough portion. The latter is called the auricle.

Entry channels are superior vena cava, inferior vena cava and coronary sinus.

Exit channel is tricuspid valve.

Right Ventricle

It forms inferior border of heart, 2/3rd of sternocostal and 1/3rd of diaphragmatic surface of heart. It is separated from the left ventricle by an IV septum. Its wall is 1/3rd the thickness of the left ventricle. It contains **3 papillary muscles** to which chordae tendinae are attached (Fig. 4.16). These in turn are attached to the cusps of 3 valves at the right AV orifice. Besides these, rest of ventricular muscle is called **trabeculae carneae**. One

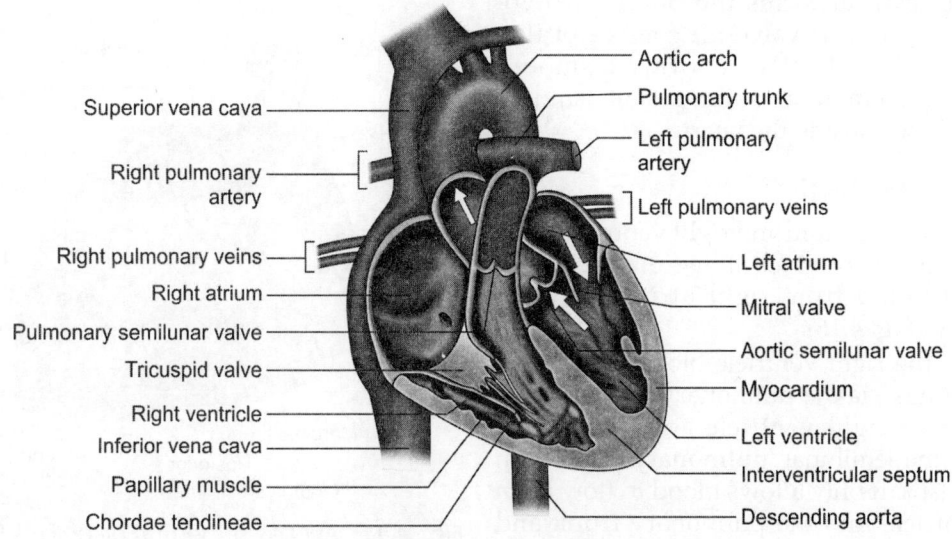

Fig. 4.16: Interior of the heart *(For colour Fig. see Plate 1)*

moderator band is present which conducts right atrioventricular bundle.

- Entry channel: Tricuspid valve
- Exit channel: Pulmonary trunk.

Left Atrium

It chiefly forms the base or posterior surface of heart.

- Entry channel: 4 pulmonary veins
- Exit channel: Bicuspid or mitral valve.

Left Ventricle

This is the thickest chamber of the heart. It forms 2/3rd of diaphragmatic surface, 1/3rd of sternocostal surface. It also forms the apex of the heart. It contains 2 strong papillary muscles and lot of trabeculae carneae.

- Entry channel: Bicuspid mitral valve
- Exit channel: Aortic opening.

Structure of the Heart

The heart is composed of three layers of tissue—epicardium (mentioned above), myocardium and endocardium.

Myocardium consists of specialised cardiac muscle. Each cardiac muscle fibre has a nucleus and one or more branches. It also has cross striations like skeletal muscle. The ends of cells and their branches are in close contact with ends and branches of adjacent cells.

Endocardium forms the lining of myocardium and heart valves. It consists of flattened epithelial cells. It forms a smooth glistening membrane which permits smooth flow of blood inside the heart.

Valves of the Heart

Between right atrium and right ventricle is the **'tricuspid valve'**, which allows unidirectional flow of blood from right atrium to right ventricle (Fig. 4.16).

From the right ventricle blood is pumped to the lungs via the pulmonary trunk. At the junction of right ventricle and pulmonary trunk is the semilunar **'pulmonary valve'** with three cusps. It only allows blood to flow from the ventricle into the pulmonary trunk and lungs.

After the blood is purified in the lungs, it returns to the left atrium which pushes the blood to the left ventricle through the **bicuspid or mitral valve'**. This also permits blood to flow only from atrium to the ventricle.

Lastly, the pure or oxygenated blood is pumped by the thick musculature of left ventricle into the ascending aorta through the **'aortic valve'** with three cusps.

Thus all the valves normally allow unidirectional flow of blood.

Blood Supply

Heart is supplied by right and left coronary arteries. These arise from the beginning of ascending aorta and are **functional end arteries.**

Right coronary artery runs in the right anterior part of atrioventricular sulcus turns posteriorly around the right border and again runs in posterior part of AV sulcus and ends by anastomosing with circumflex branch of left coronary artery.

It gives branches to right atrium, right ventricle, part of left ventricle and IV septum (posterior part). Main branches are marginal artery along the inferior border and posterior IV branch in posterior IV groove (Fig. 4.17).

Left coronary artery is larger and has a small course on the sternocostal surface. It runs in left anterior part of AV sulcus, gives a large anterior IV branch. Then it is called circumflex branch and it turns posteriorly in

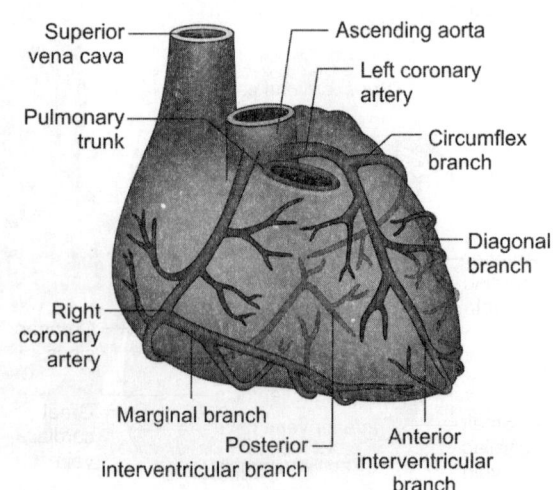

Fig. 4.17: Arteries of heart *(For colour Fig. see Plate 1)*

the AV sulcus to anastomose with right coronary artery.

Besides anterior IV branch it gives branches to left ventricle.

Venous blood is returned to the right atrium of heart via the **coronary sinus** (Fig. 4.18). It receives great, middle and small cardiac veins.

CIRCULATION OF BLOOD

Blood has to perform number of functions which are only possible if the blood is used and reused by the circulation.

Circulatory system consists of heart which acts as a pump and closed blood vessels. Blood vessels are of 3 types: (1) Arteries, (2) Capillaries, (3) Veins.

Arteries arise from the largest artery, the aorta which arises from left ventricle of heart. Arteries branch like branches of a tree.

The very small arteries are called **arterioles** which further divide to form the **capillaries.**

The wall of arteries and arterioles is made up of three layers of tissue:

1. Outer layer of fibrous tissue—tunica adventitia.
2. Middle layer of smooth muscle and elastic tissue—tunica media.
3. Inner lining of endothelium—tunica intima.

The arteries have thicker walls and contain variable amount of muscular and elastic tissue depending on their size.

Capillaries are minute channels and connect arterioles with the venules. Capillaries allow diffusion of gases, nutrients and waste products through their single layered walls. The network of capillaries is 7,000 square metres in adults.

Capillary Exchange

This difference of pressure at the arterial end of capillary forces fluid from the capillaries into tissue spaces. Blood flows slowly through the large network of capillaries from the arterial end to the venous end. At the venous end, the difference of pressure helps in sucking 9/10th of the fluid back into the venous end of capillary (Table 4.1).

The remaining 1/10th fluid is drained from tissue spaces as lymph into minute lymph capillaries which originate as blind end tubes. These lymph capillaries continue as lymph vessels and lymphatic ducts and from there to the blood stream.

Veins are thin walled tubes with relatively larger lumen. These receive the deoxygenated blood from the capillaries and venules. The two larger veins drain into right atrium of heart.

Differences between artery and vein are shown in Table 4.2.

Table 4.1: Showing pressures at arterial and venous ends of capillary

Capillary	Hydrostatic pressure	Osmotic pressure
Arterial end	35 mmHg	25 mmHg
Venous end	15 mmHg	25 mmHg

Table 4.2: Differences between artery and vein

Artery	Veins
Blood flow is in spurts	Continuous blood flow
Flow is at high pressure	At low pressure
Carries blood from heart to capillaries	Carry blood from capillary to heart
Offers resistance under pressure	Easily flattened under pressure

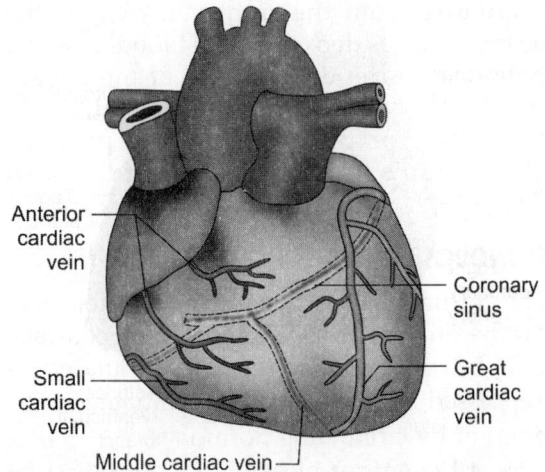

Anterior cardiac vein

Coronary sinus

Small cardiac vein

Great cardiac vein

Middle cardiac vein

Fig. 4.18: Veins of heart *(For colour Fig. see Plate 1)*

SYSTEMIC CIRCULATION

Circulation between left ventricle and right atrium through the tissues of upper limb, head, neck, brain and thorax, abdomen and lower limb is called **'systemic circulation'** (Flowchart 4.1). Aorta and its branches carry oxygenated blood from the left ventricle of heart to various tissues of the body. Oxygen is utilised by the tissues releasing carbon dioxide. The deoxygenated blood via vena cavae returns to the right atrium of the heart (Fig. 4.19).

The force with which blood is pumped out is not enough to return it to the heart by veins. Return is possible by the following factors:

1. Back flow is prevented by the valves of the vein.
2. Gravity helps in return of blood from head and neck but puts obstacles in return of blood from lower limb. Valves help to counter the effect of gravity.
3. Contraction of skeletal muscles, especially lower limbs put pressure on the veins and help in return of venous blood.

Total blood volume is 5 litres, out of which 84% is in systemic circulation and 16% in pulmonary circulation.

Out of 84%, 64% is in venous sinuses and veins, 13% in arteries and 7% in capillaries. Out of 16% blood in pulmonary circulation 7% is in heart and 9% is in lungs.

Flowchart 4.1: Circulation of blood

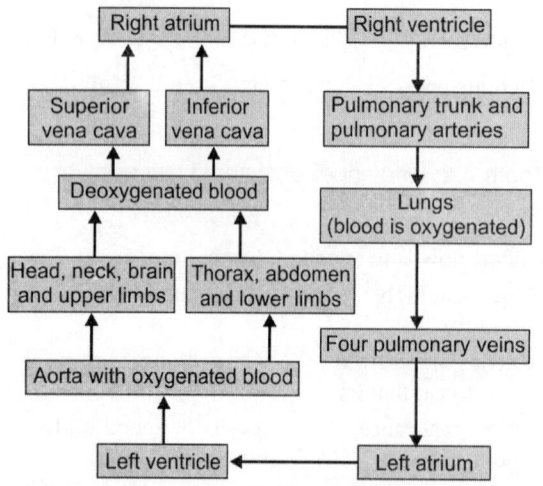

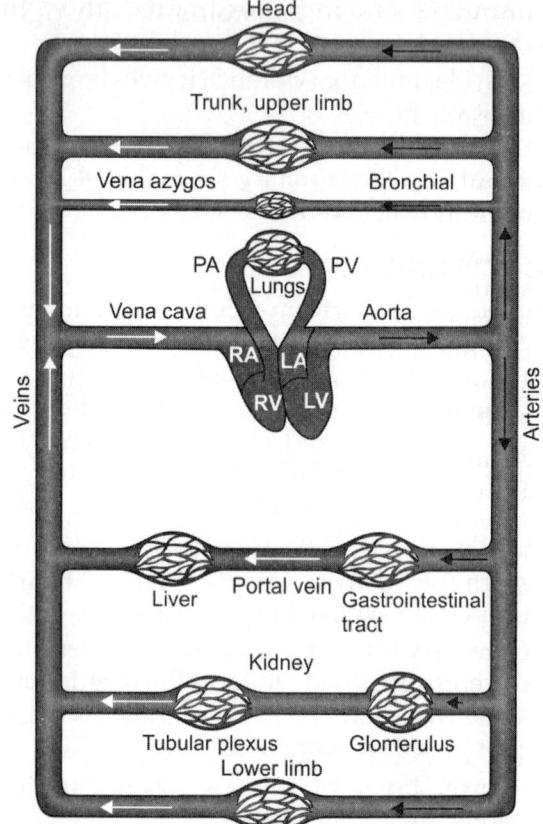

Fig. 4.19: Circulation of blood

PULMONARY CIRCULATION

Blood circulation between right ventricle and left atrium through lungs is known as **'pulmonary circulation'**. Pulmonary trunk originates from the right ventricle of the heart. It carries deoxygenated blood. The two pulmonary arteries (branches of pulmonary trunk) carry the deoxygenated blood to the lungs for purification. The purified blood returns to the left atrium of the heart (Fig. 4.19).

CONDUCTING SYSTEM OF HEART

The cardiac muscle has intrinsic system that can be automatically stimulated to contract. This intrinsic system can be stimulated or depressed by nerve impulses initiated in the brain or by circulating hormones.

Small groups of specialised neuromuscular cells in the myocardium initiate and conduct impulses causing coordinated and synchronised contraction of heart muscle.

Sinoatrial (SA) node is present in the wall of the right atrium and acts as the pacemaker of the heart because of its ability to initiate impulses more rapidly than other groups of neuromuscular cells.

Atrioventricular (AV) node is present in atrial septum near atrioventricular valves. It can initiate impulses capable of causing contraction but slower than SA node. Normally, it is stimulated by impulses that sweep over the atrial myocardium (Fig. 4.20).

Atrioventricular bundle (AVB) or **bundle of His** originates from AV node and at upper end of ventricular septum divides into **right bundle branch** and **left bundle branch (RBB and LBB)**. In the ventricular myocardium, it breaks up into the fibers called **Purkinje fibres.** Impulses from these cause contraction of ventricular myocardium.

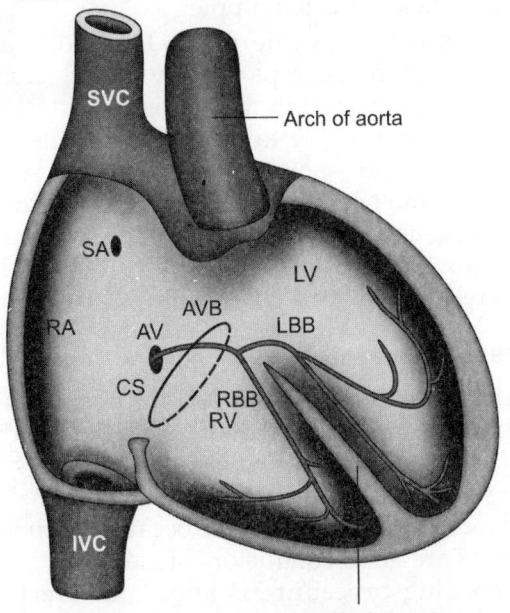

SA	: Sinoatrial node	LV	: Left ventricle
RA	: Right atrium	LBB	: Left bundle branch
AV	: Atrioventricular node	RBB	: Right bundle branch
CS	: Coronary sinus	RV	: Right ventricle
AVB	: Atrioventricular bundle		

Fig. 4.20: Conducting system of heart

Nerve Supply of Heart

Heart is supplied the parasympathetic and sympathetic nerves. These autonomic nerves arise in the **cardiovascular centre** in medulla oblongata.

The vagus nerve (parasympathetic) mainly supply the SA and AV nodes and atrial muscle. Stimulation of vagus nerve decreases the heart rate and force of heart beat.

Sympathetic nerves supply the SA node, AV node and myocardium of atria and ventricles. Its stimulation increases the heart rate and force of heart beat.

Factors Affecting Heart Rate

In addition to the autonomic nerves, heart rate is also increased by circulating adrenaline, noradrenaline and thyroxine.

The heart rate is also increased in anxiety, excitement, by exercise and by rise in body temperature.

CARDIAC CYCLE

The heart functions as a pump to maintain constant circulation of blood throughout the body.

Sequence of events from one beat to the next is known as **cardiac cycle.** Its duration is 0.8 seconds.

During each cardiac cycle, the heart contracts and then relaxes. The period of contraction is called **systole** and that of relaxation, **diastole.**

Atrial Cycle

- Atrial systole: 0.1 second
- Atrial diastole: 0.7 second.

Ventricular Cycle

- Ventricular systole: 0.3 seconds (Fig. 4.21)
- Ventricular diastole: 0.5 seconds (Fig. 4.22).

During diastole all the four cardiac chambers relax and receive blood. During systole cardiac chambers contract. Atria and ventricles contract at different timings but relax at the same time.

When auricles relax, blood enters via superior vena cava and inferior vena cava to

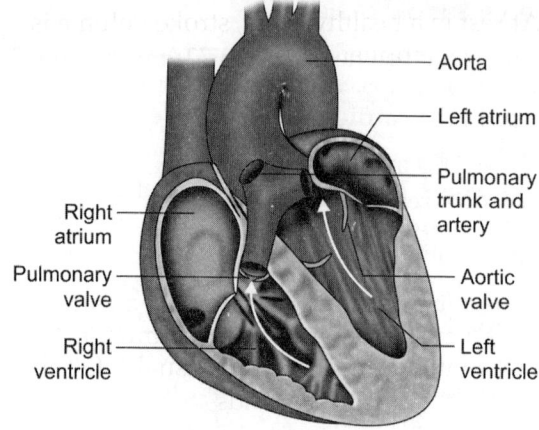

Fig. 4.21: Systole of cardiac cycle

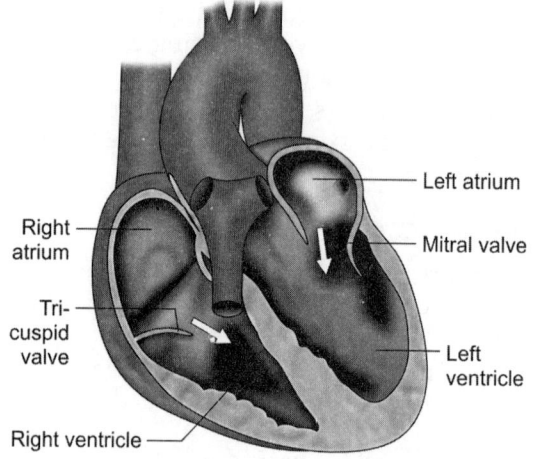

Fig. 4.22: Diastole of cardiac cycle

the right atrium and from 4 pulmonary veins into the left atrium.

Seventy percent of this blood reaching the atria enters the ventricles via the AV openings. When atria contract 30% additional blood enters the ventricles.

End diastole volume in each ventricle is 130 mL.

The left ventricle on contracting ejects blood into aorta and it enters systemic circulation. The ejected volume is 80 mL. Similarly blood from right ventricle enters the pulmonary circulation. An adequate blood pressure is required for flow of blood into the circulation.

The valves of the heart and of the great vessels open and close according to the pressure within the chambers of the heart.

The sequence of opening and closing of valves ensures that the blood flows in only one direction.

The AV valves (mitral and tricuspid) open while the ventricle is relaxed during atrial filling and systole. When ventricles contract, pressure inside ventricles increases and when it is above atrial pressure AV valves close. When the ventricular pressure rises above the pressure in aorta and pulmonary artery, the pulmonary and aortic valves open and blood flows into these vessels. When the ventricles relax pressure within them falls. First the pulmonary and aortic valves close, then the AV valves open and cycle begins again.

Heart Sounds

The sounds produced by the closure of heart valves during cardiac cycles are called heart sounds. The **heart sounds** can be easily heard with the help of a stethoscope placed a little below the left nipple.

In a cardiac cycle normally two heart sounds are heard, separated by a short pause. The first sound 'lub' is prolonged and low pitched and is due to the closure of the AV valves. It corresponds to ventricular systole. The second heart sound 'dub' is abrupt, short interval and high pitched. It is due to closure of aortic and pulmonary valves. This corresponds with atrial systole.

Electrical Events in Heart

All excitable tissues including heart show changes in electrical potentials before the mechanical events. The electrical changes in the heart can be easily recorded by electrodes placed on the body surface because the body fluids are good conductors of electricity. The recording procedure is known as **electrocardiography,** the paper on which recording is done is known as **electrocardiograph** and the recording is known as **electrocardiogram.**

The Normal Electrocardiogram (ECG)

As the cardiac impulses pass through the heart, a small proportion of these spread all the way to the surface of the body. Electrodes

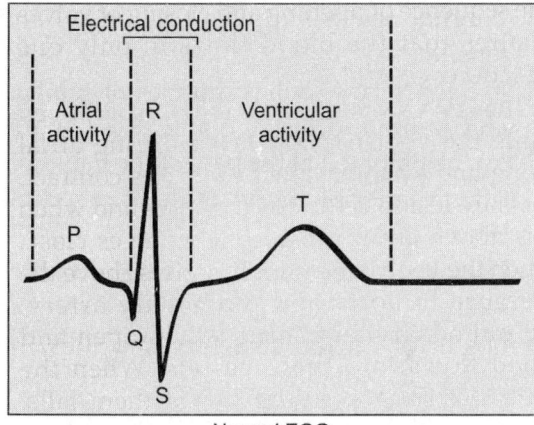

Fig. 4.23: Normal electrocardiogram

placed on the skin of the chest wall pick up the electrical potentials generated by these currents and they can be recorded. This record is known as electrocardiogram (ECG) (Fig. 4.23). A normal ECG of the heart is as follows:

Normal ECG comprises:

1. *P wave* is caused by the electrical potentials generated in the atria prior to contraction (atrial depolarisation).
2. *QRS complex* is caused by potentials generated in the ventricles prior to contraction (onset of ventricular depolarisation).
3. *T wave* is caused by potentials generated as the ventricles relax (ventricular repolarisation).

By examining the pattern, the waves and the time interval between the cycles, the physician obtains valuable information regarding the condition of myocardium and conducting system.

CARDIAC OUTPUT

Cardiac output is volume of blood ejected out from the heart per minute. **Venous return** is the volume of blood returned to the right atrium (via the vena cavae) per minute. **Stroke volume** is volume of blood pumped out by each contraction of the ventricles.

Cardiac output = stroke volume × heart rate/minute.

At rest in a healthy adult, stroke volume is 70 mL and if the heart rate is 72/minute, the cardiac output is 5 litres/minute. It can be increased up to 25 litres/minute during exercise. This increase during exercise is called the **cardiac reserve**.

PULSE

Pulse is felt by slightly compressing an artery against an underlying bone or flat muscle by the three middle fingers. It is usually felt in the radial, brachial, carotids, femorals and dorsalis pedis arteries. The subject should be seated comfortably or lying supine. The radial pulse is best felt with the subject's forearm is in mid prone position and wrist slightly flexed. The following observations are made.

i. Rate   ii. Rhythm
iii. Character   iv. Volume
v. Condition of arterial wall.

i. Rate

The rate is expressed as beats per minute. The counting is started when the subjects pulse has settled down after an initial quictency due to nervousness. The beats should be counted for at least one minute. The normal resting heart rate is 72 ± 10 beats per minute.

Causes of increase in pulse rate: Exercise, anxiety, excitement, fever, thyrotoxicosis sleep.

Causes of decrease inpulse rate: Regular athletic training, myxoedema and sleep.

ii. Rhythm

Normally the pulse beat is at regular interval and therefore regular. An irregular pulse is seen in disease conditions.

Remaining features will be dealt in clinical years.

MAJOR ARTERIES AND VEINS OF THE BODY

Arterial Supply

The largest artery is the **ascending aorta** arising from the left ventricle. Near the beginning it gives the right and left coronary arteries for the heart (Fig. 4.17).

Ascending aorta continues in an arched fashion and is called **arch of aorta** (Fig. 4.24). Its three branches are:

1. Brachiocephalic, which divides into right common carotid and right subclavian artery
2. Left common carotid
3. Left subclavian.

Blood Supply of Head and Neck

Arterial supply to the head and neck is from the common carotid arteries and the vertebral arteries, both paired. Each **common carotid artery** runs along the anterior border of sternocleidomastoid muscle. It is palpable in the neck. At the level of 4th cervical vertebra, it divides into:

1. External carotid
2. Internal carotid (Fig. 4.25A).

External carotid artery: This artery supplies structures in the head and neck through following branches:

1. Superior thyroid artery supplies the thyroid gland.

2. Lingual artery supplies the tongue and tonsil.
3. Facial artery supplies muscles of the face and submandibular gland. This artery can be palpated at the base of the mandible 2.5 cm anterior to the angle of mandible (Fig. 4.25B).
4. Occipital artery supplies posterior part of scalp.
5. Posterior auricular artery supplies the auricle.

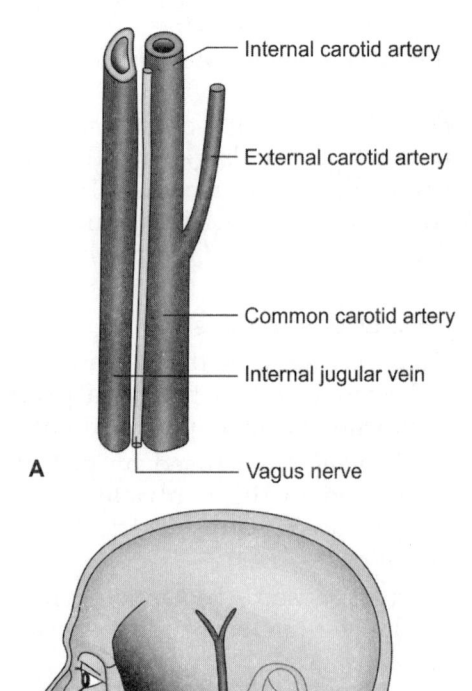

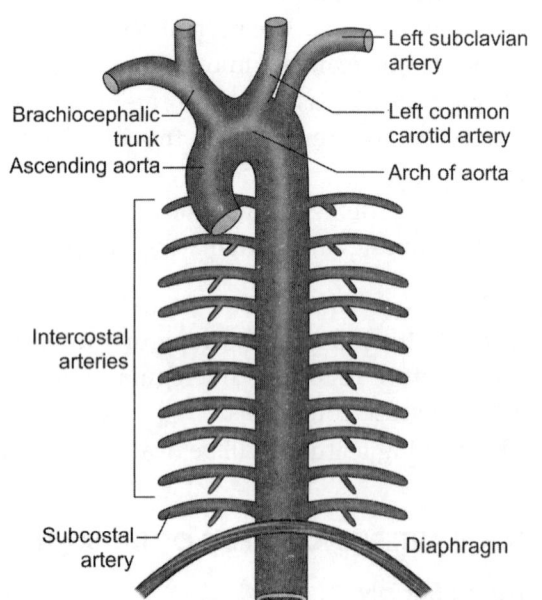

Fig. 4.24: Branches of arch of aorta and descending aorta

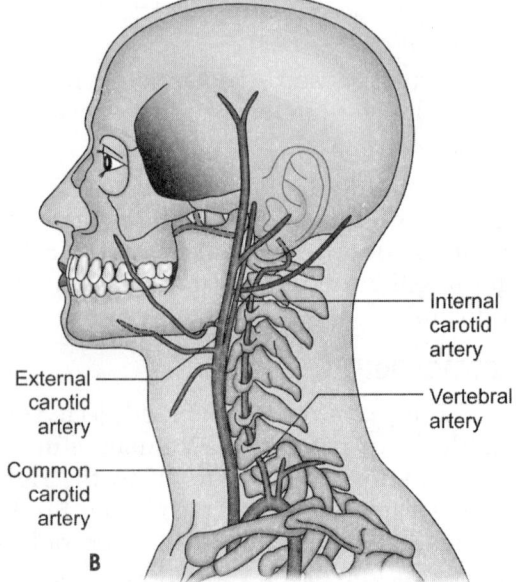

Figs 4.25A and B: (A) Arteries of head and neck and (B) branches of external carotid artery

6. Ascending pharyngeal artery supplies the pharynx and prevertebral muscles.
7. Maxillary artery supplies the muscles of mastication, 8 upper and 8 lower teeth. Its important branch is the middle meningeal artery, which supplies the meninges of the brain.
8. Superficial temporal artery supplies the scalp in front of the ear. Its pulsations can be felt here.

Internal carotid artery: It is the major contributor to the circle of Willis. It enters the cranial cavity through the carotid canal. In addition to brain it supplies eye, forehead and nose.

BLOOD SUPPLY OF BRAIN

Circle of Willis: It is the arterial anastomoses at the base of the brain in subarachnoid space to supply it. It is formed by four arteries, viz., **two internal carotid** and **two vertebral** arteries. The vertebral arteries unite to form the **basilar artery**. This artery runs on the anterior surface of pons to its upper border, where it divides into its two terminal branches, the **posterior cerebral arteries**. The internal carotid artery after entering the cranial cavity divides at the base of the brain into **anterior cerebral**, **middle cerebral** and **posterior communicating arteries**. The **posterior communicating artery** joins the internal carotid artery to posterior cerebral artery. The right and left anterior cerebral arteries are connected with each other by **anterior communicating artery**. This completes the circle of Willis (Fig. 4.26).

Branches of circle of Willis are cortical, central and choroidal.

Venous Return from the Head and Neck

Venous return from the head and neck is by superficial and deep veins. The superficial

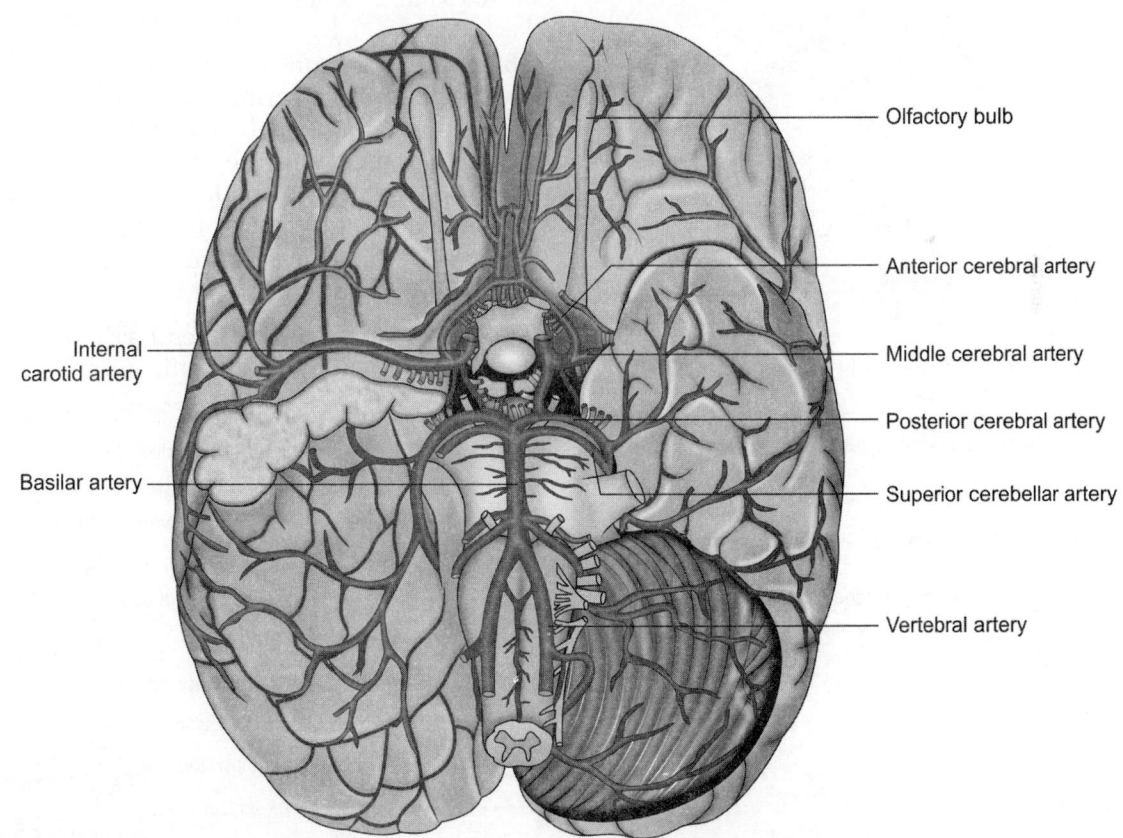

Fig. 4.26: Arteries of brain *(For colour Fig. see Plate 2)*

veins have the same nomenclature as the branches of the external carotid artery. These drain venous blood from the superficial structures of the scalp and face and unite to form the external jugular vein at the angle of the mandible. It courses downwards on the anterior surface of sternocleidomastoid muscle to join the subclavian vein behind the clavicle.

The venous blood of the brain is collected by the deep veins/venous sinuses. The main venous sinuses are:

- One superior sagittal sinus
- One inferior sagittal sinus
- One straight sinus (Fig. 4.27)
- Two transverse sinuses
- Two sigmoid sinuses.

The sigmoid sinus passes through the jugular foramen to continue as the internal jugular vein outside the cranial cavity. It

receives venous blood from tongue and thyroid gland. It runs along the anterior border of sternocleidomastoid muscle to join the subclavian vein to form the brachio-cephalic vein. The left brachiocephalic vein is longer than the right and passes obliquely behind the manubrium sterni to join the right brachiocephalic vein and forms the superior vena cava (Fig. 4.28). Superior vena cava brings deoxygenated blood from brain, head, neck and upper limbs to the right atrium of the heart.

Blood Supply of Upper Limb

Arterial Supply

The subclavian artery at the outer border of first rib enters the region of axilla. There it is known as **axillary artery.** Running through the axilla it gives branches to the muscles forming anterior, posterior, lateral and medial walls of axilla, and shoulder joint At the lower end of axilla, it changes its name to brachial artery.

Brachial artery runs through the region of arm (brachium-upper arm). It runs along with branches of brachial plexus. It also gives muscular branches to the muscles of arm, cutaneous branches to the skin of arm, articular branches to the elbow joint (Fig. 4.29).

In cubital fossa it gives terminal branches— radial and ulnar arteries.

Radial artery runs on the lateral side of the forearm, giving muscular and cutaneous

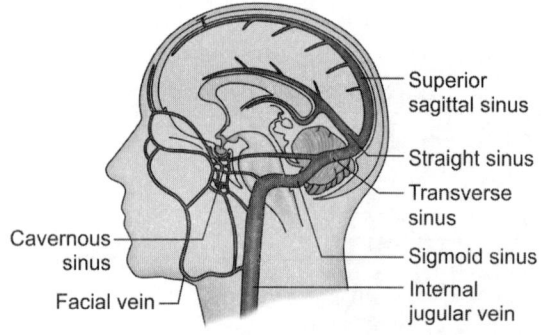

Fig. 4.27: Veins of head and neck

Superior sagittal sinus
Straight sinus
Transverse sinus
Sigmoid sinus
Internal jugular vein
Cavernous sinus
Facial vein

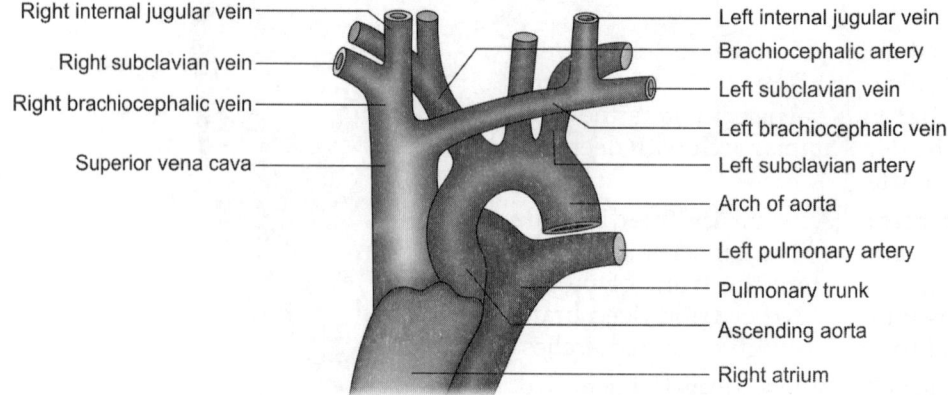

Right internal jugular vein
Right subclavian vein
Right brachiocephalic vein
Superior vena cava

Left internal jugular vein
Brachiocephalic artery
Left subclavian vein
Left brachiocephalic vein
Left subclavian artery
Arch of aorta
Left pulmonary artery
Pulmonary trunk
Ascending aorta
Right atrium

Fig. 4.28: Formation of superior vena cava

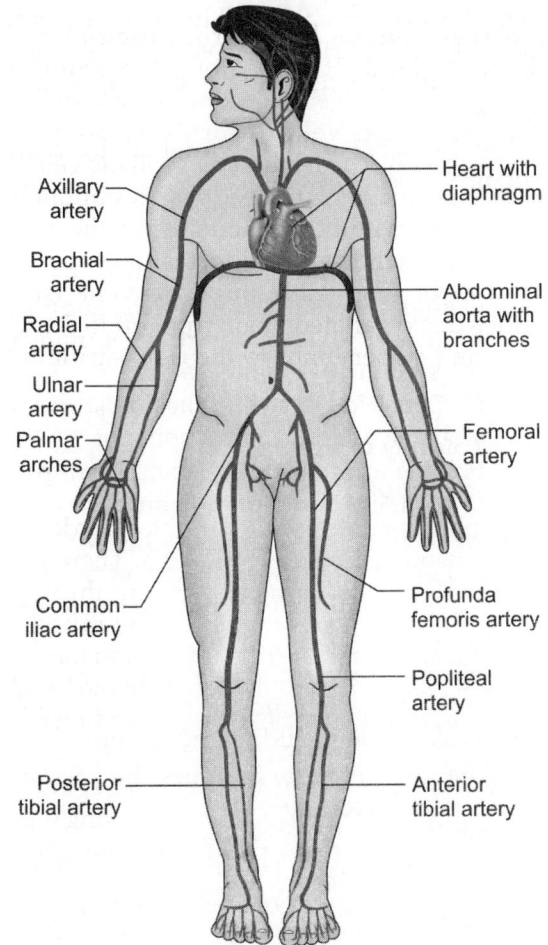

Fig. 4.29: Arterial system

tendons in the palm and all the joints in this region.

Venous Drainage of Upper Limb

Veins are in 2 sets, a superficial and a deep set.

Superficial veins can be seen through the skin. These start in the digits and form **dorsal venous plexus** on dorsum of hand. From its lateral end, **cephalic vein** starts, which runs up on the lateral side of the upper limb. It gives a communication called **median cubital vein** to the **basilic vein** (Fig. 4.30).

The cephalic vein ends in **axillary vein.**

From the medial end of dorsal venous plexus starts the **basilic vein** which ascends on the medial side of upper limb. In the upper

branches. It gives articular branches to the wrist joint. It also gives superficial palmar branch which forms the **superficial palmar arch** with the superficial branch of ulnar artery.

Radial artery continues on the lower and lateral side of forearm, where it is palpated as the **radial pulse.** Then it enters the palm to form the **deep palmar arch** with deep branch of ulnar artery.

Ulnar artery runs on the medial side of forearm amongst its muscles, giving them branches. It enters the front of palm and divides into a superficial and deep branches which form the respective palmar arches.

The palmar arches, superficial and deep supply the skin of the digits, muscles and

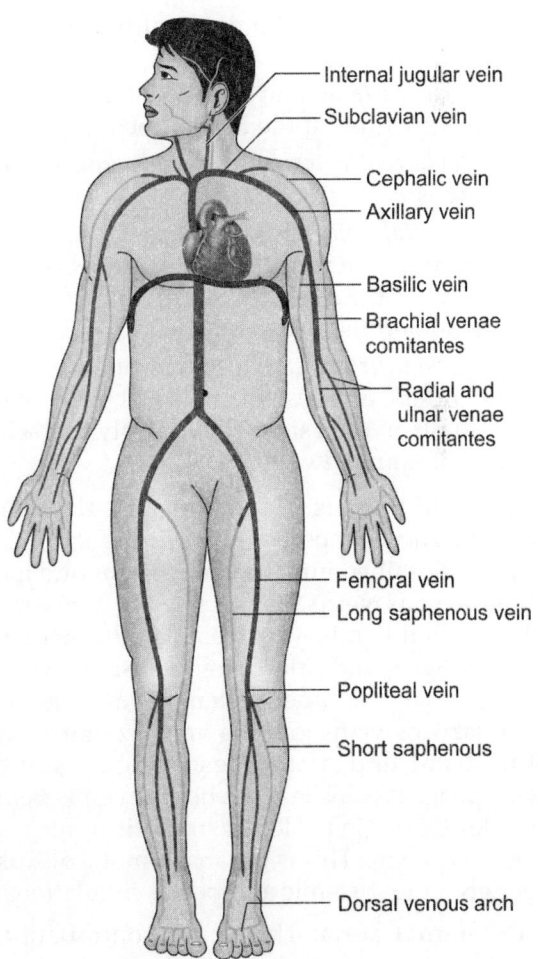

Fig. 4.30: Venous system

arm, it becomes deep and continues as the **axillary vein.**

The **deep set** of veins run along the arteries. Along small arteries there are two small veins called **vena comitantes.** Vena comitantes along palmar arches continue with radial and ulnar vena comitantes. These then end in the **brachial vein** and finally end in the **axillary vein.**

Descending Thoracic Aorta

The arch of aorta continues downwards as the descending aorta at the level of 4th thoracic vertebra. It is situated on the left and anterior surface of the bodies of vertebrae up to the 12th thoracic vertebra, where it pierces the diaphragm and continues as the abdominal aorta.

The branches of the descending thoracic aorta are:

1. *Bronchial arteries* that supply the lung tissue and structures at the root of the lungs.
2. *Oesophageal arteries* to supply the oesophagus.
3. *Intercostal arteries:* There are 11 pairs of intercostal arteries which lie in the subcostal groove of the rib. They supply the thoracic and abdominal walls (Fig. 4.24).
4. *Subcostal arteries:* There are one pair of intercostal arteries which lie just below the 12th rib on each side. They supply thoracic and abdominal walls.

Return of venous blood from the thoracic cavity: The venous blood from the thoracic cavity is drained into the **vena azygos** and the **hemiazygos veins.** Tributaries to the vena azygos and hemiazygos veins are **bronchial, oesophageal and intercostal veins.** The vena azygos joins the superior vena cava while the hemiazygos veins join the vena azygous. At the distal end of the oesophagus, some oesophageal veins join the hemiazygous vein while others join the left gastric vein to form a venous plexus. This is the anastomotic plexus between the systemic and portal circulations.

Abdominal aorta: This is the continuation of the thoracic aorta in the abdominal cavity at the level of 12th thoracic vertebra. It runs in front of the thoracic and lumbar vertebrae to the level of 4th lumbar vertebra where it divides into the right and left common iliac arteries.

The branches of the abdominal aorta are unpaired and paired.

Unpaired Arteries

1. *Coeliac trunk:* It has three branches, viz.
   a. Common hepatic artery which supplies liver, gall bladder, parts of stomach, duodenum and pancreas.
   b. Left gastric artery supplies most of the stomach and part of oesophagus.
   c. Splenic artery supplies the spleen, part of pancreas and part of stomach.
2. *Superior mesenteric artery:* Supplies whole of small intestine, ascending and part of transverse colon and part of pancreas (Fig. 4.31).
3. *Inferior mesenteric artery:* Supplies the transverse colon and descending colon, sigmoid colon including the rectum.
4. *Median sacral artery:* Supplies the sacrum, coccyx and rectum.

Paired Arteries

1. *Inferior phrenic arteries:* Supply the inner surface of the diaphragm and part of the suprarenal glands.
2. *Renal arteries:* Supply the kidneys and part of suprarenal glands.

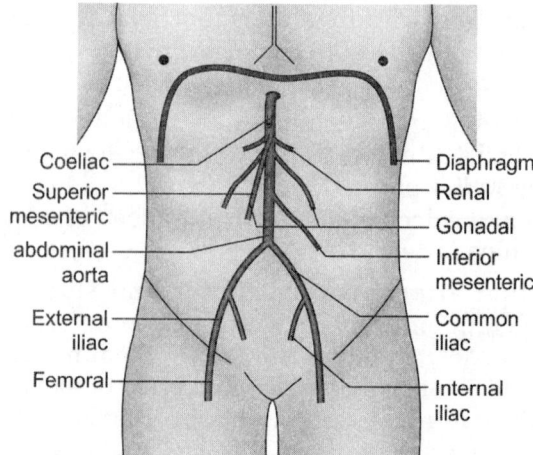

Coeliac — Diaphragm
Superior mesenteric — Renal
abdominal aorta — Gonadal
— Inferior mesenteric
External iliac — Common iliac
Femoral — Internal iliac

Fig. 4.31: Branches of abdominal aorta

3. *Suprarenal arteries:* Supply suprarenal glands.
4. *Gonadal arteries:* In males, the **testicular arteries** supply the testes and scrotum, while in females the **ovarian arteries** supply the ovaries.
5. *Lumbar arteries:* Supply the skin and muscles of the lumbar region of the back. They also supply the spinal cord and its meninges.

Thus, the abdominal aorta supplies the abdominal wall and all the viscera in the abdominal cavity.

Venous Return from the Abdominal Region

It is done is by the largest vein of the body, the inferior vena cava. The left and right iliac arteries join at the level of 5th lumbar vertebra to form the inferior vena cava (Fig. 4.32). After receiving blood from all the abdominal viscera it pierces the central tendon of the thoraco-abdominal diaphragm at the level of 8th thoracic vertebra.

The venous blood from the digestive system first enters the liver through the portal system. It then drains by two hepatic veins from the liver into the inferior vena cava.

PORTAL CIRCULATION

The portal circulation carries venous blood beginning in one set of capillaries and ends in another set of capillaries without passing through the heart (Fig. 4.19). Portal vein carries

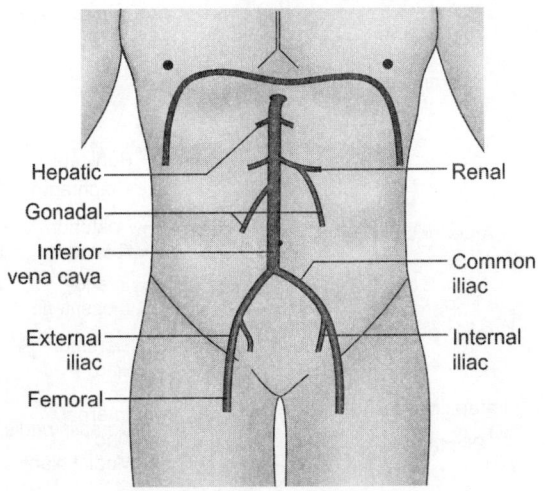

Fig. 4.32: Veins of the abdomen

blood from the abdominal part of the alimentary tract, gall bladder, pancreas and spleen and conveys it to the liver (Fig. 4.33). Here, it breaks up into sinusoids which are drained by two hepatic veins into the inferior vena cava. Blood in the portal vein is rich in nutrient material which has been absorbed in the stomach and the intestines. This is metabolised in the liver before entering the systemic circulation.

The inferior mesenteric vein drains blood from the rectum, anal canal and the desceding and sigmoid colon. The superior mesenteric vein drains blood from the small intestine, appendix, caecum and the ascending and transverse colon.

The splenic vein drains blood from part of the stomach, spleen and pancreas.

The gastric vein drains blood from the lower end of the oesophagus and part of the stomach.

The cystic vein drains blood from the gall bladder into the right branch of portal vein.

Hepatic veins drain into the inferior vena cava and act as a support for the liver.

Circulation of Blood in the Pelvis

Arterial blood supply to the pelvis is by the branches of the **right and left common iliac arteries.** These are two terminal branches of the abdominal aorta. Each divides into **internal iliac artery** and **external iliac artery** in front of the sacroiliac joint (Fig. 4.31).

The internal iliac artery supplies the organs in the pelvis, viz. the urinary bladder and rectum and gluteal muscles. Branches of this artery in the males supply the prostate gland and vas deferens. In females, the **uterine artery and vaginal artery** supply the uterus and vagina.

The external iliac artery runs downwards obliquely to pass under the inguinal ligament to enter the thigh, where it becomes the femoral artery.

Internal iliac vein drains the pelvic viscera (Fig. 4.32).

External iliac vein is the continuation of femoral vein from the lower limb. Both internal and external iliac veins join to form **common iliac**

vein on each side. Left common iliac vein crosses the median plane to join right common iliac vein to form the largest vein of the body, the **inferior vena cava.**

Inferior vena cava runs up on the posterior abdominal wall and receives renal veins, suprarenal vein and testicular or ovarian vein in the abdomen.

It passes through the thoracoabdominal diaphragm at level of 8th thoracic vertebra and opens into the **right atrium.** Thus it brings deoxygenated blood of lower limbs, pelvic viscera, kidney, etc. to the heart.

Portal Vein

Portal vein brings the deoxygenated blood from the digestive system. More than this it is responsible for conveying the products of digestion, i.e. amino acids, glucose, etc. from intestines to be deposited in the liver (Fig. 4.33). The portal vein is formed by the joining of the splenic and the superior mesenteric veins behind the neck of pancreas. It terminates by dividing into right and left branches at the porta hepatis.

Blood Supply of the Lower Limb

Arterial Supply

The chief artery of lower limb is **femoral artery.** It starts at the mid-inguinal point,

courses through the femoral triangle, then through the adductor canal and ends by changing its name to **popliteal artery.** It gives number of muscular branches to the big muscles of this region besides cutaneous branches and the articular branches to the knee joint (Fig. 4.34). The biggest branch is the **profunda femoris artery.**

Popliteal artery is so named as it runs through the popliteal fossa. It ends at the distal border of popliteus by dividing into a large posterior tibial and a smaller anterior tibial artery (Fig. 4.34).

This artery also gives branches to surrounding muscles, genicular branches to knee joint and to the skin.

Posterior tibial artery runs amongst the muscles of the back of leg (calf region) till the back of ankle where it is palpable between medial malleolus and tendocalcaneus. It gives muscular and cutaneous branches.

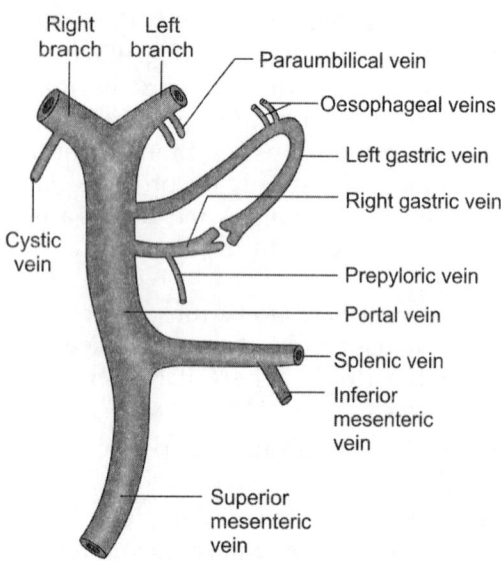

Fig. 4.33: Portal vein

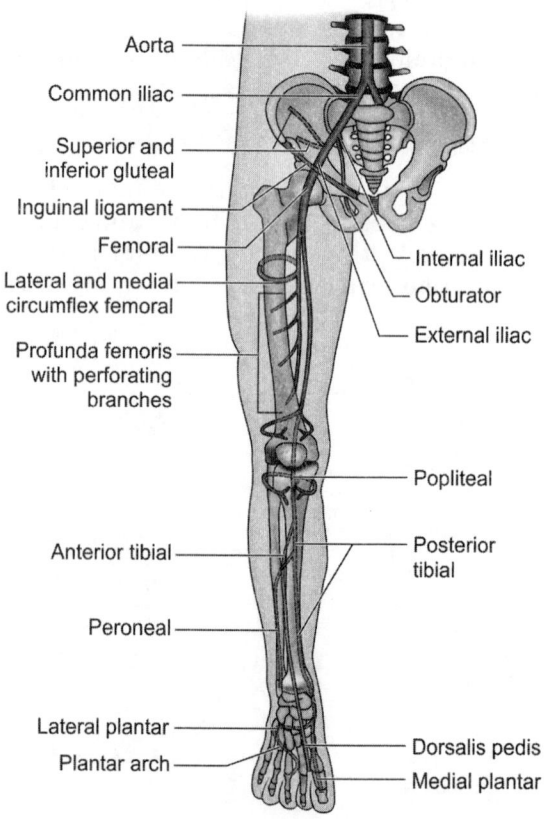

Fig. 4.34: Arteries of lower limb

Posteromedial to the ankle joint, the posterior tibial artery ends by dividing into medial and lateral plantar arteries.

Medial plantar artery supplies muscles, tendons, joints and skin of medial side of sole and 3½ medial digits.

Lateral plantar artery runs along the lateral side of sole to supply muscles, tendons, joints and lateral 1½ digits. It also forms a **plantar arch** which also supplies tendons of the sole.

Anterior tibial artery enters the anterior region of the leg, descends till the ankle joint and continues as **dorsalis pedis** artery in the dorsum of foot. Gives branches to the muscles, skin and joints of the region.

Dorsalis pedis artery runs on the dorsum of foot where it is palpable. It supples skin of dorsum of foot and digits.

Venous Drainage

Veins are in two sets, a superficial and a deep set (Figs 4.35A and B).

The superficial set is in the form of a **dorsal venous plexus** and two veins, the great and small saphenous veins. **Great saphenous** vein starts at the medial end of dorsal venous plexus, ascends in the leg and thigh to drain into the femoral vein. This vein is provided with number of valves.

The small saphenous vein starts at the lateral end of dorsal venous plexus, runs up the leg to drain into the **popliteal** vein.

The deep set of veins is in the form of vena comitantes along the plantar arch, anterior and posterior tibial arteries. These continue as the **popliteal** vein and then as **femoral** vein to continue as **external iliac** vein.

BLOOD PRESSURE

It is defined as the lateral pressure exerted by column of blood of the walls of blood vessels. Venous pressure is less than arterial pressure. Contraction of the left ventricle during systole pushes blood into the arterial system. The

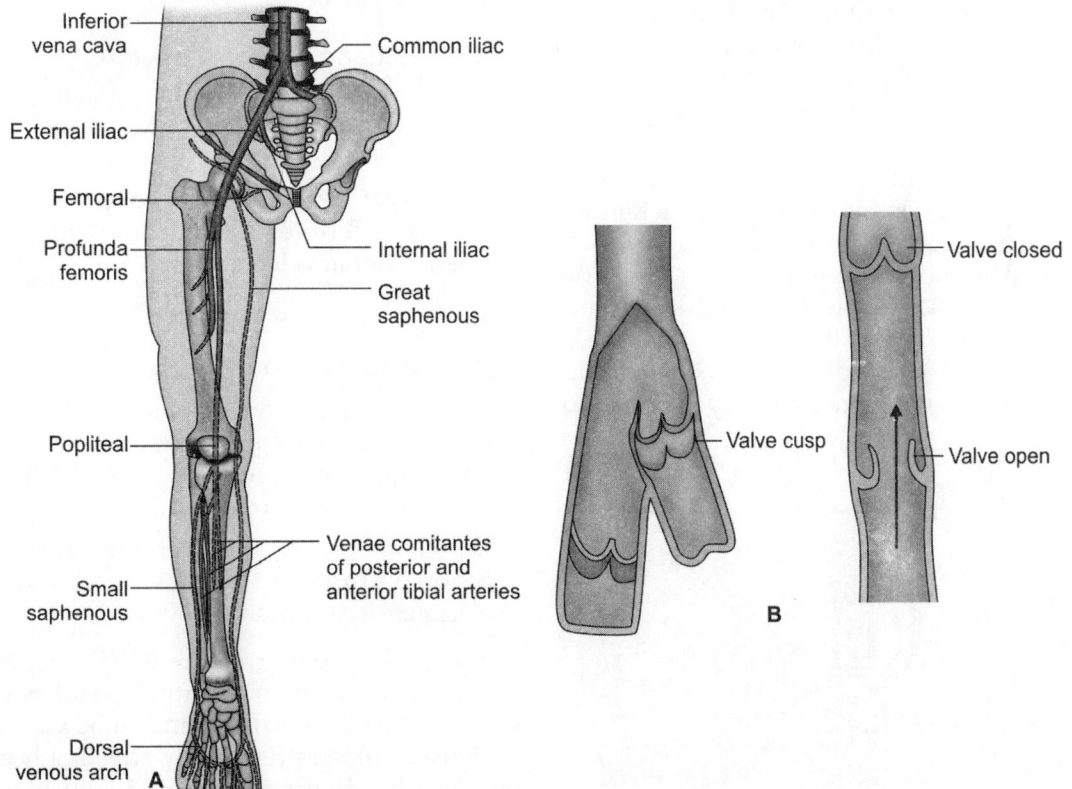

Figs 4.35A and B: (A) Veins of lower limb and (B) valves in a vein

pressure produced is called the systolic blood pressure (SBP) and is about 120 mmHg. During the diastole the pressure in the arteries is called the diastolic blood pressure (DBP). It is about 80 mmHg.

Factors affecting blood pressure are:
1. Age
2. Body built
3. Posture
4. Exercise
5. Sleep.

Blood pressure (BP) is measured by an instrument called sphygmomanometer. There are two methods by which one can record BP (Fig. 4.36).
1. Palpatory
2. Auscultatory.

Palpatory Method

i. The subject is either seated comfortably or is lying supine on the examination couch for 5 minutes. The blood pressure cuff is placed firmly around the bare arm 2.5–3 cm above the elbow joint. The instrument should be placed at the level of the heart.

ii. Feel the radial pulse. Inflate the cuff 20–30 mmHg above the point when the radial pulse disappears. Now slowly deflate the cuff (2 mm/sec) and note the reading when the radial pulse becomes palpable. This is the systolic blood pressure (SBP). The diastolic blood pressure (DBP) cannot be measured by this method.

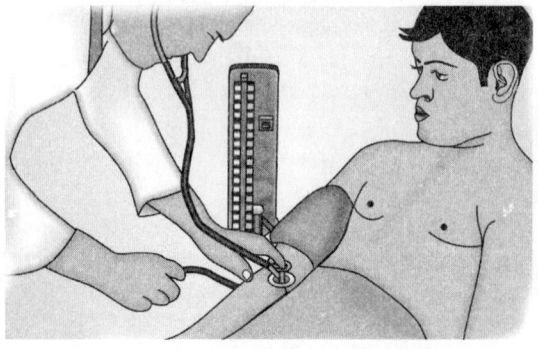

Fig. 4.36: Measurement of blood pressure

Auscultatory Method

Now place the diaphragm of the stethoscope on the brachial artery at the elbow. Inflate the cuff till 180 mmHg or SBP + 10 whichever is higher. Then, gradually deflate the cuff. Note the reading when clear sharp tapping sounds (Korotkoff's sounds) are heard. This is SBP. These sound gradually become dull and muffled and then disappear. The cuff pressure at the muffling disappearanc of the Korotkoff' sounds is recorded as the diastolic blood pressure. The blood pressure is expressed as SBP/DBP mmHg.

Normal BP in adult is 120/80 mmHg.

Arterial blood pressure maintains the essential flow of substances into and out of the organs of body. Control of blood pressure especially to the vital organs is essential to maintain homeostasis.

Blood pressure is determined by cardiac output and peripheral resistance.

Blood pressure = cardiac output × peripheral resistance.

Factors Influencing Blood Pressure

1. *Cardiac output:* It depends upon volume of blood ejected (stroke volume) and heart rate.
2. *Peripheral resistance:* It depends on tone of arterioles. It is also affected by elasticity of arteriolar wall.

Regulation of Blood Pressure

Blood pressure is controlled in two ways:
1. *Short-term control,* on a moment to moment basis. It involves mainly baroreceptor reflex and also chemoreceptors, higher centres and circulating hormones.
2. *Long-term control,* involves regulation of blood volume by kidneys and renin-angiotensin-aldosterone system.

The **cardiovascular centre** (CVC) in pons and medulla sends sympathetic and para-sympathetic nerves to heart and blood vessels. It regulates blood pressure by affecting heart rate and by dilating or constricting blood vessels.

Baroreceptors

These are nerve endings sensitive to pressure changes, present in arch of aorta and carotid sinus. These are important for short term control of BP. High BP increases baroreceptor activity which increases parasympathetic activity and decreases sympathetic activity which causes dilatation of blood vessels leading to fall in BP. If pressure decreases in arch of aorta and carotid sinus, sympathetic activity is increased. This leads to increase heart rate and vasoconstriction of blood vessels, causing rise in BP.

Chemoreceptors

These are nerve endings situated in carotid and aortic bodies. These respond to changes in levels of CO_2, O_2 and pH of blood. Discharge from these affect the cardiovascular centre.

Higher Centres

Higher centres, e.g. hypothalamus, cerebral cortex also help in regulating BP.

Renin-Angiotensin-Aldosterone System

In response to decreased renal blood flow, enzyme renin is secreted by renal tubular cells. Renin converts angiotensinogen (a plasma protein produced by liver) to angiotensin I. Angiotensin converting enzyme (ACE) produced by lungs converts angiotensin I to angiotensin II, which stimulates secretion of aldosterone. It also causes vasoconstriction and increases BP.

CLINICAL ASPECTS

Arteries

Arteries carry the oxygenated blood from the heart to all the tissues. These are subjected to following diseases.

Atheroma

Due to accumulation of cholesterol and other lipid compounds in tunica intima patchy changes develop in large and medium sized arteries. These plaques grow in size and may cause narrowing and occlusion of an artery. Most commonly it affects the arteries of heart,
brain, kidneys and lower limbs. Predisposing factors for development of atheroma are heredity, increasing age, hypertension, diabetes mellitus, smoking, fat rich diet, obesity, etc.

The arteries may be partially or completely blocked by plaques. This may reduce or completely block the blood supply. Narrowing due to partially blocked artery leads to inadequate blood supply and cramp like ischaemic pain develops. Complete occlusion of an artery leads to tissue degeneration and death of tissue **(infarction).**

The plaque may get dislodged and travels in the blood vessel. Such a moving plaque is called **embolus.** This embolus circulates in the blood till it blocks an artery distally, causing small infarcts (areas of dead tissue).

Arteriosclerosis

The walls of the arteries show degenerative changes and lose their elasticity. It is mostly associated with hypertension and ageing. The walls of arteries are infiltrated with fibrous tissue and thicken.

Hypertension

It is the sustained elevation of systemic arterial pressure. Usually, it is of unknown cause in 85–90% of all cases. It is a systemic disease and affects many systems of the body. Hypertension leads to many problems including brain haemorrhage, myocardial infarction and heart failure. It must be treated continuously with drugs.

Veins

Superficial Thrombophlebitis

The superficial veins of the limb get inflamed due to intravenous fluid infusion and thrombosis occurs. It usually heals well, as thrombus resolves completely and does not form an embolus.

Deep Vein Thrombosis

In case of immobility due to any reason, damage to vessel wall and change in viscosity of blood, the venous blood may clot in the deep veins. The venous thrombus fragment may become detached and travel through the heart to lodge in pulmonary artery or one of its branches. It causes infarction of lung tissue. Massive pulmonary embolism may lead to sudden collapse and death.

Varicose Veins

Occur in lower limb due to incompetent valves of the superficial veins or of the perforators. These occur more often in obese old females who stand for long hours, especially doctors, nurses and others. The backward flow of blood occurs in veins due to incompetent valves. The veins lose their elasticity, become elongated and tortuous.

Heart

Congenital Abnormalities

1. *Patent foramen ovale* is due to non-closure of the foramen between the right and the left atria.
2. *Patent interventricular foramen* is due to non closure of the foramen between the right and the left ventricles. This has more serious implications than patent foramen ovale, as there is more pressure of blood in the ventricles.
3. *Patent ductus arteriosus:* The ductus arteriosus in foetal life connects the left pulmonary artery to the arch of aorta beyond its left subclavian branch. Normally, it closes soon after birth. If it does not close, the condition is called **patent ductus arteriosus** which can lead to heart failure.
4. *Fallot's tetralogy:* Four defects are present. These are:
   - Patent interventricular foramen
   - Aorta arising from both the ventricles
   - Pulmonary stenosis
   - Right ventricular hypertrophy.

   It leads to 'blue baby' and growth retardation in young children.
5. *Coarctation of aorta:* When the aorta just beyond the ductus gets narrowed, the condition is called coarctation of aorta. This leads to high blood pressure in upper limbs and lower pressure in lower limbs.

Acquired Abnormalities

1. *Diseases of valves:* The four valves of the heart may be stenosed (narrowed) or incompetent leading to regurgitation. The conditions thus are:
   i. Mitral (bicuspid) stenosis or regurgitation
   ii. Tricuspid stenosis or regurgitation
   iii. Pulmonary stenosis or regurgitation
   iv. Aortic stenosis or regurgitation.
2. *Heart failure:* It results when the cardiac output is unable to maintain the circulation of sufficient blood to meet the needs of the body. It may affect either side of the heart but eventually it leads to failure of the other half also.
   i. *Right-sided heart failure:* The right ventricle is not able to push the blood in the lungs. The blood gets congested in the right atrium, superior and inferior venae cavae resulting in ascites (fluid in peritoneal cavity) and **oedema** (swelling in the limbs).
   ii. *Left-sided heart failure:* The left ventricle is not able to pump blood in the systemic arteries. It may be due to high blood pressure and aortic valve disease. This failure results in congestion of blood in lungs and **dyspnoea** (difficulty in breathing).
3. *Angina pectoris:* The blood supply to the myocardium is less than its actual requirement due to narrowing of coronary artery by atheromatous plaque. The subject feels pain in the chest radiating to medial side of left arm on exertion or even at rest.
4. *Myocardial infarction:* When one of the branches of either coronary artery gets blocked, the muscle supplied by it gets anoxic, leading to its infarction, i.e. an area of dead tissue. This is a serious condition and immediate treatment is necessary. The two coronary arteries and their branches are functional end arteries. In case of blockage

of one, the other cannot compensate for the loss of blood supply.

5. *Heart block:* When appropriate impulses from SA node do not reach the ventricles, there is heart block. It may be complete and has serious outcome.

6. *Bacterial endocarditis:* It is subacute or acute bacterial infection of the endocardium or heart valves or both. It is caused usually by streptococci or staphylococci bacteria. Infection of valves lead to their destruction followed by healing by fibrosis, which distorts their shape leading to stenosis and/or incompetence. Heart failure may develop.

Ascites

Accumulation of excessive fluid in the peritoneal cavity.

Pleural Effusion

Accumulation of excess fluid in the pleural cavity.

Shock

In shock, there is inadequate blood flow to the body tissue. The decreased blood flow leads to reduction in delivery of oxygen, nutrients, hormones and electrolytes to body tissues and decreased removal of metabolic wastes.

There is reduction in circulating blood volume, blood pressure and cardiac output.

Points to Remember

1. Systemic circulation starts from left ventricle, goes to most of the tissues of the body and returns to right atrium of heart.
2. Pulmonary circulation starts from right ventricle, goes to lungs and returns to left atrium of heart.
3. Some arteries in the body are superficial and are palpated to count heart rate. These are radial, commmom carotid, facial and superficial temporal, etc.
4. Normal functioning valves are responsible for unidirectional flow of blood especially in lower limb.
5. Hypertension or high blood pressure must be controlled, or it may lead to haemorrhage, or aneurysm of the arteries.
6. Lymph vessels also carry cancer cells from the original site of disease to nearby or distant regions.
7. Lymphatic system forms the first line of defense of the body.

MCQs

1. **Which vessels show valves?**
   (a) Capillaries
   (b) Arteries
   (c) Veins of neck
   (d) Veins of lower limb

2. **Which is the thickest layer in veins?**
   (a) Tunica intima
   (b) Tunica media
   (c) Tunica adventitia
   (d) All tunics are of same thickness

3. **Which is the thickest layer in the arteries?**
   (a) Tunica intima
   (b) Tunica media
   (c) Tunica adventitia
   (d) All layers of equal thickness

4. **Anaemia is diagnosed by:**
   (a) Decreased number of RBC
   (b) Incareased number of RBC
   (c) Decreased number of WBC
   (d) Increased number of WBC

5. End arteries are present in:
 (a) Skeletal muscle (b) Bone
 (c) Retina   (d) Middle ear

6. Splenomegaly commonly occurs in:
 (a) Malaria   (b) Cirrhosis of liver
 (c) Anaemia   (d) Elephantiasis

7. Thoracic duct drains the following areas except:
 (a) Left upper limb
 (b) Left lower limb
 (c) Right lower limb
 (d) Right upper limb

Respiratory System

Respiratory system consists of organs which provide the pathway for supply of oxygen to the body and expulsion of carbon dioxide from the body to the surrounding atmosphere. Oxygen is required for the chemical reactions releasing energy used for the proper functioning of the cells.

Respiration involves exchange of gases and is a twofold process:

1. **External respiration** is the exchange of gases between the blood and the alveoli of the lungs.
2. **Internal respiration** is the interchange of gases in the tissues.

ORGANS OF RESPIRATION

Organs of respiration include organs which help in the mechanism of respiration. These are as follows:

- Nose: External nares, nasal cavity and posterior nares
- Paranasal sinuses
- Nasopharynx
- Larynx
- Trachea and bronchi (Fig. 5.1)
- Lungs in the pleural cavity
- Respiratory muscles: The diaphragm and intercostal muscles.

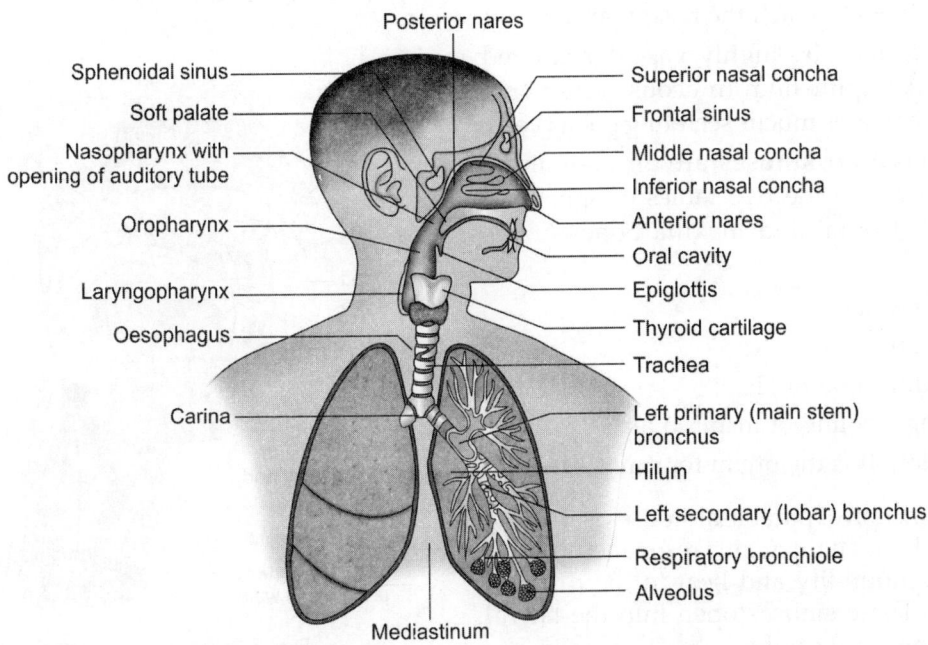

Fig. 5.1: Components of the respiratory system

Nose

It is comprised of a pair of external nares, through which air is inhaled in and exhaled out. Nose is the prominence on the face in between and below the eyes. It is made of small flat **nasal bones** and **nasal cartilages.** The lower lateral part is made up of fibrous tissue and is called the 'ala' of the nose.

The nasal cavity is divided into two halves by a nasal septum formed by **ethmoid, vomer and septal cartilage.** Roof is formed by **nasal, frontal, ethmoid and sphenoid bones.** Floor is formed by **hard palate and soft palate.** In the lateral wall of each cavity, there are three **conchae** or projections of bone, which divide the cavity into **meatuses.** The frontal, ethmoid, sphenoid and maxillary bones have air sinuses (*see* Fig. 3.4). Their openings are present in the meatuses. In sinusitis, there is excessive drainage of fluid from the nasal cavity.

The **nasolacrimal duct** draining the lacrimal fluid (tears) also drains into the nasal cavity, while in crying the tears also drain out from the nasal cavity.

The nasal cavity posteriorly shows two **posterior nasal apertures.** The air passes through them to reach the nasopharynx.

- Nose is lined by highly vascular ciliated columnar epithelium (mucous membrane) which contains mucus secreting goblet cells.

Paranasal air sinuses are air containing spaces between the two tables of sphenoid, ethmoid, frontal and maxilla bones of the skull.

Functions of nose:

- Filtration of air
- Humidification of air
- Heating/cooling of inspired air
- Olfaction: It is the organ for sense of smell.

The function of paranasal sinuses is to make the skull bones lighter, give resonance to voice and give humidity and heat to the dry and cold air. These sinuses open into the lateral wall of the nasal cavity.

Nasopharynx

It is the upper most part of pharynx. The posterior nasal apertures open in it. There is also an opening of the **auditory tube** or **Eustachian tube,** in its lateral wall, from the anterior wall of the middle ear. This tube equalises the pressure on the two sides of the tympanic membrane.

On the posterior wall of nasopharynx **pharyngeal tonsils** (adenoids) are present. These consist of lymphoid tissue. They are prominent in children up to 14 years of age and there after they gradually atrophy.

Air passes from nasopharynx into the larynx. Air and fluids/food cross each other in the lower part of pharynx (Fig. 5.2). If one shouts or laughs aloud while eating/drinking, the food/fluid may enter the larynx. This produces a protective bout of cough as food/fluid is forbidden inside the larynx/trachea. Pharynx also functions in speech, giving the voice its individual characteristic note.

Larynx

It is also called 'voice-box' and extends from 3rd cervical to 6th cervical vertebrae. It is made up of cartilages and membranes.

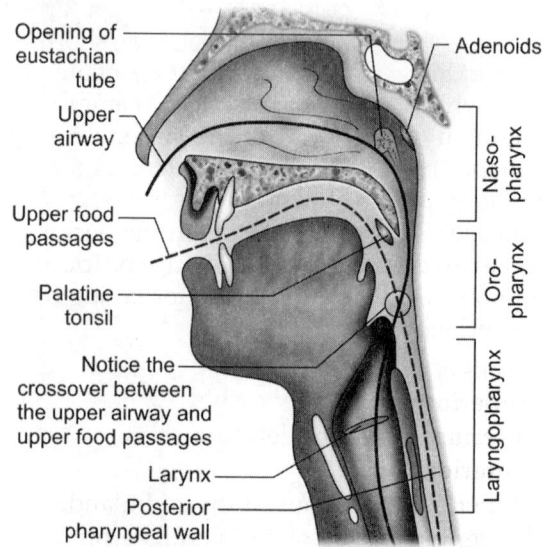

Fig. 5.2: Parts of pharynx

Cartilages of the larynx are:
- Thyroid (1)
- Cricoid (1)
- Epiglottis (1)
- Arytenoids (2).

Membrane of the larynx is folded to form **two vocal cords**. There are muscles which move these cords. Vibrations of these vocal cords produce voice.

Thyroid cartilage is very prominent in males and is called 'Adam's apple'.

Inlet of larynx acts as a sphincter preventing fluid/food from entering the larynx, trachea and lungs. Larynx at the level of 6th cervical vertebra continues as trachea.

Relations of larynx:
- **Superior:** The root of the tongue and hyoid bone
- **Inferior:** It is continuous with the trachea
- **Anterior:** The muscles attached to the hyoid bone
- **Posterior:** The laryngeal part of pharynx
- **Lateral:** The lobes of thyroid gland.

Trachea and Bronchi

Trachea is a musculocartilaginous tube extending from 6th cervical vertebra to 4th thoracic vertebra where it divides into two **primary bronchi** one each for the right and left lungs. The right bronchus is wider, shorter and is in line with trachea. Right bronchus is 2.5 cm while left bronchus is 5 cm in length. It contains hyaline cartilage incomplete rings (C-shaped) to keep the tube patent as air is constantly passing in and out of lungs.

On each side of the trachea in the neck lie the **carotid sheath** containing palpable common carotid artery with internal jugular vein and vagus nerve.

Relations of trachea:
- **Superior:** Larynx
- **Inferior:** Right and left bronchus
- **Anterior:**
  Upper part—isthmus of thyroid gland
  Lower part—arch of aorta and sternum
- **Posterior:** Oesophagus
- **Lateral:** Lungs and lobes of thyroid gland.

Lungs

Lungs are two voluminous cone-shaped organs occupying most of the thoracic cavity leaving a small space for the heart. Each lung is enclosed in a serous pleural cavity. The **pleural cavity** contains serous fluid which helps in expansion and contraction of the lung.

Pleura: It is a closed serous sac which encloses the lung. It has two layers. The **parietal pleura** which lines the inner surface of the chest wall and thoracic surface of the diaphragm. It is reflected at the **hilum** to become the **visceral pleura**. The visceral pleura lines the outer surface of lung and its fissures (Figs 5.3 and 5.4).

The pleural cavity: It is a potential space between the two pleurae. They are separated by a thin film of serous fluid, sufficient to prevent friction between them during breathing.

Parts of Lung

- *Apex:* It is rounded and rises into the root of neck about 2.5 cm above the level of the middle third of clavicle. It is related with blood vessels and nerves of the neck (Fig. 5.5).

- *Base* is concave and closely related with the upper surface of diaphragm.

- *Costal surface:* It is convex and related with the costal cartilages, ribs and intercostal muscles. This surface has impressions of the ribs.

- *Medial/mediastinal surface:* It is concave and has the hilum. The structures which leave and enter from the root of each lung are:
  - Bronchus/bronchi
  - Pulmonary artery
  - Pulmonary veins
  - Bronchial artery and bronchial vein
  - Lymphatic vessels
  - Nerves

- The lung has a **thin anterior border** and a **thick posterior border**

- Table 5.1 shows the differences between right and left lungs.

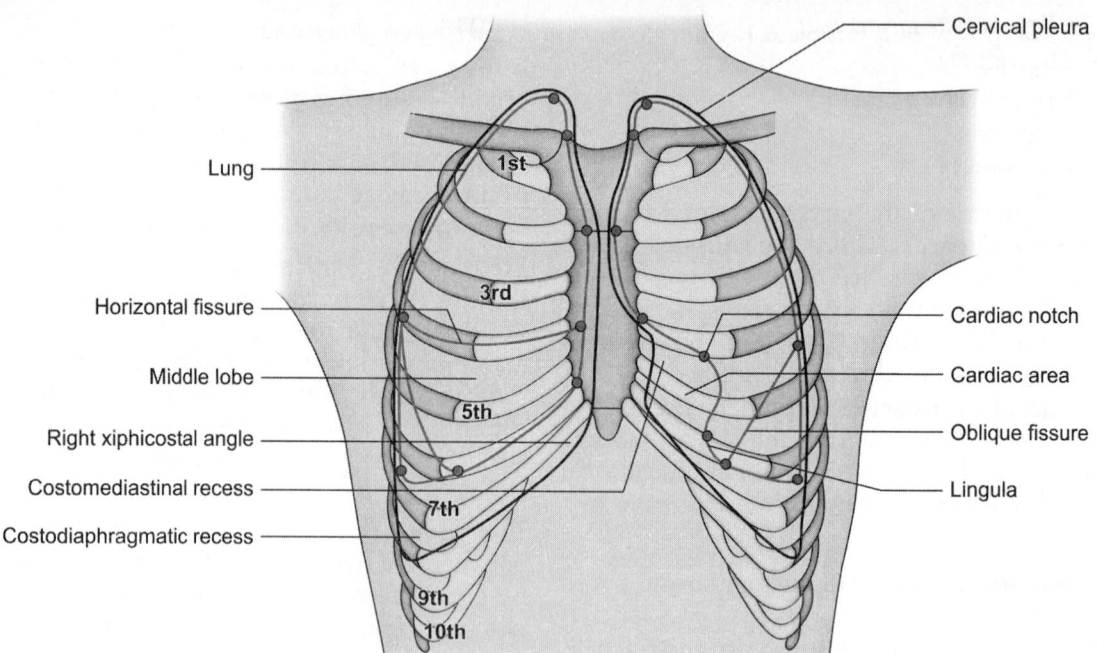

Fig. 5.3: Surface marking of the parietal pleura and visceral pleura/lung—anterior aspect

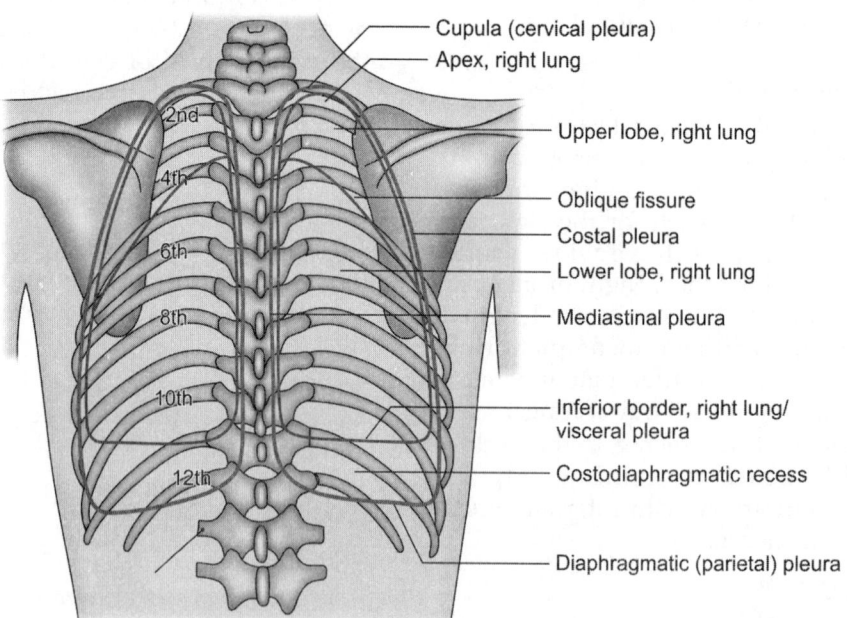

Fig. 5.4: Surface marking of the parietal pleura and visceral pleura/lung—posterior aspect

Lungs are made up of two portions, a conducting portion and a respiratory portion.

Conducting portion: The primary bronchus enters the lung at the **hilum** (Fig. 5.6). In the **right lung** it divides into **three secondary bronchi** for each of the **three lobes of the right lung,** i.e. upper, middle and lower separated by the oblique and horizontal fissures

Table 5.1: Differences beween the right and the left lungs	
Right lung	*Left lung*
1. It has 2 fissures and 3 lobes	1. It has one fissure and 2 lobes
2. Anterior border is straight	2. Anterior border is interrupted by the cardiac notch
3. Larger and heavier, weights about 700 gm	3. Smaller and lighter weighs about 600 gm
4. Shorter and broader	4. Longer and narrower

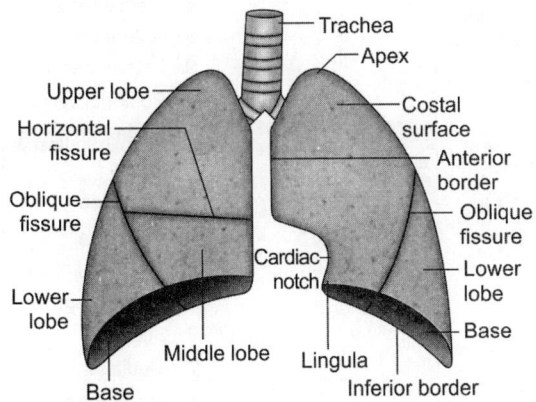

Fig. 5.5: Lungs

(Fig. 5.5). The three secondary bronchi divide into **10 segmental bronchi. Left lung** contains two lobes, i.e. upper and lower lobes, separated by oblique fissure. So, there are only **two secondary bronchi.** But, the **segmental bronchi** are **10** in this lung also, five for upper and five for lower lobe (Fig. 5.7).

Each segmental bronchus divides repeatedly till its diameter becomes 1.0 mm. At this level, it is called the **terminal bronchiole,** with no cartilage plates or glands in it.

Respiratory portion: Terminal bronchiole divides further and forms **respiratory bronchiole, alveolar sac,** and finally the **alveoli.** Here, the wall becomes thinner. Alveoli are lined by two types of cells. **Type I** cells are the sites for exchange of gases. **Type II** cells secrete **phospholipid surfactant**. This keeps the alveoli patent. In this portion, the exchange of gases occurs. So, it is called the respiratory portion.

Hilum of lung contains bronchus/bronchi, one pulmonary artery, two pulmonary veins, nerve plexuses, lymph vessels and lymph nodes (Fig. 5.6).

Bronchi conduct air to and from lungs. Pulmonary artery carries deoxygenated blood from the right ventricle for purification into the lungs. The oxygenated blood is returned via four pulmonary veins (two from each lung) to left atrium (Fig. 5.10).

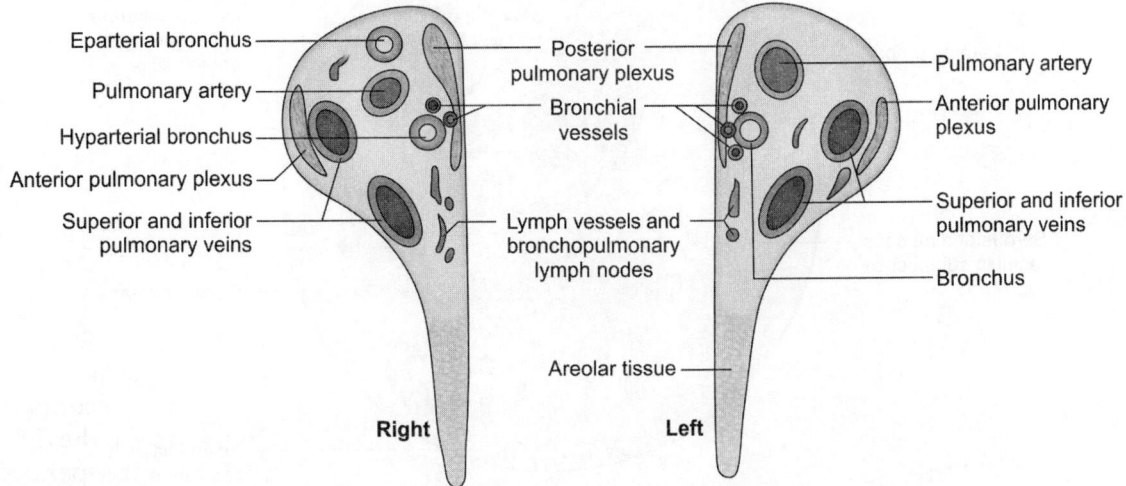

Fig. 5.6: Structures passing through the hila of right and left lungs

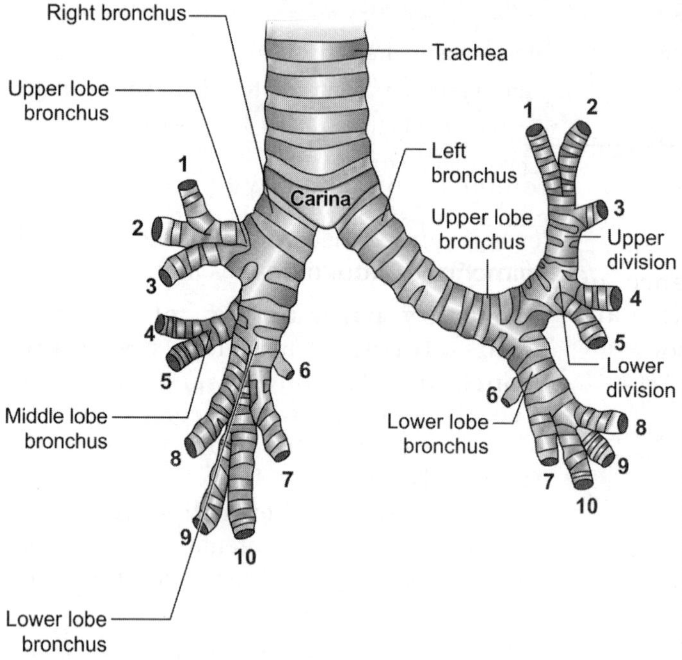

Right Lung	
Lobes	Segments
A. Upper	1. Apical
	2. Posterior
	3. Anterior
B. Middle	4. Lateral
	5. Medial
C. Lower	6. Superior
	7. Medial basal
	8. Anterior basal
	9. Lateral basal
	10. Posterior basal
Left Lung	
A. Upper	1. Apical
• Upper division	2. Posterior
	3. Anterior
• Lower division	4. Superior lingular
	5. Inferior lingular
B. Lower	6. Superior
	7. Medial basal
	8. Anterior basal
	9. Lateral basal
	10. Posterior basal

Fig. 5.7: Bronchopulmonary segments of the lungs

Histology of Trachea

The trachea is lined by **pseudostratified ciliated columnar epithelium.** The cells are of varying height, giving a false appearance of more than one layer of cells. Deep to the epithelium are mucus and serous glands.

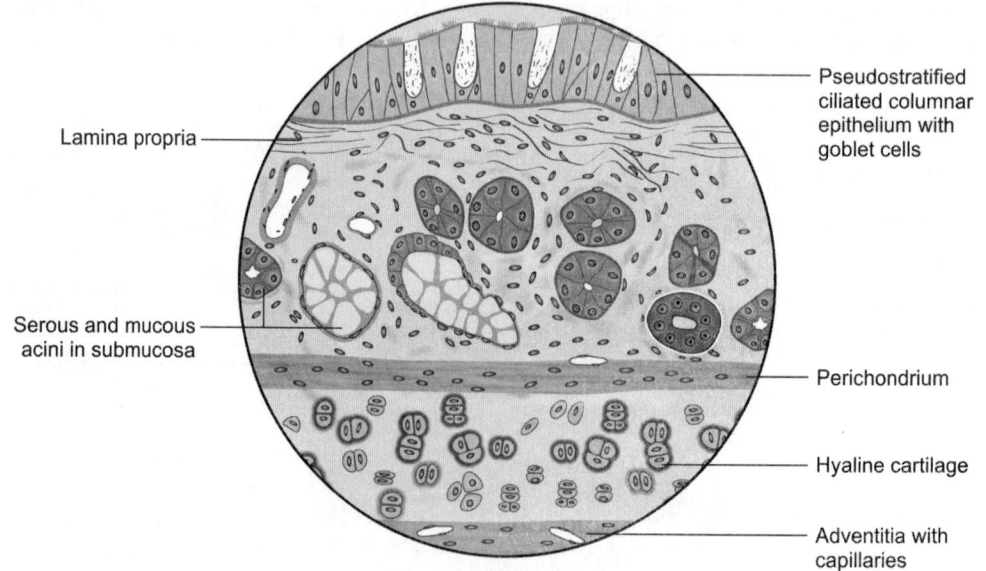

Fig. 5.8: Histology of trachea

The main bulk is formed by the **C-shaped hyaline cartilages** to keep it permanently patent. Cartilage cells lie in groups of two and four each within the matrix, fibres are not visible. At the ends of C-shaped cartilage are the smooth muscle fibres.

Outermost layer is connective tissue with arterioles (Fig. 5.8).

Histology of Lung

Lung is characterised by presence of numerous thin walled alveoli. These are mostly lined by a single layer of squamous cells, **type I pneumocyte**. Some cuboidal cells are present, these are **type II pneumocyte**. Type II cells produce serous fluid **surfactant**, which prevent the alveoli from collapsing by decreasing surface tension. Secretion of surfactant begins in 35th week of fetal life. Its presence in newborn babies facilitates expansion of lungs and the establishment of respiration.

Between the alveoli are fine capillaries for exchange of gases. CO_2 is taken from blood and O_2 is given to the blood, thus oxygenating it.

Besides the alveoli and capillaries there are intrapulmonary bronchi and bronchioles.

Intrapulmonary bronchi are lined by pseudostratified ciliated columnar cells, with glands beneath the epithelium. Cartilage is seen as small plates with smooth muscle fibres in between; outermost is thin connective tissue layer (Fig. 5.9).

Bronchioles are dilated spaces lined by columnar epithelium with no cartilage or gland, only smooth muscle fibres are present.

Pulmonary Circulation

Pulmonary artery divides into two, one branch carrying deoxygenated blood to each lung. Within the lung tissues, the pulmonary artery, divides and redivides into a dense capillary network around the walls of alveoli. The exchange of gases between air in the alveoli and blood in the capillaries takes place here. The pulmonary capillaries join up, forming **two pulmonary veins** in each lung. They leave the lung at hilum and carry oxygenated blood to heart (Fig. 5.10).

Respiratory Movements

Respiratory movements are inspiration and expiration. The diameter of thoracic cage which increse during inspiration are anteroposterior, transverse and vertical.

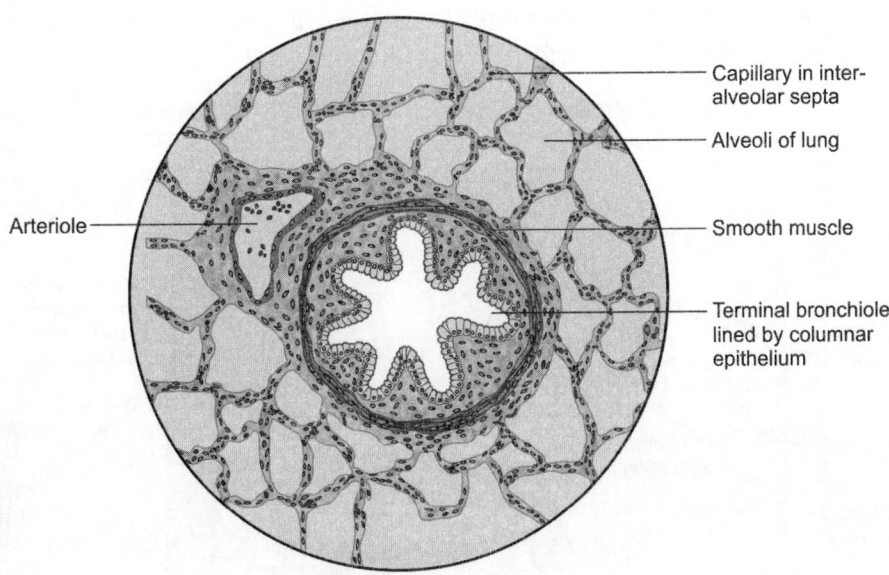

Fig. 5.9: Histology of lung

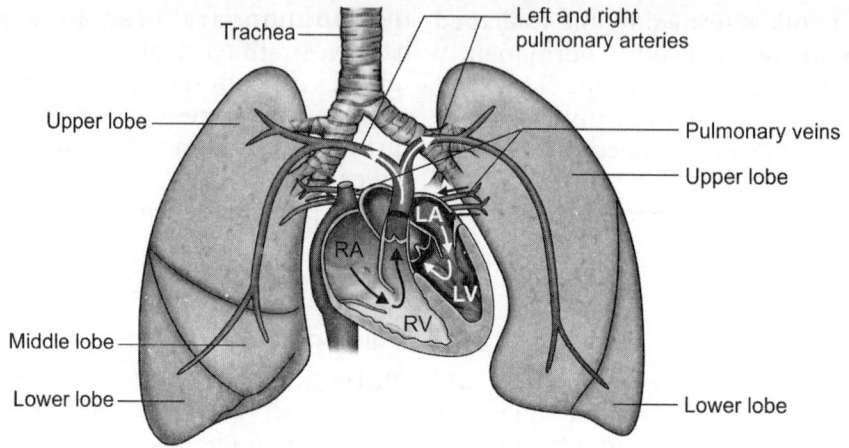

Fig. 5.10: Flow of blood between heart and lungs

The anteroposterior diameter is increased: Mainly by he pump-handle movements of the sternum brought about the elevation of the vertebrosternal second to sixth ribs (Fig. 5.11).

The transverse diameter is increased: Mainly by the bucket-handle movements of the seventh to tenth vertebrochondral ribs (Fig. 5.12).

The vertical diameter is increased by descent of the diaphragm as it contracts. This is called *piston mechanism.* During inspiration, the diaphragm contracts and it comes down by 2 cm. It facilitates in inspiration of at least

400 mL of air during each contraction. It is aided by relaxation of muscles of anterior abdominal wall. During expiration, abdominal muscles contract and diaphragm is pushed upwards.

In females, respiration is thoracoabdominal and in males it is abdominothoracic type.

Respiratory muscles

For quite inspiration—diaphragm, external intercostal muscles.

Deep inspiration—erector spinae, scalene muscles, pectoral muscles.

For expiration—passive process.

Forced expiration—muscles of anterior abdominal wall.

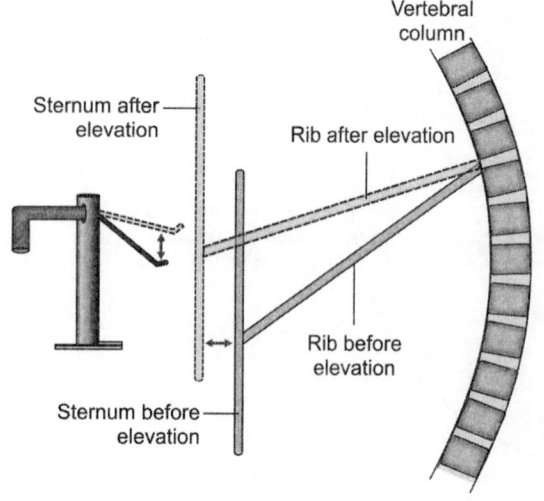

Fig. 5.11: Pump-handle movement

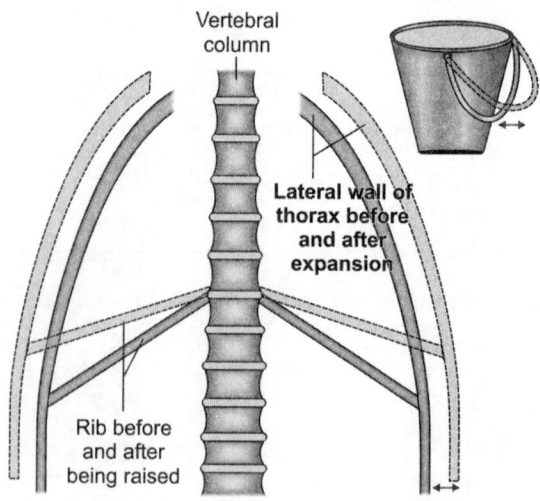

Fig. 5.12: Bucket-handle movement

Respiratory Movements during Different Types of Breathing

Inspiration

1. *Quiet inspiration*
   a. The anteroposterior diameter of the thorax is increased by elevation of the second to sixth ribs. The first rib remains fixed.
   b. The transverse diameter is increased by elevation of the seventh to tenth ribs.
   c. The vertical diameter is increased by descent of the diaphragm.
2. *Deep inspiration*
   a. Movements during quiet inspiration are increased.
   b. The first rib is elevated directly by the scaleni, and indirectly by the sterno-cleidomastoid.
   c. The concavity of the thoracic spine is reduced by the erector spinae.
3. *Forced inspiration*
   a. All the movements described are exaggerated.
   b. The scapulae are elevated and fixed by the trapezius, the levator scapulae and the rhomboids, so that the serratus anterior and the pectoralis minor muscles may act on the ribs.
   c. The action of the erector spinae is appreciably increased.

Expiration

1. *Quiet expiration:* The air is expelled mainly by the elastic recoil of the chest wall and pulmonary alveoli, and partly by the tone of the abdominal muscles.
2. *Deep and forced expiration:* Deep and forced expiration is brought about by strong contraction of the abdominal muscles and of the latissimus dorsi.

MECHANISM OF RESPIRATION

The respiratory cycle consists of inspiration, expiration and diffusion of gases. In normal quiet breathing, there are about 15 complete respiratory cycles per minute.

Diaphragm and intercostal muscles are respiratory muscles. Respiration results from differences between atmospheric and intrapulmonary pressures, as mentioned below.

Before inspiration, intrapulmonary pressure equals atmospheric pressure, at about 760 mmHg. Intrapleural pressure equals 756 mmHg (Fig. 5.13).

During inspiration, the diaphragm and external intercostal muscles contract, enlarging the thorax vertically, horizontally and anteroposteriorly (Fig. 5.14).

As the thorax expands, intrapleural pressure decreases and the lungs expand to fill the enlarging thoracic cavity.

The intrapulmonary atmospheric pressure gradient pumps air into the lungs until the two pressures are equal (Fig. 5.15).

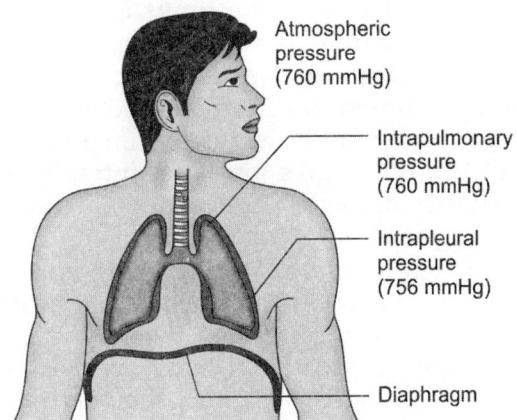

Atmospheric pressure (760 mmHg)

Intrapulmonary pressure (760 mmHg)

Intrapleural pressure (756 mmHg)

Diaphragm

Fig. 5.13: Before inspiration

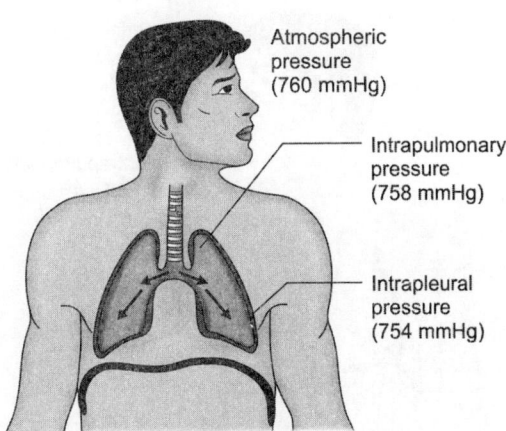

Atmospheric pressure (760 mmHg)

Intrapulmonary pressure (758 mmHg)

Intrapleural pressure (754 mmHg)

Fig. 5.14: Beginning of inspiration

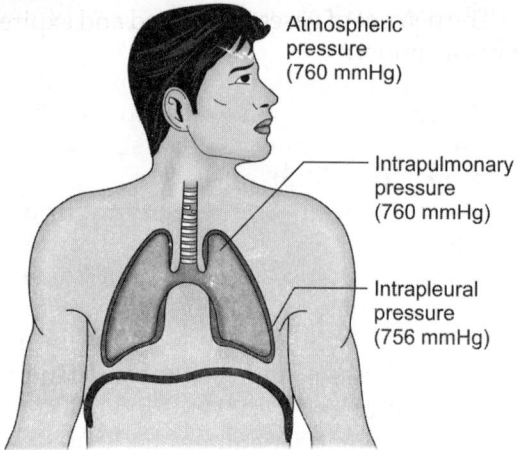

Fig. 5.15: End of inspiration

During normal expiration, the diaphragm slowly relaxes and the lungs and thorax passively return to resting size and position.

During forced or deep expiration, contraction of abdominal muscles and internal intercostals reduce thoracic volume. Lungs and thorax compression raises intrapulmonary pressure above atmospheric pressure, forcing the air to be expelled (Fig. 5.16).

The chest wall expands during normal inspiration due to simultaneous contraction of intercostal muscles and the diaphragm. During deep breathing, these muscles are assisted by muscles of neck, shoulders and abdomen. The process of inspiration is active, as it requires expenditure of energy for muscle contraction. Expiration is due to relaxation of intercostal muscles and diaphragm and elastic recoil of the lungs. Expiration is passive as it does not require expenditure of energy.

LUNG VOLUMES (Fig. 5.17)

Dead space: It is constituted by air which does not participate in diffusion, i.e. air present in nose, trachea and bronchial tree. Normally is 150 mL.

Tidal volume: Volume of gas inspired or expired in each breath during normal quiet respiration. It is 400–500 mL (10 mL/kg).

Alveolar ventilation: It is the volume of air that moves into and out of alveoli per minute.

Alveolar ventilation = (tidal volume – anatomical dead space) × respiratory rate
= (500 – 150) × 15 = 5.25 litres/minute.

Inspiratory reserve volume: It is the maximum volume of gas which a person can inhale from end inspiratory position. It is 2,400–2,600 mL.

Inspiratory capacity: It is the maximum volume which can be inhaled from end expiratory position, i.e. it is inspiratory reserve volume + tidal volume. It is 2,500 (IRV) + 500 (TV) = 3,000 mL.

Expiratory reserve volume: Maximum volume of gas that can be exhaled after normal expiration. It is 1,200–1,500 mL.

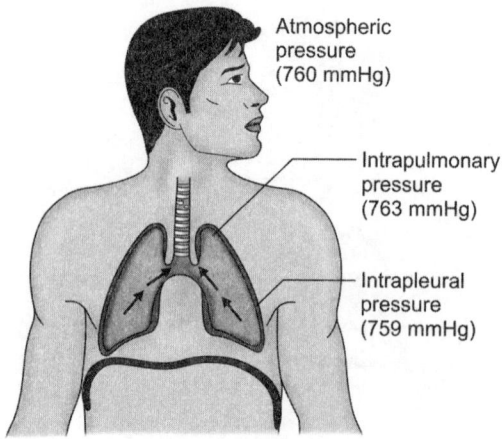

Fig. 5.16: Forced expiration

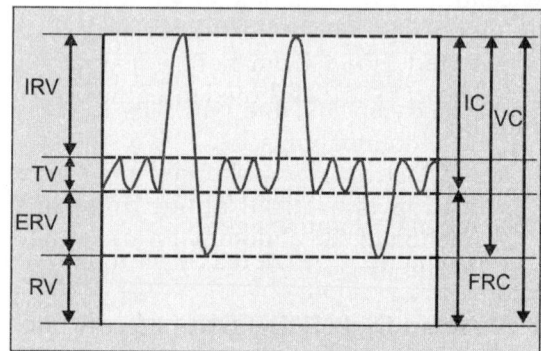

Fig. 5.17: Lung volumes. TV: tidal volume; IRV: inspiratory reserve volume; IC: inspiratory capacity; ERV: expiratory reserve volume; RV: residual volume; FRC: functional residual capacity; VC: vital capacity; TLV: total lung volume. All these lung volumes are approximately 5% less in females (except residual volume)

Vital capacity: It is the maximum amount of gas that can be exhaled after maximum inhalation, i.e. it is IRV + TV + ERV. It is 4,200 to 4,500 mL (75–80 mL/kg).

Residual volume: It is volume of gas still present in lungs after maximal expiration. It is 1,200–1,500 mL.

Maximum breathing capacity: Maximum volume of air that can be breathed/minute. It is 120–170 litre/mm (normally it is measured for 15 seconds and expressed as litre/min.)

Minute volume: It is tidal volume × respiratory rate. It is 500 × 12 = 6,000 mL/min

Total lung volume: IRV + TV + ERV + RV It is 5,500–6,000 mL.

Functional residual capacity (FRC): It is the volume of gas in lungs after end expiration. It is ERV + RV. It is 2,400–2,600 mL.

Lung function tests are based on lung volumes. They are useful in diagnosis and monitoring of respiratory system diseases.

GAS EXCHANGE IN LUNGS

The alveoli of lungs have basement membrane which is in close contact with the capillary wall. Gas exchange takes place through capillary wall and alveolar cell membrane. Gases diffuse from higher concentration to lower concentration. In the lungs, the oxygen concentration is more, letting it diffuse into the blood through the capillary wall. The oxygenated blood from here is carried to the left heart to be distributed to all the tissues of the body.

The deoxygenated blood from the tissues is carried to the right heart and is recirculated to the lungs for more oxygen.

Gas exchange is promoted by the following factors:

1. Alveolar epithelium, made of very thin epithelial cells
2. Pressure of air in the alveolus
3. Basement membrane of epithelial cells
4. At places alveolar epithelium fuses with the capillary wall
5. Alveolar epithelium is separated from capillary wall by a narrow space

The percent of gases in inspired and expired air is as under:

Gas	Inspired air %	Expired air %
Oxygen	21.0	16.0
Carbon dioxide	0.04	3.5
Nitrogen	79.0	79.0
Water vapour	Variable	6.2

External Respiration

It is the exchange of gases by diffusion between the alveoli and the blood in capillaries. Total area for gas exchange in lungs is about 70–80 square metres. Venous blood reaching the lungs has high levels of CO_2 and low levels of O_2. By diffusion O_2 diffuses from alveoli into the blood and CO_2 diffuses into alveoli from blood along concentration gradient till equilibrium is reached.

Internal Respiration

It is the exchange of gases by diffusion between blood in capillaries and body cells. Blood reaching the tissues has higher concentration of O_2 and lower concentration of CO_2 than tissues. Because of this difference in concentration, gaseous exchange occurs. O_2 diffuses from blood stream through capillary wall into tissues. CO_2 diffuses from cells into bloodstream in capillaries.

Effect of Exercise on Respiration

Exercise accelerates the function of the respiratory and cardiovascular systems. During exercise, increased cardiac output increases the blood flow to the lungs. This is called as pulmonary perfusion which rises about five times. The O_2 diffusion capacity increases three times during maximal exercise.

Muscles consume large amounts of O_2 when they contract during exercise and produce large amounts of CO_2. Pulmonary ventilation increases up to 30-fold from the resting state.

Neural changes that bring excitatory impulses into the inspiratory area in the medulla oblongata cause the abrupt increase in ventilation at the start of exercise.

At the end of exercise, pulmonary ventilation abruptly decreases. This is followed by a gradual decline to the resting level.

TRANSPORT OF GASES IN BLOOD STREAM

O_2 and CO_2 transport is essential for internal respiration. O_2 is transported in blood in chemical combination with haemoglobin as oxyhaemoglobin (98.5% of blood O_2) or in solution in plasma water (1.5% of blood O_2). Oxyhaemoglobin is unstable compound and it releases O_2 into tissues under certain conditions.

CO_2 is waste product of metabolism and is expelled by the lungs. It is transported as bicarbonate ions in plasma (70% of blood CO_2), combined with haemoglobin as carbaminohaemoglobin (23%) and dissolved in plasma (7%).

REGULATION OF RESPIRATION

The regulation of respiration is considered under two headings:

1. Mechanism of rhythmic breathing: It is regulated by neural mechanisms.
2. Regulation of depth of breathing: It is under chemical control.

Rhythmic Breathing

It is controlled by respiratory centre—group of neurons present bilaterally in medulla oblongata and pons.

1. *In the medulla,* there is an inspiratory centre, i.e. collection of neurons that fire during inspiration and expiratory centre, i.e. neurons that fire during forced expiration.
2. *In the upper pons* there is pneumotaxic centre situated bilaterally. These neurons have an inhibitory influence on the inspiratory centre in the medulla. This centre regulates the rate of breathing.
3. *Hering-Breuer reflex:* There are stretch receptors in the wall of smooth muscle of bronchi and bronchioles. The impulses from these receptors reach the medulla oblongata via the vagus nerve.

    Over inflation of lungs stimulates the stretch receptors and cause inhibition of discharge from the inspiratory centre. This helps to slow the respiratory rate.

4. *Irritant receptors:* These are present between the epithelial cells. These receptors get stimulated by irritant gases or dust particles. Activation of receptors causes coughing, and increased mucus secretion.

Chemical Control of Respiration

The chemical control of respiration regulates pulmonary ventilation according to the metabolic requirements. In the body, few chemoreceptors are present which respond to changes in pH, pO_2 and pCO_2.

Breathing is stimulated either by a decrease in pH or pO_2 and an increase in pCO_2. The chemoreceptors are able to maintain the arterial pCO_2/pO_2 and pH within the normal range.

The peripheral chemoreceptors are present in the aortic and carotid bodies. The aortic bodies are two or more located in the arch of the aorta. The carotid body is located at the bifurcation of common carotid artery. The **central chemoreceptors** are present on the surface of medulla oblongata.

The sensitivity of chemoreceptors to raised arterial CO_2 concentration is most important factor in maintaining homeostasis of blood gases.

BASAL METABOLIC RATE

When a person is at rest and if his/her digestive system is also at rest (12–18 hours after the last meal) then the basal metabolic activities like respiration, heart beat, formation of urine, sweat and maintenance of body temperature will go on.

The minimum energy required to maintain the above mentioned basal activities is called **basal metabolic rate** (BMR). Energy is derived from the oxidation of food resulting in the production of carbon dioxide. O_2 consumption is calculated in the morning time 12–18 hours after last meal. The person is in complete physical and mentally relaxed state.

BMR is expressed in kilocalories/hour/ sq metre of body surface area (BSA), i.e. kcal/

h/m^2 BSA. Average normal BMR in adult male is 40 kcal/h/m^2 BSA. In adult female, it is 37 kcal/h/m^2 BSA.

Factors Affecting BMR

1. **Sex:** Males have higher BMR.
2. **Age:** Children have higher BMR. It declines gradually to adult level by the age of 18 years. After 60 years it falls slightly.
3. **Body surface area:** BMR is directly related to body surface area, which can be calculated from height and weight of the person.
4. **External temperature:** Cold weather increases BMR.
5. **Endocrine glands:** Thyroxine increases BMR. In hyperthyroidism, BMR is high and in hypothyroid conditions it is low.
6. **Sleep:** During sleep it falls.
7. **Body temperature:** For each 1°C rise of body temperature, BMR increases by 14%.
8. **Effect of proteins:** Protein intake enhances BMR.
9. **Physical activity:** BMR is directly proportional to the activity of the person.
10. **Anxious and tense person:** These conditions increase BMR.
11. **Pregnancy:** During late pregnancy BMR increases.
12. **Reading and mental activities:** These do not effect BMR.

CLINICAL ASPECTS

Nose

- The nasal bone often gets **fractured** as the two nasal bones form the prominence of the nose.
- The nasal septum may be **deviated** to one or other side, causing asymmetry in the size of nasal cavity. Picking of the lower part of nasal septum may cause bleeding from the nose, called as the **epistaxis.**
- **Nasal cavity** is prone to **common cold.** It is caused by the rhinovirus and is a mild, but irritating disease. One is not too ill, but not too well as well. It takes about one week for cold to be alright.

- **The paranasal sinuses** are draining into the nasal cavity. The infection from the nasal cavity reaches the sinuses to cause **sinusitis.** Maxillary sinusitis does not heal fully as it is not able to drain completely Postural drainage is advised in addition to other treatment.
- Infection of palatine tonsils is called **'tonsillitis'.** Infection of nasopharyngeal tonsil is called **'adenoids'.** The adenoids obstruct normal passage of air, so the child breathes through the mouth.

Tracheostomy

Tube is put through an artificial opening made in the trachea.

Foreign body enters commonly in the right bronchus as it is shorter, wider and in line with the trachea.

Diphtheria

It is caused by the bacteria *C. diphtheriae.* The membrane formed in the disease obstructs the air passage and is a serious condition.

Bronchitis

The bacterial infection associated with common cold extends down into the trachea and the bronchi, causing 'bronchitis'. It may be acute or may become chronic. The infection may extend further down into the lungs causing **bronchopneumonia.** Bronchitis is common in smokers.

Pneumonia

Develops due to colonisation of the lungs by microorganisms. It may develop due to impaired coughing, damage to ciliary epithelium of respiratory tract, pulmonary oedema and decreased resistance to infection.

Lobar pneumonia results from infection of one or more lobes of lung by *Streptococcus pneumoniae.* It is treated by antibacterial drugs.

Bronchopneumonia results from spread of infection from bronchi to terminal bronchioles and alveoli.

Asthma

This starts as an allergic process with superadded inflammatory reaction. Person finds expiration rather difficult, due to bronchospasm (contraction of bronchial muscle) and excessive secretion of mucus in the bronchial tree.

Tuberculosis

This is extremely common in our country due to poor hygiene, malnutrition and living in overcrowded colonies. Tuberculosis (TB) is caused by *Mycobacterium tuberculosis*. Cough of more than 3–4 weeks of duration should be investigated for TB. The patient also develops weight loss, malaise, haemoptysis (expectoration of blood stained sputum).

It needs treatment for 6–8 months under medical supervision. TB may spread from lungs to intestine also.

Cancer of the Lung

Cancer of the bronchi is common in active or passive smokers. In smokers, the cancer of lung is far more common than non smokers. The cancer cells may spread to lung tissue, liver, brain and bones. It is usually fatal.

Pneumothorax

There is air present in the pleural cavity. It may occur spontaneously or as a result of trauma. **Spontaneous pneumothorax** may occur because of unknown cause or is secondary to pleural rupture due to lung disease, e.g. emphysema, asthma, tuberculosis.

In **traumatic pneumothorax,** fractured rib may penetrate into the pleura, allowing air to enter the pleural cavity, causing collapse of the lung and respiratory distress.

Haemothorax

Presence of blood in the pleural cavity is called haemothorax. It may be secondary to injury to the chest or erosion of blood vessel by a malignant tumor.

Pleural Effusion

It is excess of fluid in pleural cavity. It may be caused by increased hydrostatic pressure, increased capillary permeability or decreased plasma osmotic pressure. It usually occurs in TB lungs.

*Words used in relation to **exchange** and transport of oxygen and carbon dioxide.*

1. *Eupnoea* means normal quite breathing.

2. *Pulmonary ventilation* means the movement of air in and out of the lungs. It is also called breathing.

3. *Hypoventilation* means slow and shallow breathing.

4. *Hypoxia* means decreased amount of oxygen in the tissues.

Points to Remember

1. Respiratory system is for exchange of carbon dioxide of the body with oxygen.
2. Soft palate prevents bolus of food from entering into the nasal cavity.
3. Right lung has 3 lobes while left lung has 2 lobes only.
4. There are 10 segmental bronchi in both right and left lungs.

MCQs ?

1. **Which of these body systems is involved in the removal of carbon dioxide?**
   (a) Respiratory system
   (b) Digestive system
   (c) Urinary system
   (d) Nervous system

2. **Normal tidal volume in adult is about:**
   (a) 300 ml
   (b) 500 ml
   (c) 1200 ml
   (d) 3600 ml

3. **Muscles used in quiet respiration are all except:**
   (a) Internal intercostal muscle
   (b) External intercostal muscle
   (c) Diaphragm
   (d) Sternocleidomastoid

4. **The actual gas exchange with blood occurs in the:**
   (a) Bronchi
   (b) Respiratory bronchioles
   (c) Terminal bronchioles
   (d) Alveolar ducts and alveoli

Urinary System

Waste products are products not required by the body. These have to be eliminated. Gases like carbon dioxide and nitrogen are expelled through expiration. Solid waste products of food including fibres are expelled through the anal canal. Some amount of water and a few salts are removed as sweat from the skin.

The various metabolic waste products, salts, urea, uric acid and water are expelled as urine by the urinary system.

COMPONENTS OF URINARY SYSTEM

Urinary system comprises various organs. These are 2 kidneys, 2 ureters, one urinary bladder and single urethra (Fig. 6.1).

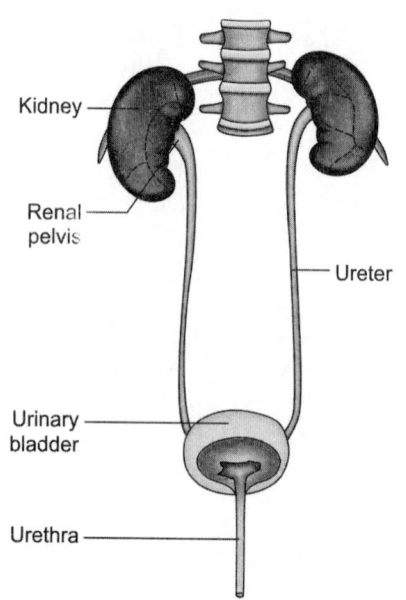

Fig. 6.1: Urinary system

Urinary system plays a vital part in maintaining homeostasis of water and electrolyte concentrations within the body. The kidneys produce urine that contains metabolic waste products.

Kidneys

The two bean-shaped kidneys lie behind the peritoneum on each side of posterior abdominal wall from 12th thoracic vertebra to 3rd lumbar vertebra. Each kidney is about 11 cm long, 6 cm wide, 3 cm thick and weighs 150 g.

Hilum lies at level of 1st lumbar vertebra. Upper ends are medial while lower ends are lateral. Hilum is present in the middle of the medial border. Structures present at the hilum are renal vein, renal artery and pelvis of ureter from before backwards (Fig. 6.2).

Right kidney is little lower, because of the huge liver present on the right side.

Supports of the Kidney

These are (from within outwards) renal capsule, perirenal fat, renal fascia, pararenal fat and vessels at the hilum. These support the kidney and keep it in position.

Relations

Posterior relations are similar on two sides except that left kidney is related to 11th and 12th ribs, and right kidney only to 12th rib. Diaphragm is related in the **upper part**. The **lower part** is related to muscles of the posterior abdominal wall.

Anterior relations are different on the two sides.

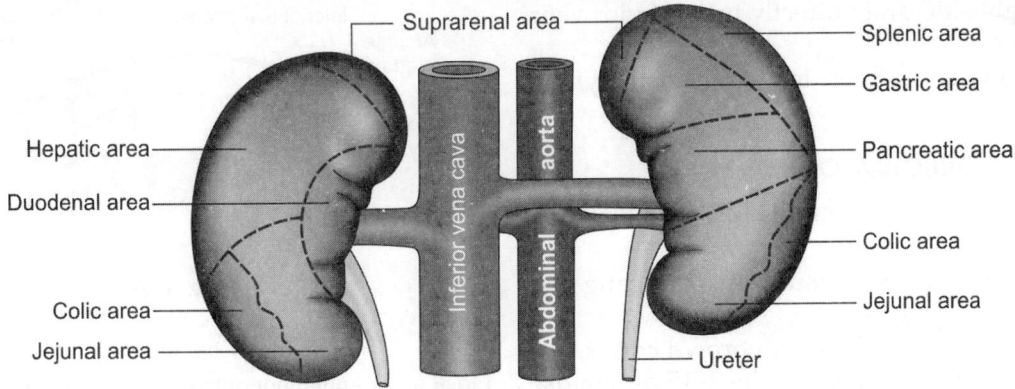

Fig. 6.2: Anterior relations of kidneys

1. *Right kidney* is related to suprarenal on its upper pole, to duodenum at its hilum, liver on the upper part, ascending colon along lateral border and coils of intestine.

The *Left kidney* is related to suprarenal on the upper pole, spleen along upper lateral border, pancreas across the kidney and stomach between pancreas and spleen. Along the lateral border is the descending colon and at the lower pole and adjacent area are the coils of intestine (Fig. 6.2).

2. *Renal pelvis* emerges from the hilum. This is a reservoir for urine and soon narrows and changes its name to ureter. Anterior to renal pelvis is renal artery and anterior most is the renal vein. VAP (vein, artery, pelvis) from before backwards.

Blood Supply and Lymphatic Drainage

The paired **renal arteries** arise from abdominal aorta at right angles at the level of second lumbar vertebra. Each artery divides into 5 segmental arteries which after repeated divisions reach the glomeruli (Fig. 6.3).

The single **renal vein** lies in front of the artery and drains into inferior vena cava.

The right vein is 2.5 cm long while the left one is 7.5 cm long.

Into the left renal vein, the left gonadal and left suprarenal veins also drain. Same veins

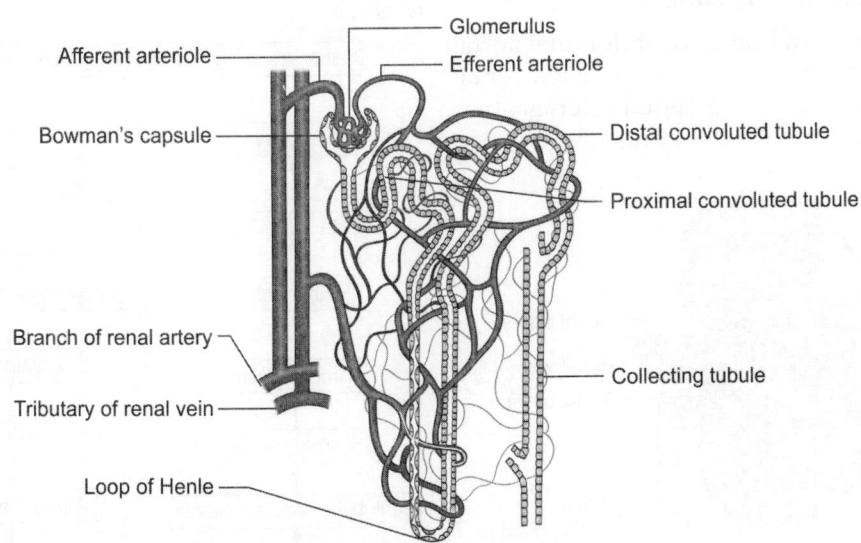

Fig. 6.3: Blood supply of kidney

of right side drain directly into inferior vena cava.

Lymphatics drain into para-aortic lymph nodes.

GROSS STRUCTURE OF KIDNEY

Longitudinal section of kidney reveals the following structures:

1. The **fibrous capsule** surrounding the kidney (Fig. 6.4).
2. The peripheral reddish brown **cortex** between the capsule and the 8–15 pyramids.
3. The inner **medulla** comprised of triangular renal pyramids. **Lobe** of the kidney is comprised of a pyramid and the cortical tissue capping it.
4. The **renal pelvis** containing the expanded end of the ureter (pelvis of ureter) which divides into 2–3 major calyces. Each major calyx further divides into 2–3 minor calyces. Each minor calyx is indented by the apex of the pyramid of the renal medulla.

Urine formed in the kidney passes through a papilla at the apex of a pyramid into a minor calyx, then into a major calyx before passing through the pelvis into the ureter. Peristalsis of the smooth muscle in the walls of the calyces propels urine through the pelvis and ureters to the bladder.

BLOOD SUPPLY OF THE KIDNEY

The renal artery, a branch of abdominal aorta is the only artery to the kidney. Each renal artery divides into 5 segmental arteries after entering the hilum (Figs 6.4 and 6.5).

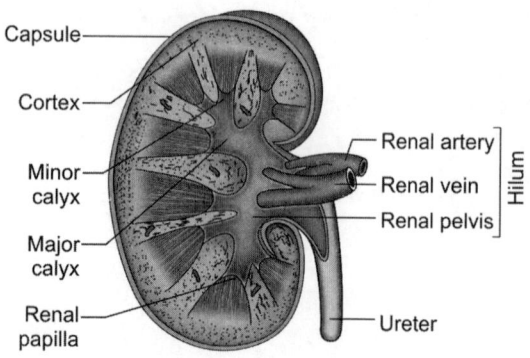

Fig. 6.4: Longitudinal section of the kidney

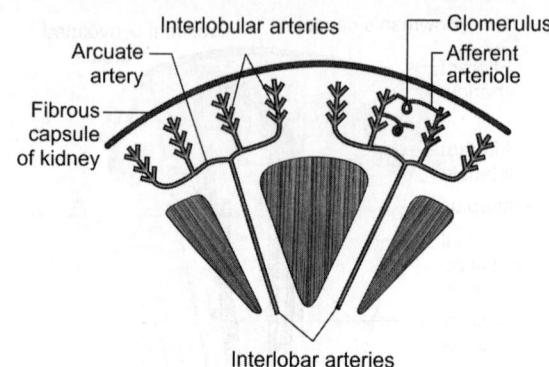

Fig. 6.5: Arrangement of the arteries in the kidney

Course of renal artery and vein is shown in Flowchart 6.1.

NEPHRON

It is the structural and functional unit of kidney. There are 1–1.3 million nephrons in each kidney (Fig. 6.6).

Structure and Functions of Nephron

There are two types of nephrons in each kidney: (1) cortical and (2) juxtamedullary. Their differences are as follows.

Cortical Nephron
1. 85% are located in cortex.

Flowchart 6.1: Showing course of renal artery and renal vein

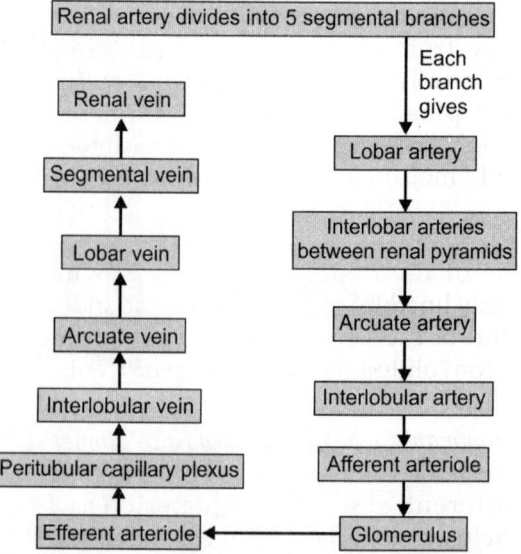

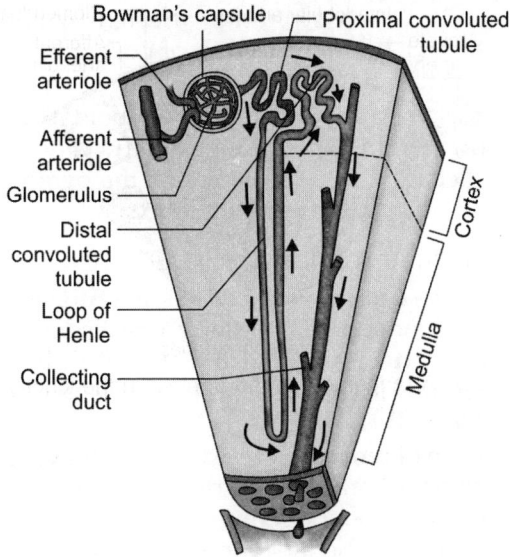

Efferent arteriole

Afferent arteriole

Glomerulus

Distal convoluted tubule

Loop of Henle

Collecting duct

Bowman's capsule — Proximal convoluted tubule

Cortex

Medulla

Fig. 6.6: Nephron

2. Short loop of Henle and rate of filtration is slow.

3. Less concentrated urine is formed.

Juxtamedullary Nephron

1. 15% located at the junction of cortex and medulla.

2. Long loop of Henle and rate of filtration is high.

3. Highly concentrated urine is formed.

Approximately 2 million nephrons present in both the kidneys filter blood plasma in their glomeruli. The ultrafiltrate which is formed is free from blood cells and proteins but contains all the other constituents present in blood plasma. This tubular fluid passes through various portions of renal tubule. It is greatly modified and urine is formed.

Parts of the Nephron

Parts of the nephron are—(1) Bowman's capsule lined by epithelial cells and indented by tuft of capillaries (glomerulus), (2) proximal convoluted tubule, (3) loop of Henle and (4) distal convoluted tubule.

1. *Bowman's capsule contains the glomerular capillaries.* These are interposed between afferent and efferent arterioles. This helps to maintain high hydrostatic pres-

sure in the capillaries required for huge glomerular filtration.

The glomerulus consists of fenestrated type of capillaries. The epithelial cells of inner layer of Bowman's capsule are called **podocytes** as these possess feet like processes which rest on the outer aspect of basement membrane. The **glomerular membrane** consists of:

1. Endothelial cells of capillaries.

2. Basement membranes fused.

3. Podocyte epithelial cells of Bowman's capsule.

From the blood in the capillaries the fluid passes through fenestra of endothelial cells, basement membranes and slits between network of podocytes.

2. *Proximal convoluted tubule* (PCT) constitutes major portion of the nephron and bulk of renal parenchyma. The tubule is lined by single layer of epithelial cells that show prominent brush border at the luminal surface and a large number of mito-chondria in the cytoplasm.

Because of brush border the cells are able to reabsorb 70% water and electrolytes including 100% reabsorption of glucose and amino acids from the filtrate. The necessary energy is provided by large number of mitochondria.

3. *Loop of Henle:* It consists of thick descending segment followed by a thin descending segment. The latter forms a loop with a thin ascending segment in the medulla and a thick ascending segment that enters back in the cortex.

The thin segment of loop of Henle is lined with squamous epithelial cells with few microvilli and mitochondria. The thick descending segment of loop of Henle resembles PCT structurally and func-tionally. In the same way, the thick ascend-ing segment of loop of Henle resembles distal convoluted tubule (DCT). Each thick ascending segment of loop of Henle returns to the cortex and comes in contact with the glomerulus between the afferent and efferent arterioles. The epithelial cells of this part of tubule are close together with crowded nuclei and are named **macula densa** (Fig. 6.7).

The loop of Henle penetrates the medulla to a varying degree. The loops arising from the glomeruli in the deeper part of the cortex (juxtamedullary glomeruli) descend deeper into the medulla than the superficially placed glomeruli. By the time the filtrate enters the descending limb of loop of Henle, its water content has been reduced by 70%. At this point, the filtrate contains high amount of sodium. As the filtrate moves along the loop of Henle, osmosis draws even more water into extracellular spaces, thus the filtrate is further concentrated.

4. *Distal convoluted tubule* (DCT) is lined by epithelial cells. These cells contain large number of mitochondria only and the brush border is absent. 10–20% water and electrolytes are reabsorbed from DCT.

DCT reabsorption is affected by anti-diuretic hormone (ADH) of posterior lobe of pituitary gland.

Collecting tubule is lined by cuboidal cells and it joins the collecting duct. Many collecting ducts pass through the pyramid and open into the minor calyx.

Juxtaglomerular Apparatus (JGA)

It is composed of modified cells at the junction of distal convoluted tubule, where it comes in close contact with afferent arteriole of glomerulus in that region. It consists of three types of cells:

1. *Juxtaglomerular (JG) cells:* These are myo-epitheloid cells formed due to proliferation of vascular smooth muscle cells of afferent arteriole at the junction where it comes in contact with DCT. These JG cells release a proteolytic enzyme **renin** in response to low blood volume, hypoxia and low blood pressure and help to regulate blood pressure (Fig. 6.7).

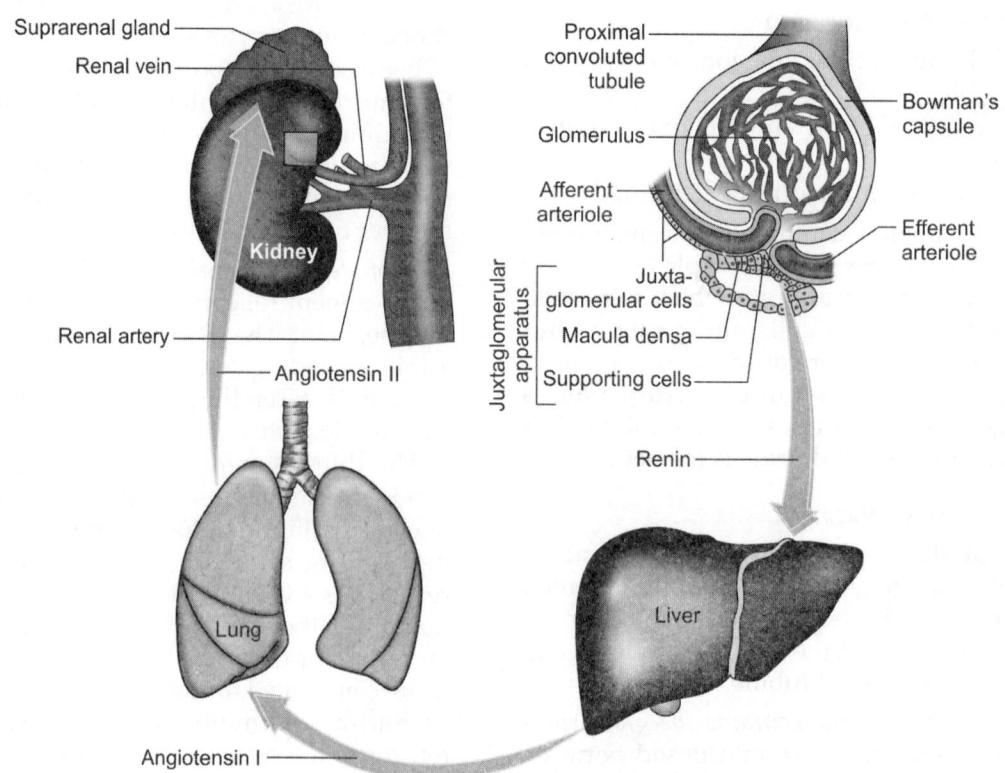

Fig. 6.7: Regulation of blood pressure by the juxtaglomerular apparatus

2. *Macula densa cells:* These are crowded large columnar cells in the inner lining of DCT at the point where it comes in contact with the afferent arteriole. These are sensitized due to low sodium in tubular fluid and stimulate the JG cells to release renin.
3. *Supporting cells:* These are present between JG cells and macula densa cells. These cells may contract and regulate the glomerular filtration.

FUNCTIONS OF KIDNEY

1. Maintenance of internal body environment (milieu interior) by regulating the volume and composition of blood and extracellular fluid.
2. Urine formation and elimination of waste products of metabolism in dissolved form in urine, e.g. urea, uric acid, creatinine and various electrolytes, e.g. Cl^-, K^+, HCO_3^-, H^+.
3. Regulation of blood pressure through renin-angiotensin aldosterone mechanism (Fig. 6.8).
4. Renal erythropoietic factor helps in increasing the number of circulating red blood cells whenever there is anaemia or less number of red blood cells.
5. Synthesis of vitamin D by converting dietary vitamin D_3 to 1, 25 DHCC (dihydrocholecalciferol). In this form, vitamin D can be utilised to prevent rickets.

6. Maintenance of pH of blood (acid–base balance) by excreting acidic or alkaline urine.

Ureters

Each ureter is a smooth muscle tube about 25 cm long, lined by transitional epithelium or urothelium. It does not allow absorption of urine.

Ureter passes behind the peritoneum of posterior abdominal wall over the psoas major muscle. It lies opposite the transverse processes of lumbar vertebrae.

At the division of common iliac artery into internal and external iliac arteries, the ureter enters the pelvis and lies on the side wall of pelvis in front of the internal iliac artery. On reaching the pelvic floor, it turns medially and forwards to enter the urinary bladder (Figs 6.8 and 6.9)

Ureter shows **three main constrictions**, at pelvi-ureteric junction, while crossing the pelvic brim and at the entry into the bladder. Ureteric stones are more liable to get impacted at these sites of constriction.

Ureter is supplied by blood through small branches of renal, gonadal and iliac arteries. Veins follow the arteries and drain into respective veins.

Lymph vessels drain into adjacent abdominal and pelvic lymph nodes.

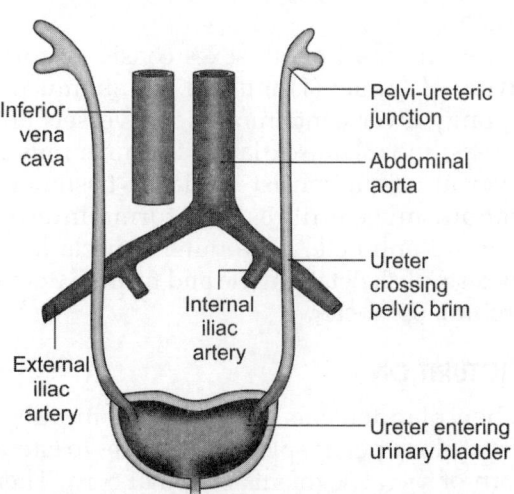

Fig. 6.8: Main constrictions of ureter

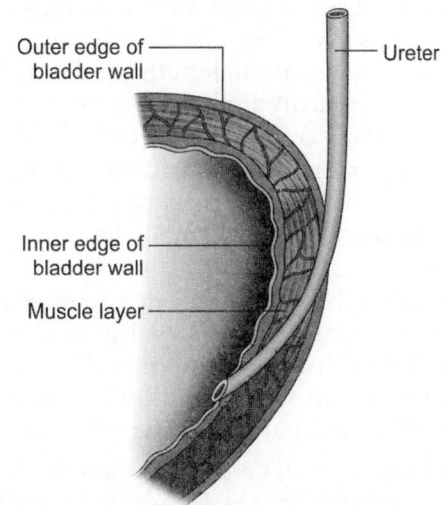

Fig. 6.9: Opening of ureter into the urinary bladder

Nerve supply is from both sympathetic and parasympathetic fibres. Pain is carried along sympathetic nerves. These enter spinal cord via T11–12 and Ll–2 nerves.

The ureters consist of three layers of tissue: (1) fibrous tissue (outer), (2) muscular layer (middle) of smooth muscle, and (3) mucosa (inner) lined by transitional epithelium. The ureters convey urine from the kidneys into the bladder by peristaltic contraction of the smooth muscle layer.

Urinary Bladder

Urinary bladder is the temporary store house for urine. Its capacity is 250–500 mL. Its mucous membrane is lined by urine proof transitional epithelium.

Situation and Surfaces

It is situated in front part of the pelvis, behind the pubic symphysis. In adult, it is entirely a pelvic organ, but a distended bladder is an abdominal organ. In a child, up to 2–3 years due to small size of pelvis, bladder is an abdominal organ.

It consists of a superior surface, two inferolateral surfaces and a posterior surface or base.

The base is related posteriorly to rectum in male and to vagina in female.

The lower part of the base is **trigone** of the bladder. At its upper part, the two orifices are the openings of ureters, and at the lowest part of trigone lies the **internal urethral orifice**. The region of internal urethral meatus at the lowest part of trigone is called the neck of the bladder.

The superior surface and inferolateral surfaces are related to coils of intestine. In female, body of uterus normally lies on top of the bladder.

The **arterial supply** is from superior and inferior vesical branches of internal iliac artery. **Veins** drain into internal iliac veins. **Lymphatics** run with the blood vessels to internal iliac and para-aortic lymph nodes.

The bladder wall consists of three layers:
1. An outer layer of loose connective tissue,
2. Middle layer of smooth muscle and
3. Elastic tissue. The smooth muscle is known as detrusor muscle. The inner layer is lined with transitional epithelium.

Female Urethra

It is a straight tube 4 cm long, lying in front of vagina between the internal urethral meatus and the external urethral meatus. Urethra is lined by urine proof transitional epithelium. Almost the whole length of urethra is surrounded by sphincter urethrae, which maintains urinary continence. Catheter can be easily passed in females.

Male Urethra

Male urethra is 15–20 cm long and has 4 parts: (1) **preprostatic**; (2) **prostatic** which is 3 cm long when it courses through the prostate gland; (3) **membranous** (narrowest and shortest) and (4) a **spongy part** passing through corpus spongiosum of penis to open at external urethral orifice at the tip of the glans penis.

Spongy urethra takes a right angled turn to continue up as membranous urethra. This fact must be remembered while passing a catheter through the male urethra, a difficult process.

The male urethra provides a common pathway for the flow of urine and semen, the combined secretions of the male reproductive organs.

The urethra in both sexes consist of three layers of tissue: (1) mucosa, (2) submucosa (spongy layer containing blood vessels and nerves) and (3) muscle layer. The inner muscle layer at origin consist of elastic tissue and smooth muscle fibres and forms internal urethral sphincter. The outer muscle layer consists of skeletal muscle and forms external urethral sphincter.

MICTURITION

When bladder gets full, afferent impulses travel along pelvic splanchnic nerves to lateral horn of sacral segments of spinal cord. Their fibres pass back to the bladder muscle in same nerves to cause contraction of its detrusor muscle and relaxation of internal urethral sphincter.

Autonomic stretch reflex is typical of infant. The fibres pass through the spinal cord. After training, brain keeps external sphincter closed till the appropriate time of passage of urine. External sphincter is supplied by branch of pudendal nerve (S2, 3, 4 segments). Feeling of full bladder is conveyed by parasympathetic nerves to spinal cord and then via posterior column of spinal cord to brain.

In very old age, cerebral control may be lost. If spinal cord is injured above sacral level, afferent impulses cannot reach the brain, external sphincter relaxes automatically and bladder is emptied.

If sacral segments are destroyed, bladder muscle gets paralysed, bladder becomes abnormally distended, resulting in overflow incontinence.

Catheterisation of bladder may result in urinary infection.

FORMATION OF URINE

The three steps in urine formation are:
1. Glomerular filtration
2. Tubular reabsorption
3. Tubular secretion.

1. *Renal blood flow* is 1,200 to 1,300 mL/minute. Out of this 125 mL/minute is filtered and is known as **glomerular filtrate.** It contains water, electrolytes, glucose, amino acids and waste products of metabolism, e.g. urea, uric acid and creatinine. The volume of filtrate formed by both kidneys each minute is called **glomerular filtration rate (GFR).** In a normal adult the GFR is about 125 mL/min. Most of the filtrate is reabsorbed with less than 1%, i.e. 1–1.5 litres, excreted as urine. Renal blood flow is inherently **autoregulated,** i.e. it is maintained at a constant pressure across a wide range of systolic blood pressure. But, at systolic blood pressure below 80 mmHg autoregulation fails.

2. *Tubular reabsorption:* As this filtrate passes through PCT, there is reabsorption of 70% of water and electrolytes and 100% reabsorption of glucose and amino acids, which are useful to our body. 10–20% water and electrolytes are reabsorbed from DCT and collecting tubule (CT) to the blood. Thus, the tubules reabsorb into the blood those filtrate constituents needed by the body to maintain fluid and electrolyte balance and pH of the blood. Active transport of substances is carried on against concentration gradient at carrier sites in epithelial membrane using chemical energy. Glucose, amino acids, sodium, potassium, calcium, phosphate and chloride are reabsorbed by active transport.

3. *Tubular secretion:* Many electrolytes, e.g. H^+, Cl^-, K^+, HCO_3^-, and water are secreted from blood into tubular fluid. Certain substances not required by the body and foreign materials are cleared by secretion into convoluted tubules and excreted from the body in the urine.

Composition of Urine

Composition of urine depends on the amount of substances secreted and absorption of water and electrolytes. Most of the water from the glomerular filtrate is reabsorbed by PCT. Decreased water reabsorption results in diuresis or dilute urine formation.

Volume of urine varies from day-to-day depending on the intake of fluids, food, temperature of the surroundings, humidity excessive sweating and during different time of a day.

Scanty urine formation (less than 400 mL per day in adults) is known as **oliguria;** complete absence of urine formation is called as **anuria.**

Normal physical characteristics of urine:
- **Colour:** Normal urine has amber colour.
- **Specific gravity:** 1,010–1,030. Specific gravity indicates relative proportion of solids to water. Normal urine contains 95% water and 3% solids.
- **Odour:** mildly aromatic
- **Volume:** 1,500–2,000 mL/day.
- **Turbidity:** Transparent when freshly passed, becomes turbid after standing

- **pH:** 5.0–8.0, averge 6.0.
- **Water:** 97%.
- **Solids:** 3%. Solids are minerals and waste products of metabolism.

CLINICAL ASPECTS

Congenital Anomalies

1. *Pelvic kidney:* Kidney develops in the pelvic region and then ascends to lumbar region. If it does not ascend, the condition is called pelvic kidney. Such a kidney may cause problem during pregnancy as the renal vessels or ureter may get pressed by the enlarging uterus.

2. *Polycystic kidney:* If the excretory and collecting parts of kidney do not join each other properly, multiple cysts are formed in the kidneys. These cysts are present at the junction of distal convoluted and collecting tubules. These cysts gradually enlarge and cause destruction of nephrons due to pressure. Chronic renal failure usually develops.

Infective Disorders

1. *Acute glomerulonephritis:* This is a inflammatory condition of the glomerulus. This is either due to bacterial infection or immune reaction to toxins of bacteria, especially *Streptococcus haemolyticus*. It may become a chronic condition if untreated. It may affect all the glomeruli (diffuse) or some glomeruli (focal). The patient presents with haematuria (passage of blood in urine), proteinuria (passage of proteins in urine), hypertension, fluid retention, anuria or oliguria. There may be chronic renal failure due to irreversible destruction of nephrons.

2. *Acute pyelonephritis:* This condition is due to acute bacterial infection of the pelvis or calyces of kidney causing small abscesses in the kidney. This condition may also become chronic in nature.

3. *Cystitis:* Inflammation of urinary bladder is called 'cystitis' and that of urethra is known as 'urethritis'.

Renal Dialysis and Renal Transplant

If both kidneys are not functioning, renal dialysis is done repeatedly before the kidney can be transplanted. Dialysis can be done by two ways: (1) **haemodialysis** and (2) **peritoneal dialysis** (Figs 6.10 and 6.11). Kidney from blood relation is accepted better. Life is prolonged by some years if the grafted kidney is taken up well by the host.

Renal Calculi

When some components of urine get precipitated to form crystals, the condition is

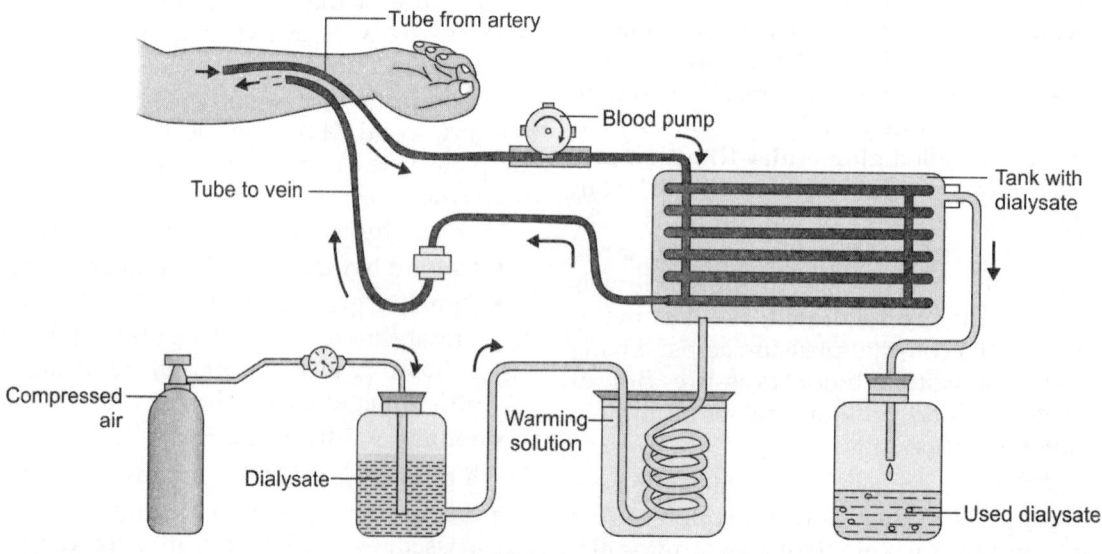

Fig. 6.10: Haemodialysis

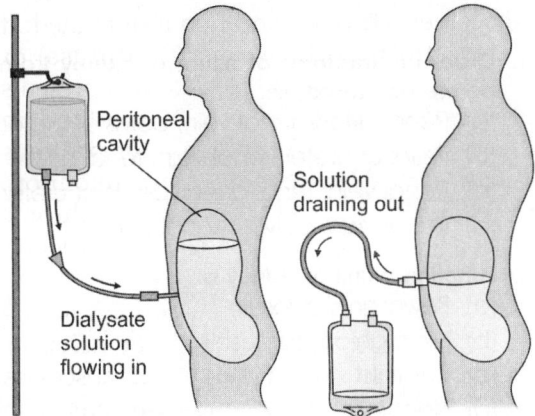

Fig. 6.11: Peritoneal dialysis

called 'renal calculus'. If the calculus is small, these pass down into the ureter, as ureteric calculi. Sometimes, renal calculus may become big to become one large stone in the renal pelvis. Pain in renal stone is present in 'renal angle' between the 12th rib and the lateral border of erector spinae muscle. In ureteric stone pain extends from 'loin to the groin'. Drinking more water is the key to prevent calculi formation.

Tumours

1. Hypernephroma is a malignant tumour of tubular epithelium.
2. Nephroblastoma is highly malignant tumour in children.
3. Papilloma arise from the transitional epithelium of urinary bladder.

Hydronephrosis

It is the dilatation of renal pelvis and calyces caused by accumulation of urine. It occurs due to obstruction to the passage of urine. Both the kidneys are affected if the abnormality is in the urethra or the bladder. Obstruction above bladder affects only one kidney. There is destruction of nephrons due to increase pressure.

Urinary Incontinence

There is involuntary passage of urine due to defective voluntary control of external urethral sphincter.

Nephrotic Syndrome

At occurs in a variety of conditions. In children, the most common cause is minimal change glomerulonephritis. The main clinical features are excessive proteinuria, hypoalbuminaemia (decreased serum albumin due to its leakage from glomerular membrane), generalised oedema and hyperlipidaemia.

Acute Renal Failure

There is sudden and severe reduction in glomerular filtration rate and kidney function. It is reversible over days or weeks when treated.

Oedema

It is defined as excessive accumulation of tissue fluid, which causes swelling. It may be present in the superficial tissues or in lungs (pulmonary oedema).

It may occur due to:
1. Increased venous hydrostatic pressure
2. Increased small vessel permeability
3. Decreased plasma osmotic pressure
4. Impaired lymphatic drainage.

Points to Remember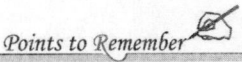

1. Right kidney is lower than the left as bulky liver pushes it down.
2. Structures in hilum of kidney from before backwards are renal vein, renal artery and pelvis of ureter
3. Kidney is supported by perirenal fat, renal fascia and pararenal fat.
4. Adequate water intake will prevent formation of renal stone.

MCQs

1. **Blood vessels entering the glomerulus is known as:**
   - (a) Afferent
   - (b) Efferent
   - (c) Renal artery
   - (d) Renal vein

2. **Length of female urethra:**
   - (a) 2 cm
   - (b) 3 cm
   - (c) 4 cm
   - (d) 6 cm

3. **Order of structures of hilum of kidney from before backwords is:**
   - (a) Renal artery, renal vein, pelvis of ureter
   - (b) Pelvis of ureter, renal vein, renal artery
   - (c) Renal vein, renal artery, pelvis of ureter
   - (d) Renal vein, pelvis, reanal artery

4. **Functional unit of kidney is:**
   - (a) Bowman's capsule
   - (b) Malpighian carpuscles
   - (c) Pyramid
   - (d) Nephron

Muscular System

The muscle tissue is specialised for the purpose of contraction. By means of contraction, movements are performed. Muscles constitute about 50% mass of total body weight.

The muscle tissue has four properties that enable it to function:

1. *Electrical excitability:* Muscle has property to respond to certain stimuli by producing electrical signals such as action potentials.
2. *Contractility:* It is the ability of muscle tissue to contract when stimulated by an action potential.
3. *Extensibility:* It is the ability of muscle to stretch without being damaged.
4. *Elasticity:* It is the ability of muscle tissue to return to its original length and shape after contraction or extension.

CLASSIFICATION

There are three types of muscles:

1. Skeletal or striated or striped or voluntary
2. Smooth/unstriped or involuntary
3. Cardiac.

Skeletal Muscle

As the name suggests this type of muscles are attached to the bone or skeleton. These are supplied by spinal or somatic nerves and are under the control of the will (voluntary muscles). These are most numerous in the body. The histology of skeletal muscle fibre shows transverse striations, so these are called striped muscles as well, e.g. biceps brachii, deltoid, etc. (*see* Fig. 2.19).

These are most numerous in the body. They are responsible for causing movements at various joints of bones, e.g. shoulder joint, hip joint, knee joint, etc. The movements of these muscles are under the control of the will.

Each muscle fibre is a single cell with multiple peripheral nuclei. The myofibrils of muscle cell have alternate light and dark bands and these myofibrils are "in register" form so that the whole muscle fibre shows alternate dark and light striations.

Each skeletal muscle fibre is encircled by a connective tissue layer called **endomysium**. Many muscle fibres are bound together in a bundle in connective tissue sheath called **perimysium**. Many bundles are encircled by another sheath of connective tissue called **epimysium** (Fig. 7.1).

These muscle fibres are richly supplied by cranial/spinal nerves. The termination of nerve in the skeletal muscle fibre is known as **neuromuscular junction**. When a muscle contracts it shortens thereby resulting in movement.

Smooth Muscle

These muscle fibres do not show striations and hence are called smooth muscle. These muscles are supplied by autonomic nerves and are not under the control of the will (involuntary muscles). These are present in the wall of the viscera of the body like stomach, intestines, ureter, uterus, etc. (*see* Fig. 2.20).

These are involuntary and unstriped, and situated in the walls of the organs like stomach, intestine, ureter, uterus, vas

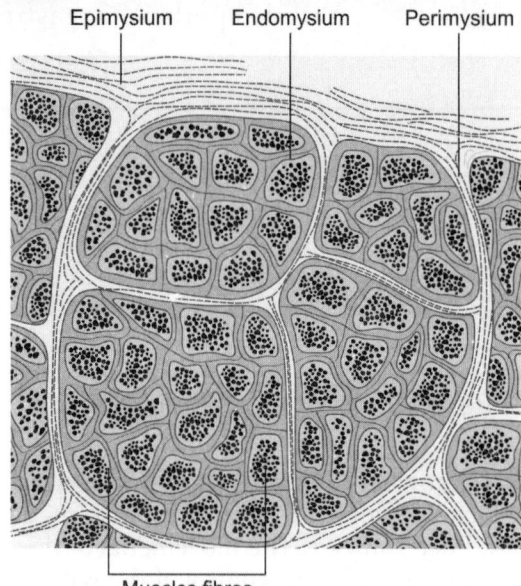

Epimysium   Endomysium   Perimysium

Muscles fibres

Fig. 7.1: Structure of striated muscle

deferens, trachea, bronchi, etc. These muscles are under the control of autonomic nervous system, though these have inherent power of contraction as well.

Each muscle fibre is spindle-shaped with a central elongated nucleus. The transverse striations are not seen in these muscle fibres.

Cardiac Muscle

These muscle fibres are only found in the heart. They are striped or striated and are supplied by autonomic nerves like the smooth muscle. This type has properties of both skeletal as well as smooth muscle (*see* Fig. 2.21).

It is the muscle of the heart. It has partial features of both striated and smooth muscles. The cardiac muscle is made of short cylindrical fibres which branch and unite with the adjacent fibres. The junction of the two fibres is marked by an **intercalated disc.**

Cardiac muscle is controlled by autonomic nerves though there is the characteristic property of autorhythmicity.

Functions of Muscles

- Skeletal muscles are used for moving the various joints used in walking, writing, eating, etc.
- Diaphragm is the chief muscle of respiration.

- Muscles of the larynx are used in talking.
- Smooth muscles of the digestive system are used to propel the food forwards for digestion and absorption.
- Smooth muscles of the urinary bladder contract to expel the urine from it. The smooth muscle of the sphincter of urinary bladder relaxes (opens) to push the urine outside.
- Cardiac muscle/myocardium pumps the oxygenated blood from the heart into the arteries and receives the venous (deoxygenated) blood.

SKELETAL MUSCLE FIBRE

Each muscle fibre is enclosed by a cell membrane called as **sarcolemma.** Within the sarcolemma, like other cells, it bounds the cell cytoplasm, known as **sarcoplasm** with the organelles. In the sarcoplasm are parallel arranged myofibrils.

Myofibrils are variable in numbers in each muscle fibre. Each myofibril is divisible into individual filaments. Each filament is made up of contractile proteins. The contractile mechanism in each muscle depends on proteins myosin, actin, tropomyosin and troponin. Each myofibril shows two alternate **light** and **dark bands.** In the centre of light band there is a narrow dark line-Z line, to which protein filaments are found attached. The Z line produces the effect of striations of muscle fibres. The area between two adjacent Z lines is called **sarcomere,** which is the contractile or functional unit of skeletal muscle (Fig. 7.2). The sarcoplasm besides myofibrils also contains mitochondria [which generates chemical energy adenosine triphosphate (ATP) from glucose], glycogen and myoglobin (O_2 binding protein).

A myofibril has repeating series of sarcomeres and each sarcomere consist of thin filaments of actin and thick filaments of myosin.

MUSCULAR CONTRACTION AND FATIGUE

During muscular contraction the thick and thin filaments maintain their normal length. Shortening of the muscle results from sliding

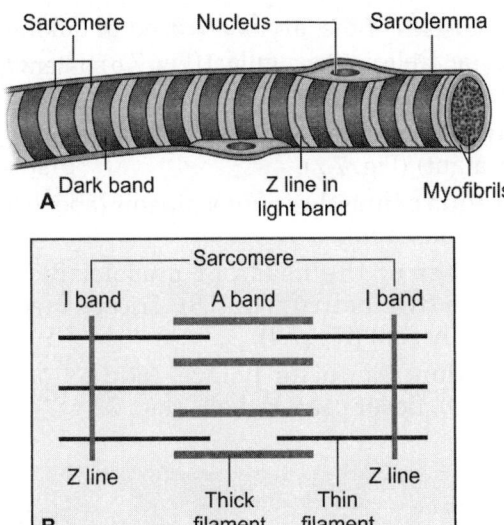

Fig. 7.2: Organisation within a skeletal muscle fibre

of the actin filaments over the myosin filaments (Fig. 7.2).

Motor Unit

A motor neuron and all the muscle fibres innervated by it constitutes motor unit. The number of muscle fibres in motor unit varies. Eye and finger muscles have only 6–60 muscle fibres in a motor unit. These cause fine and precise movements. Muscles of leg have 1,000 or so muscle fibres in one unit as the movement required is gross.

Muscle Fatigue

When a person is doing heavy exercise, almost all of oxygen is utilised within a minute or so to provide energy by oxidation of nutrients. Then, muscle glycogen is converted to lactic acid in anaerobic metabolism and accumulates in body fluids. This causes fatigue.

After the exercise is over, breathing still continues rapidly for few minutes to repay the O_2 debt during exercise and conversion of lactic acid to glucose and then to glycogen in muscles.

Muscle Tone

It is a state of partial contraction of muscles. It is achieved by contraction of a few muscle fibres at a time. In skeletal muscle, tone is essential for maintenance of posture. Smooth muscle tone is also important in gastro-intestinal tract and blood vessels.

Classification of Muscles According to Functions

Prime movers (agonist): It is the main muscle causing a desired movement. For example, brachialis causing flexion of the elbow joint (Fig. 7.3).

Antagonist: A muscle causing a movement opposite to the prime mover is called antagonist. For example, triceps brachii is antagonistic to brachialis (Figs 7.3 and 7.4).

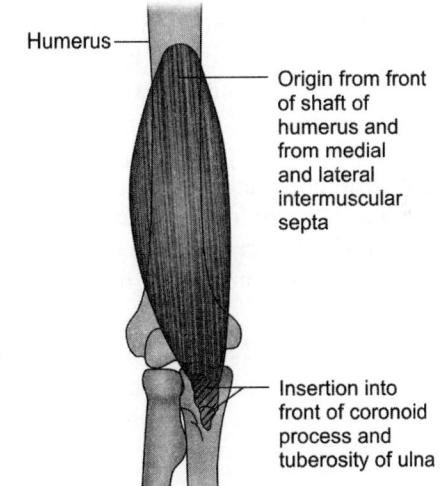

Fig. 7.3: Brachialis

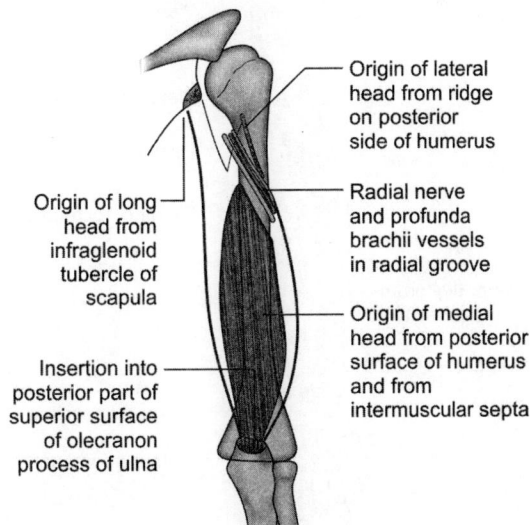

Fig. 7.4: Triceps brachii

Synergists: Muscles helping the prime movers are called synergists (Fig. 7.5). These at times prevent undesired movements at the proximal joints.

Fixators: Muscles which fix a part so that a prime mover works efficiently. For example, trapezius fixes the shoulder girdle to the trunk so that deltoid can act efficiently to abduct the shoulder joint.

Classification of Muscle Contractions

1. *Isometric contractions:* In this type, the length of the muscle fibres does not change. The amount of tension increases during the contraction process. Muscles of the back contract isometrically to maintain the length of the muscle. Thus, they are responsible for the maintenance of posture.
2. *Isotonic contractions:* Here, the amount of tension produced by the muscle is constant during the contraction process, but there is decrease in the length of muscle fibres. Muscles of the arm, forearm and leg show isotonic contraction during movements of the joints.

Combinations of isotonic and isometric contractions are mostly seen in the muscles where muscle shortens some distance and the degree of tension increases.

Nomenclature of the Muscle

Shape: Deltoid (triangular) (Fig. 7.6) trapezius (trapezium shape).

Direction of muscle fibres: Rectus abdominis (straight) (Fig. 7.7).

Position of muscles: Supraspinatus (above the spine of scapula).

Number of the heads of muscle: Biceps brachii (two heads) (Fig. 7.8). Triceps brachii (three heads) (Fig. 7.4).

Function: Adductor pollicis (adduction of thumb), flexor carpi radialis (Fig. 7.5).

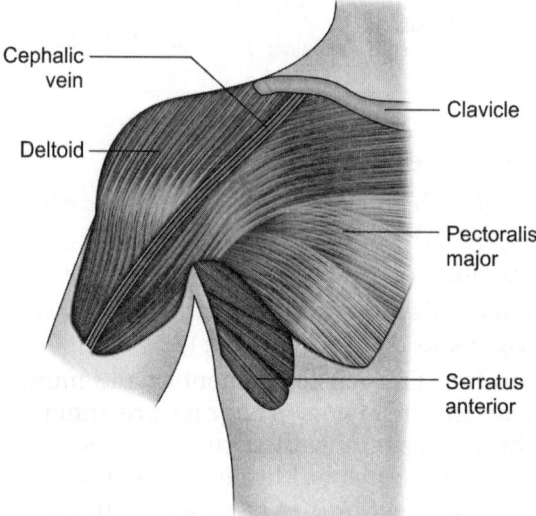

Fig. 7.6: Pectoralis major and deltoid

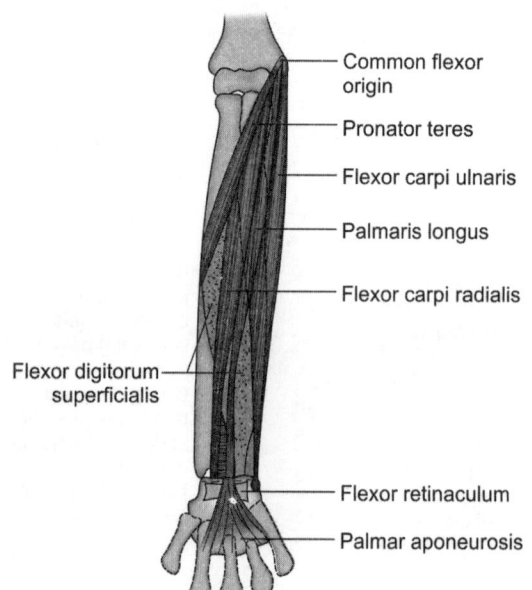

Fig. 7.5: Muscles of the forearm—superficial group

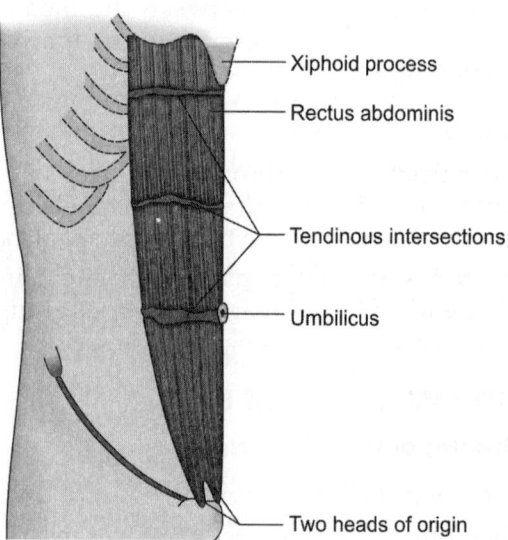

Fig. 7.7: Rectus abdominis

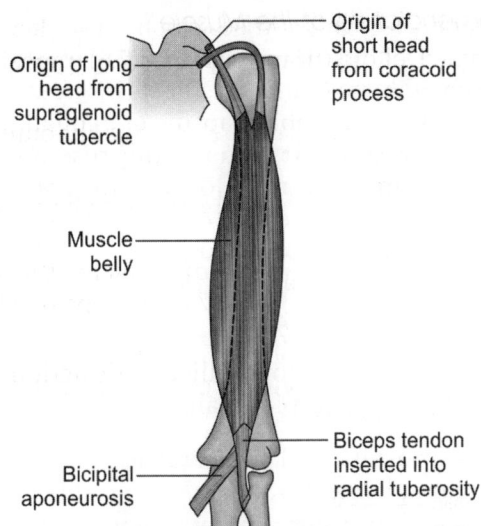

Fig. 7.8: Biceps brachii

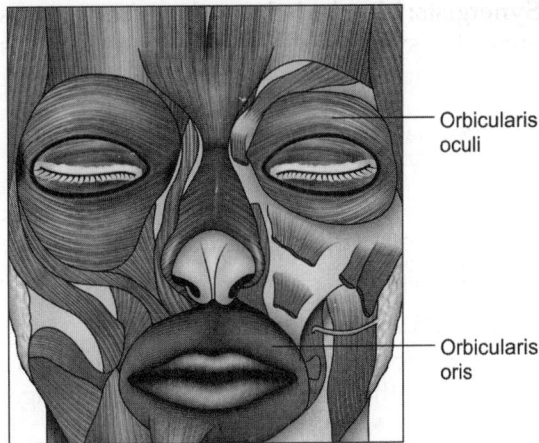

Fig. 7.9: Muscles of the face

Parts of the Skeletal Muscle

Origin: The more fixed part of the muscle.

Insertion: The more movable part of the muscle.

Belly: Thickness of the muscle fibres between origin and insertion (Fig. 7.8).

Tendon: Fibrous component of the muscle near the insertion. Tendons are inelastic fibrous bands that bind the muscles to the bones. They are cord like in shape (Fig. 7.8).

Aponeurosis: An opened up or flattened tendon. For example, bicipital aponeurosis in the cubital fossa lies between the median cubital vein and the termination of brachial artery (Fig. 7.8).

Fascia

Superficial fascia: Fibrous tissue deep to the dermis containing cutaneous vessels and lymph vessels including the mammary gland.

Deep fascia: The dense fascia enclosing groups of muscles, separating various groups of muscles and enclosing blood vessels.

CHIEF MUSCLES OF THE BODY

Muscles of Head and Neck

Muscles of the Face and Scalp

These are small muscles which get inserted into the skin of face and are known as muscles of facial expression (Fig. 7.9). The various groups are:

Orbicularis oculi: Around the orbital opening.

Nasal muscle: Around the opening of nose.

Orbicularis oris: Around the opening of mouth.

Platysma: In the superficial fascia of neck.

Auricularis muscles: Present in the external ear and have no function in human beings.

Occipitofrontalis: Situated between occipital bone and skin of forehead and is united by aponeurosis.

Some of the muscles of the cheek/face are zygomaticus major (smiling muscle) and buccinator for blowing out the air from vestibule of the mouth (whistling muscle).

All these muscles are supplied by the facial nerve (VII cranial nerve). Paralysis of this nerve results in facial paralysis.

Muscles of Mastication

There are four muscles of mastication. These are:

Temporalis: It arises from temporal fossa of the skull and is inserted into the coronoid process and ramus of the mandible (Fig. 7.10). It acts on temporomandibular joint causing its elevation and retraction.

Masseter: It originates from the deep aspect of zygomatic arch and gets inserted into outer surface of ramus including the angle of mandible (Fig. 7.11). It elevates the mandible.

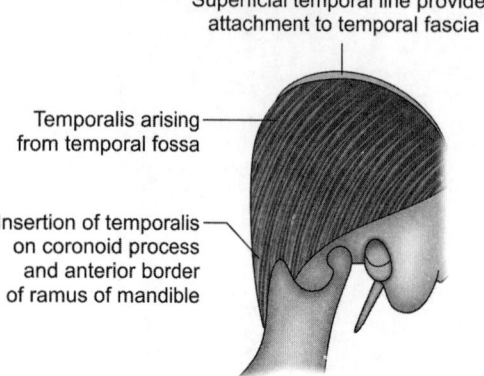

Fig. 7.10: Temporalis

Superficial temporal line provides attachment to temporal fascia

Temporalis arising from temporal fossa

Insertion of temporalis on coronoid process and anterior border of ramus of mandible

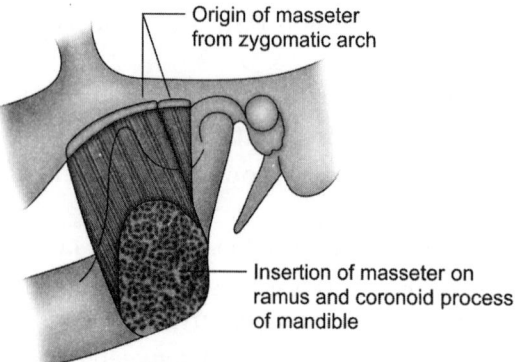

Origin of masseter from zygomatic arch

Insertion of masseter on ramus and coronoid process of mandible

Fig. 7.11: Masseter

Medial pterygoid: It arises from medial surface of lateral pterygoid plate (wing-shaped) of the sphenoid bone. It is inserted into inner aspect of the angle of mandible (Fig. 7.12). It causes elevation, protraction and side-to-side movement of the temporo-mandibular joint.

Lateral pterygoid: Arises chiefly from lateral surface of the lateral pterygoid plate of sphenoid bone (Fig. 7.12). It gets inserted into the neck of mandible, capsule of joint and its articular disc. It causes depression of temporomandibular joint and thus is responsible for opening of the mouth while eating, drinking and laughing, etc. It also causes protraction and side to side movements of the joint.

All the muscles of mastication are supplied by mandibular division of trigeminal nerve (V cranial nerve).

Temporalis and masseter are tested by clenching the teeth.

Medial and lateral pterygoids are tested by moving the chin to right and left sides.

Muscles Which Move the Head

Sternocleidomastoid: Strong key muscle of the head and neck. Takes origin from clavicle and sternum, passes obliquely upwards in the neck to get inserted into the mastoid process of the temporal bone (Fig. 7.13). When the muscle of the right side contracts, it turns the chin to the left side. It is also called **chin-turning muscle**. Its nerve supply is by spinal accessory nerve (XI cranial nerve).

Other muscles which move the head are splenius capitis, semispinalis capitis and longissimus capitis. Nerve supply is by posterior rami of the cervical nerves.

Muscles of the Neck

Sternocleidomastoid: Has been described earlier.

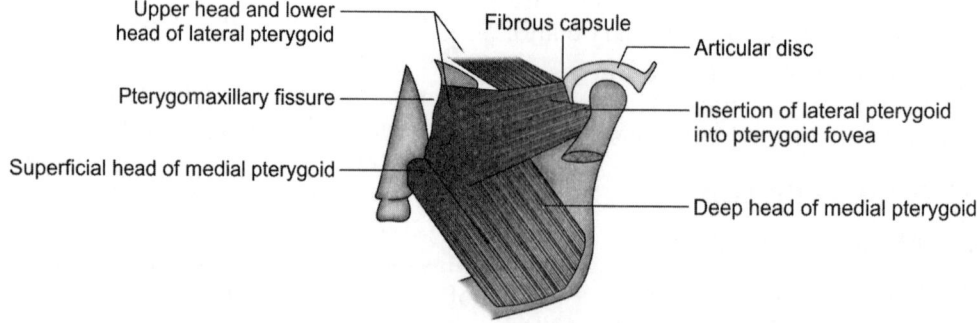

Upper head and lower head of lateral pterygoid

Pterygomaxillary fissure

Superficial head of medial pterygoid

Fibrous capsule

Articular disc

Insertion of lateral pterygoid into pterygoid fovea

Deep head of medial pterygoid

Fig. 7.12: Medial and lateral pterygoid

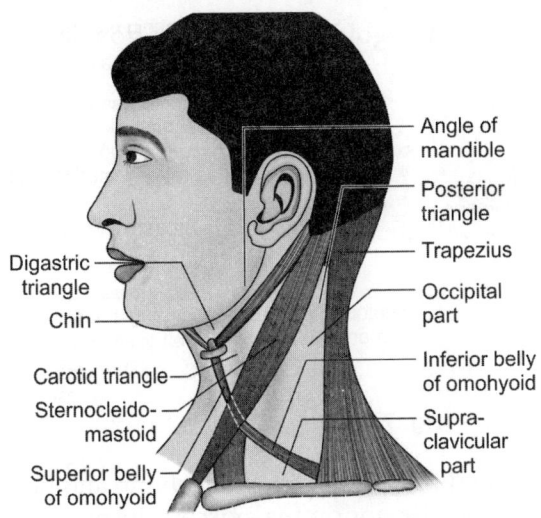

Fig. 7.13: Muscles of the neck

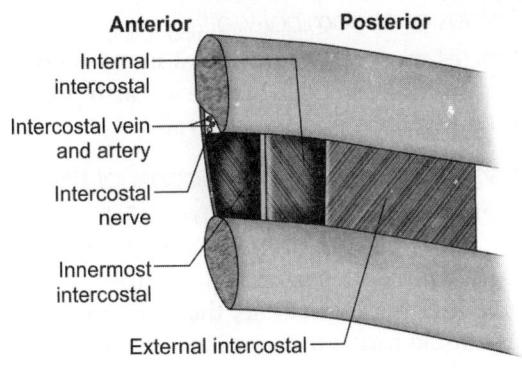

Fig. 7.14: Intercostal muscles

Trapezius: It arises from occipital bone, ligamentum nuchae, spines of 7th cervical vertebra and all thoracic vertebrae. The muscle is inserted into lateral one-third of clavicle, acromion process and spine of scapula.

The upper fibres cause shrugging of the shoulder, middle fibres retract the scapula and lower fibres help serratus anterior in 90–180° abduction of shoulder joint. It is supplied by spinal root of accessory nerve and is also called "shrugging muscle".

Prevertebral muscles: These small muscles lie between bodies and transverse processes of cervical vertebrae. These cause flexion of neck and are supplied by branches of cervical plexus.

Muscles of Trunk

Trunk comprises thorax and abdomen.

Muscles of Thorax

Muscles of thorax are situated in the intercostal spaces between the adjacent ribs and the adjacent costal cartilages. There are 12 pairs of ribs and 11 intercostal spaces. Each space contains the **external intercostal muscle, internal intercostal muscle and the innermost intercostal muscle** (Fig. 7.14). All these are respiratory muscles and keep thoracic wall intact. They are supplied by intercostal nerves and vessels. These lie in the subcostal groove lie between the internal and the innermost intercostal muscles (Fig. 7.15).

Muscles of the Back

The muscles of the back are strong muscles and they maintain erect posture. These overlap each other and have multiple origins and insertions. The muscles are **erector spinae/ sacrospinalis.** These start from sacrum and reach the skull.

The deeper group comprises of **semispinalis, multifidus, interspinalis,** etc. They are supplied by the dorsal primary rami of the various spinal nerves.

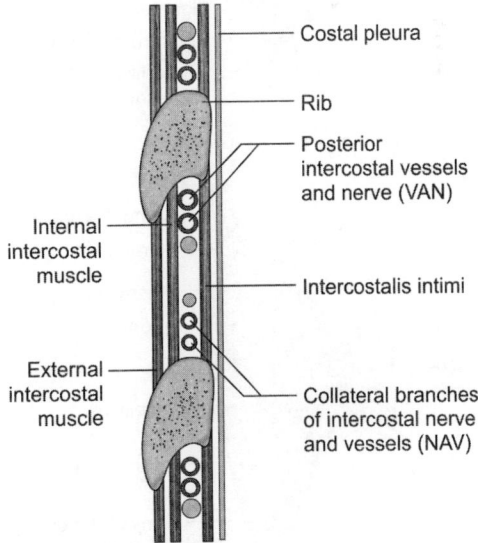

Fig. 7.15: Intercostal nerves and vessels in subcostal groove

Muscles of Abdominal Wall

Muscles are present in layers in the antero-lateral abdominal wall. These are also present in the posterior abdominal wall.

Muscles of Anterolateral Abdominal Wall

External oblique: Arises from 5th to 12th ribs and is inserted into linea alba, iliac crest (Fig. 7.16). Between anterior superior iliac spine and pubic tubercle, the aponeurosis of the muscle forms the inguinal ligament.

Internal oblique: Arises from inguinal ligament, iliac crest, lumbar fascia and gets inserted into linea alba and cartilages of lower 4 ribs (Fig. 7.17).

Transversus abdominis: Arises from inguinal ligament, iliac crest and inner aspect of 7th to 12th ribs (Fig. 7.18). This is also inserted into the linea alba.

These muscles compress the abdominal cavity and are muscles of expiration. They also

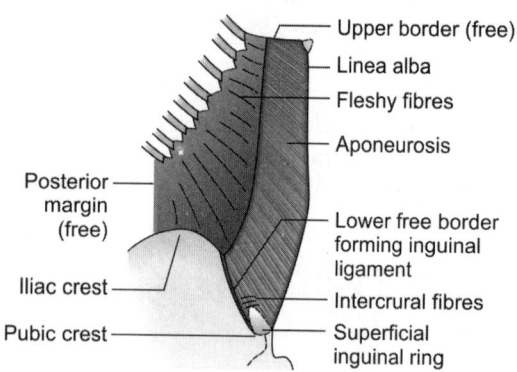

Fig. 7.16: External oblique

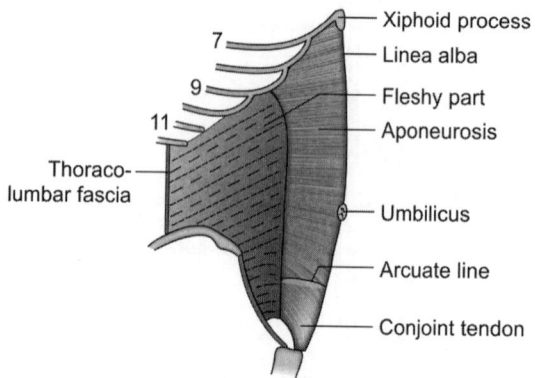

Fig. 7.17: Internal oblique

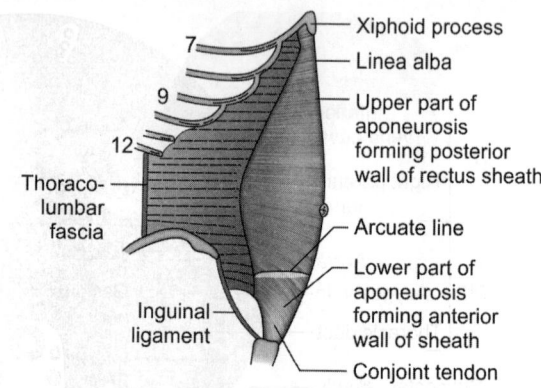

Fig. 7.18: Transversus abdominis

flex and rotate the vertebral column and help to keep the abdominal viscera in position. Nerve supply is by thoracic 6th to thoracic 12th nerves.

Rectus abdominis: Arises from the pubic bones and gets inserted into cartilages of 7th, 6th and 5th ribs. The paramedian muscle lies on each side of linea alba (Fig. 7.7). It is chief flexor of the vertebral column and is supplied by the lower 6 or 7 thoracic nerves.

Rectus sheath: Aponeurosis of external oblique, internal oblique and transversus abdominis enclose the rectus abdominis muscle forming the rectus sheath (Fig. 7.19). The sheath keeps the rectus muscle in proper position.

Muscle between Thorax and Abdomen

Diaphragm: Diaphragm is a dome shaped thin musculotendinous structure separating the thoracic cavity above from the abdominal cavity below. It arises from inner aspects of 7th to12th ribs and xiphoid process, and bodies of lumbar vertebrae. The fibres from all around converge to be inserted into a triangular tendinous portion (Fig. 7.20).

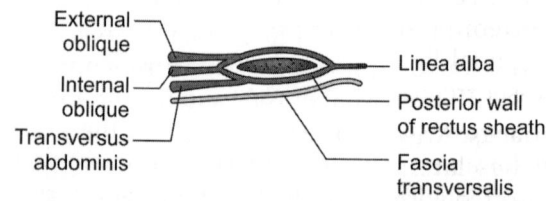

Fig. 7.19: Upper 3/4th of anterior abdominal wall

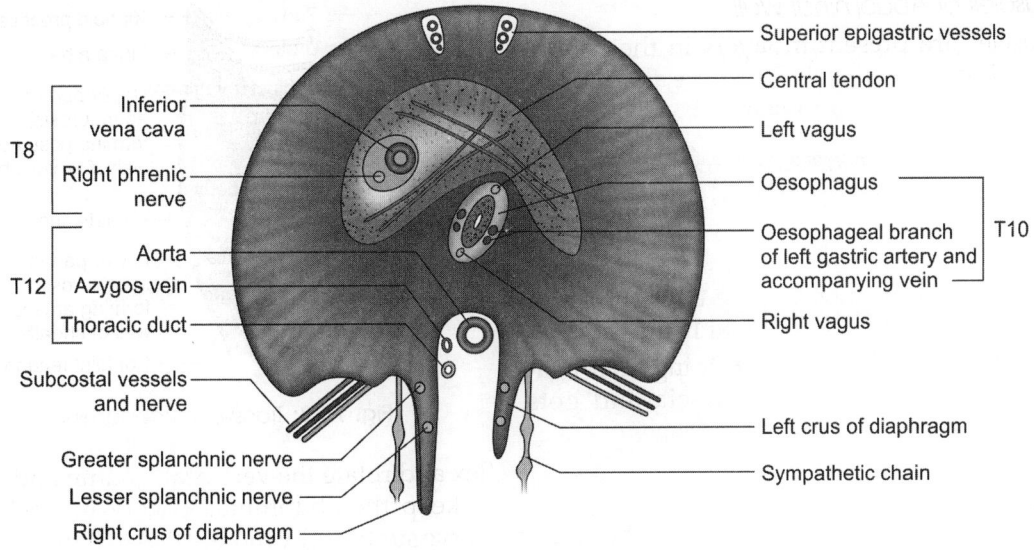

Fig. 7.20: Diaphragm

Diaphragm contracts during inspiration enlarging the vertical diameter of the thoracic cavity. This results in intake of oxygenated air. The domes get flattened during inspiration. Diaphragm relaxes during expiration, the domes rise decreasing the vertical diameter of thoracic cavity. This leads to expulsion of deoxygenated air. The diaphragm is responsible for 60% of quiet respiration. Motor nerve supply is from phrenic nerves on each side. Intercostal nerves give sensory fibres.

Openings in the diaphragm at various levels (Fig. 7.20):

Thoracic 8: Opening for the inferior vena cava.

Thoracic 10: Opening for oesophagus and vagus nerve.

Thoracic 12: Opening for aorta, thoracic duct and vena azygous.

Muscles of the Posterior Abdominal Wall

Psoas major: Arises from bodies and transverse processes of all five lumbar vertebrae. It passes downwards under the inguinal ligament and gets inserted into the lesser trochanter of femur.

Iliacus: Arises from iliac fossa of the hip bone. It lies lateral to the psoas major and gets inserted with it into the lesser trochanter. Both these muscles cause flexion of the trunk on the

thigh, including flexion of thigh on trunk. They are supplied by the lumbar nerves and femoral nerve.

Quadratus lumborum: Arising from iliac crest, this muscle passes upwards to get inserted into the inner aspect of 12th rib. It causes lateral flexion of vertebral column. Nerve supply is by the lumbar nerves.

Muscles of Pelvic Cavity

The pelvic cavity is formed by sacrum and both the hip bones. Its inlet is continuous with abdominal cavity. The outlet is guarded by muscles or the pelvic diaphragm. There are openings in the pelvic diaphragm. In females, there are three openings one each for urethral orifice, vaginal orifice and for anal canal. In males, there are two openings. These are for urethral orifice and anal canal. Pelvic diaphragm supports these various openings.

Pelvic diaphragm is comprised of **levator ani** in anterior part and **coccygeus** in posterior part. Levator ani is divisible into pubo-coccygeus and iliococcygeus (Fig. 7.21). Coccygeus arises from ischium and is inserted into coccyx. The muscles of the pelvic diaphragm support all the viscera of abdomen and pelvis. They also support and regulate the various openings in it. Nerve supply is from 4th and 5th sacral nerves.

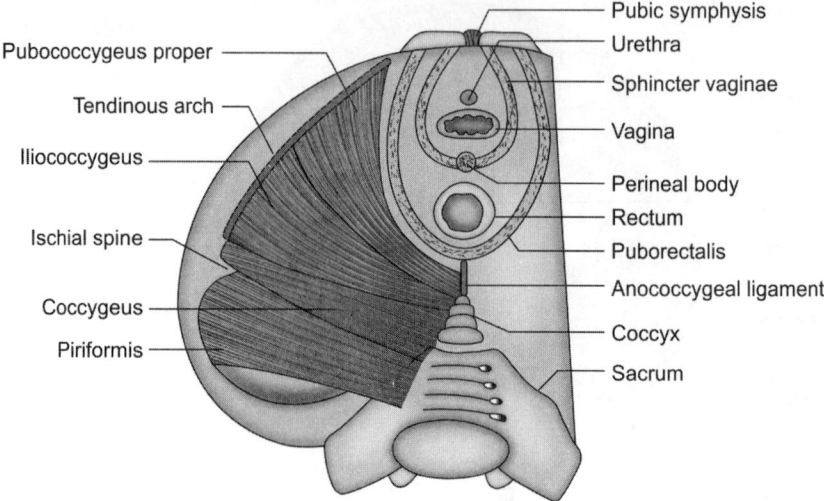

Fig. 7.21: Levator ani

Muscles of the Upper Limb

Muscles for Shoulder Girdle Movements

Trapezius: It has been described earlier.

Levator scapulae: It lies along upper part of the medial border of scapula. It elevates the scapula in shrugging of the shoulder. It is supplied by nerve to rhomboids.

Rhomboids minor and major: They lie along the rest of the medial border of scapula. These muscles cause retraction of scapula. They are supplied by nerve to rhomboids.

Serratus anterior: Arises from upper 8 ribs to be inserted into medial border and inferior angle of scapula on its costal aspect. It keeps the scapula in contact with chest wall and causes protraction of scapula. It helps trapezius in overhead abduction of shoulder. It is supplied by nerve to serratus anterior (Fig. 7.6).

Pectoralis minor: It is a triangular muscle between 3rd and 5th costochondral junctions and coracoid process of scapula. It causes depression of the shoulder girdle. It is supplied by pectoral nerves.

Muscles Acting on the Shoulder Joint

Pectoralis major: Arises from clavicle, sternum, 2nd to 6th costal cartilages and is inserted into lateral lip of intertubercular sulcus of humerus (Fig. 7.6). It causes flexion, adduction and medial rotation of shoulder joint.

Latissimus dorsi: It is a wide muscle connecting lower limb bones with upper limb bones. Arises from iliac crest, spines of thoracic 7–12 vertebrae and lower 3 ribs to get inserted into the floor of the inter-tubercular sulcus.

It causes extension, adduction and medial rotation of shoulder joint. Nerve supply is by a branch from posterior cord of brachial plexus.

Teres major: Lies between inferior angle of dorsal surface of scapula and medial lip of intertubercular sulcus. Actions and nerve supply same as latissimus dorsi.

Deltoid: Very important triangular muscle giving rounded shape to the shoulder (Fig. 7.6). Arises from lateral part of clavicle, lateral surface of acromion and spine of scapula. It is inserted in the deltoid tuberosity on the lateral surface of humerus.

Middle fibres of deltoid are very strong as these are multipennate and cause abduction of shoulder joint from 0 to 90°. Anterior fibres cause flexion and posterior fibres cause extension of the shoulder joint. It is supplied by axillary nerve, a branch of posterior cord of brachial plexus. Intra-muscular injections are given in the middle of this muscle.

Muscles of Rotator Cuff

These are **supraspinatus, infraspinatus, teres minor** and **subscapularis**. The tendons of these four muscles fuse with the capsule of shoulder joint and stabilise the weak shoulder joint.

Muscles of the Arm

Front of arm contains three muscles. These are coracobrachialis, brachialis and biceps brachii. All these muscles are supplied by musculo-cutaneous nerve.

Biceps brachii: As the name suggests it comprises of two heads, the long head and short head (Fig. 7.8). These arise from parts of scapula, pass across the whole length of humerus and are inserted into radial tuberosity of the radius.

The muscle is a flexor of the elbow joint. It causes supination of forearm when the elbow is semiflexed. It is also responsible for screwing movements.

Brachialis: Lies deep to biceps brachii muscle. It arises from most of the anterior aspect of humerus, passes across the elbow joint to get inserted into anterior surface of coronoid process of ulna (Fig. 7.3). It is the chief flexor of elbow joint.

Triceps brachii: Back of arm contains one big muscle, the **triceps brachii**. This muscle is composed of three heads, *long* arising from scapula, *lateral* and *medial*, both from posterior surface of humerus (Fig. 7.4). All three heads join to be inserted into superior surface of olecranon process of ulna.

Triceps brachii is the only extensor of the elbow joint. Each of the heads of the muscle is supplied by branches of radial nerve.

Muscles of Forearm

There are two compartments in the forearm, i.e. flexor compartment on the front (Figs 7.5 and 7.22) and extensor compartment on its back.

Muscles of the flexor compartment: The muscles of the flexor compartment are arranged in two groups, superficial and deep.

Out of eight muscles, there are two pronators of forearm, three flexors of wrist and

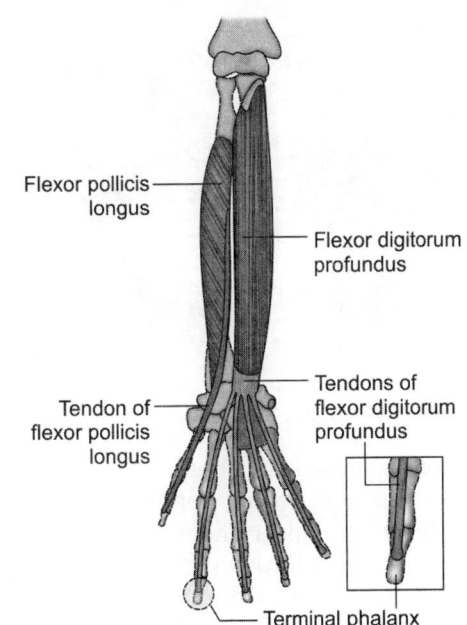

Flexor pollicis longus

Flexor digitorum profundus

Tendon of flexor pollicis longus

Tendons of flexor digitorum profundus

Terminal phalanx

Fig. 7.22: Muscles of the forearm—deep group

three flexors of the metacarpophalangeal and interphalangeal joints of all the five digits. One and a half muscles are supplied by ulnar nerve and six and a half are supplied by the median nerve.

Muscles of extensor compartment: These are a total 12 muscles. Two are short and do not reach the wrist. One reaches the lower end of radius and nine reach the five digits. These long nine muscles cause extension of the wrist and the other joints in the hand. All the muscles of the extensor compartment are supplied by radial nerve.

Muscles of Hand

Muscles are present only in the palm. There are only tendons on the dorsum of hand.

Muscles of the Palm

These are grouped as follows (Fig. 7.23):

Muscles of thenar eminence: These are present on the thumb side. They are responsible for the movements of the thumb and are supplied by median nerve.

Muscles of hypothenar eminence: These are present on the little finger side. These cause movements of the little finger and are supplied by ulnar nerve.

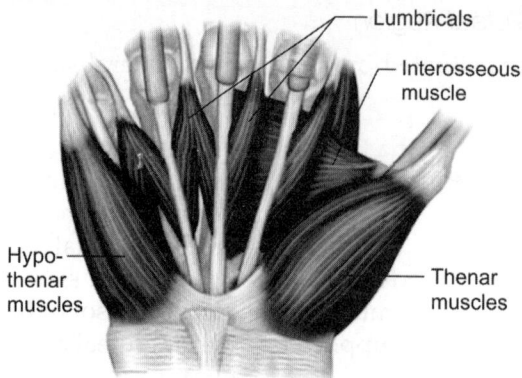

Fig. 7.23: Muscles of palm

Interossei muscles: These are present in between the metacarpal bones and make up the bulk of the palm. There are four palmar and four dorsal interossei and are responsible for abduction and adduction of 2nd to 5th digits. Nerve supply is by ulnar nerve.

Palm also contains long flexor tendons which reach up to the middle and distal phalanges. These cause flexion of the digits and are supplied by median nerve in the forearm.

Muscles of Lower Limb

Lower limb includes the muscles of:
1. Thigh region
2. Gluteal region
3. Leg region
4. Sole region.

Muscles of Thigh

These are in three well-defined groups as:
a. Extensor or anterior
b. Flexor or posterior
c. Adductor or medial.

Extensor/anterior compartment: Contains a huge **quadriceps femoris,** comprising of four heads. They are **vastus lateralis, vastus intermedius, vastus medialis and rectus femoris**

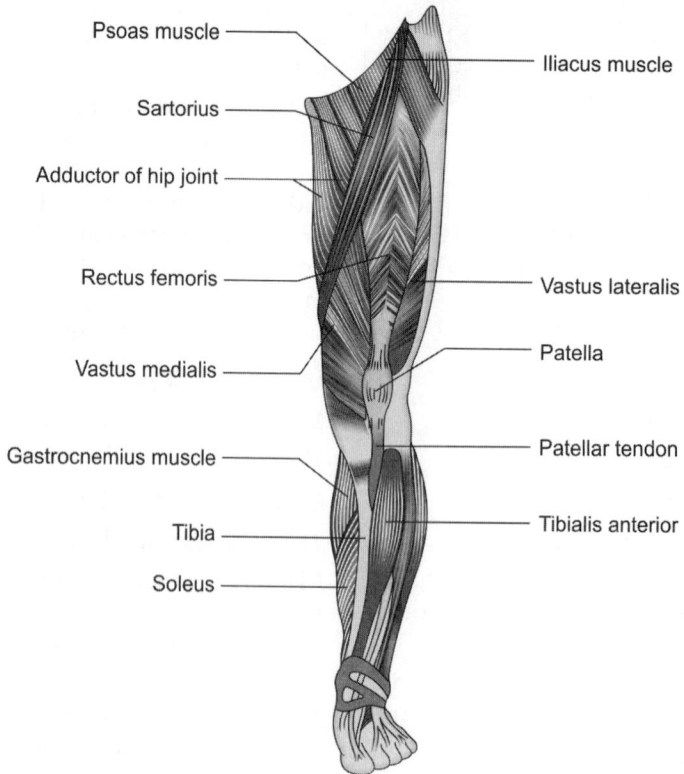

Fig. 7.24: Muscles of lower limb—anterior aspect

(Fig. 7.24). These heads arise from the femur and are inserted into patella and tibial tuberosity. This muscle is the extensor of knee joint. There is one more muscle, **Sartorius** in this compartment. It is the longest muscle of the body. It flexes the hip joint. All the muscles of this compartment are supplied by branches of femoral nerve.

Flexor/posterior compartment: Contains four muscles called hamstrings (Fig. 7.25). These are **biceps femoris, semitendinosus, semimembranosus** and **part of adductor magnus.** These cause flexion of the knee joint and are supplied by thick sciatic nerve.

Adductor/medial compartment: Contains four muscles. These are **adductor longus, adductor brevis, adductor magnus** and **gracilis.** They cause adduction of thigh at hip joint and are supplied by obturator nerve.

Gluteal Region

It is situated on the back and lateral side of thigh. The various muscles are.

Gluteus maximus: Arises from sacrum, coccyx and part of iliac crest (Fig. 7.25). It gets inserted into gluteal tuberosity at back of upper part of femur and into the iliotibial tract (a part of deep fascia on the lateral side of thigh). This muscle is the chief extensor of hip joint and is supplied by inferior gluteal nerve.

Gluteus medius and gluteus minimus: These two muscles arise from different areas of gluteal surface of hip bone. They are inserted into lateral aspect and anterior aspect of greater trochanter of femur. The chief action of the two muscles of one side (the right side) is to support the opposite/unsupported (left side) lower limb when it is in the air. The left

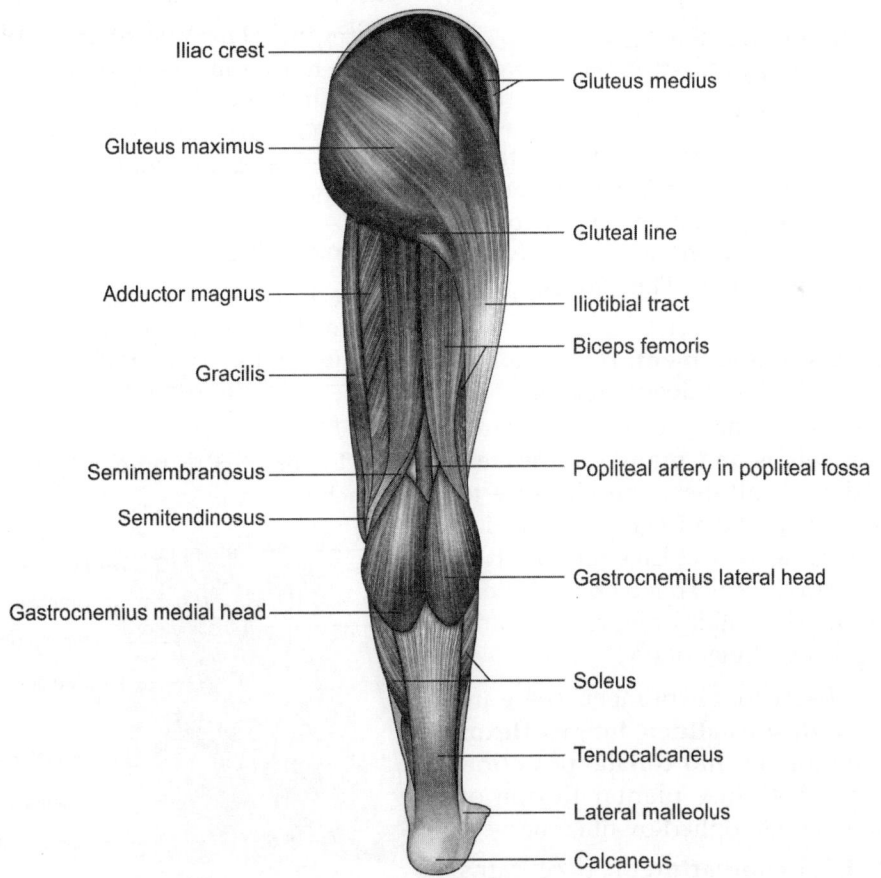

Fig. 7.25: Muscles of lower limb posterior aspect

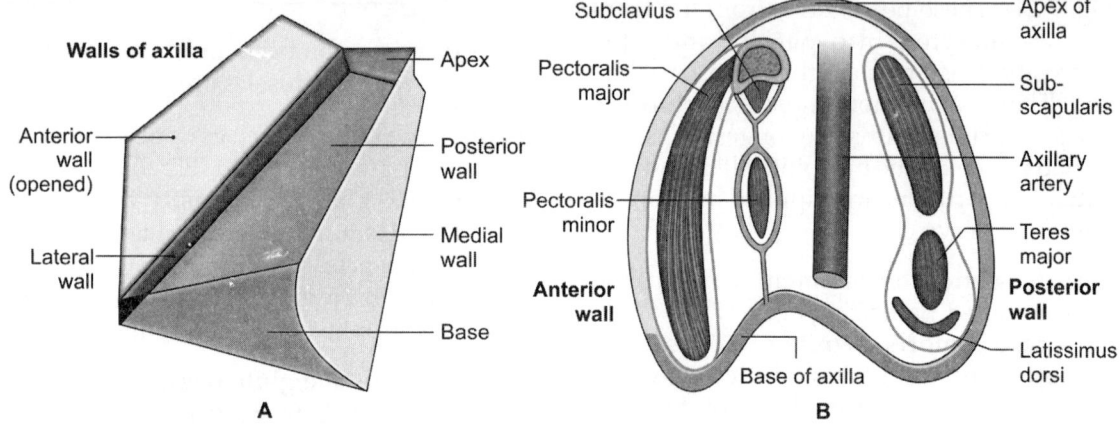

Figs 7.26A and B: Axilla—(A) diagrammatic view of axilla and (B) anterior and posterior walls of axilla

side muscles support the right lower limb when it is in the air for walking forwards.

Muscles of Leg Region

There are three compartments in the leg. These are:

1. **Extensor or anterior** (Fig. 7.24)
2. **Flexor or posterior** (Fig. 7.25)
3. **Peroneal or lateral.**

Extensor/anterior compartment: Contains four muscles. These are **tibialis anterior, extensor hallucis longus, extensor digitorum longus and peroneus tertius.** These cause dorsiflexion of ankle joint. They are supplied by deep peroneal nerve.

Flexor/posterior compartment: This compartment has superficial and deep muscles.

  i. *Superficial muscles* are two heads of **gastrocnemius, soleus and plantaris muscles.** The tendons of all these muscles fuse to form the strongest tendon in the body, i.e. **tendocalcenous or Achilles tendon.** It is inserted into the calcaneous bone. These muscles help in walking and running and are supplied by tibial nerve.

  ii. *Deep muscles* are four in number. These are **popliteus, flexor hallucis longus flexor digitorum longus and tibialis posterior.** These muscles cause plantar flexion of ankle joint and supplied by tibial nerve.

Peroneal/lateral compartment: It contains only two muscles, **peroneus longus and**

peroneus brevis. They cause eversion of the foot and are supplied by superficial peroneal nerve.

(**Note:** Tibialis anterior and tibialis posterior cause inversion of the foot).

Sole region: The sole of the foot contains muscles in four layers with nerves and blood vessels between the layers. Most of the muscles (15) are supplied by lateral plantar and only four get nerve supply from medial plantar nerve.

Anatomical Spaces

Axilla: It is a pyramidal shaped space between the medial side of arm and lateral side of upper part of thoracic cage (Figs 7.26A and B).

It contains:

• The lower part of brachial plexus and its branches

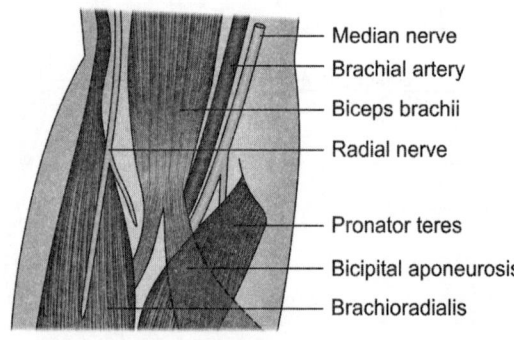

Fig. 7.27: Cubital fossa *(For colour Fig. see Plate 2)*

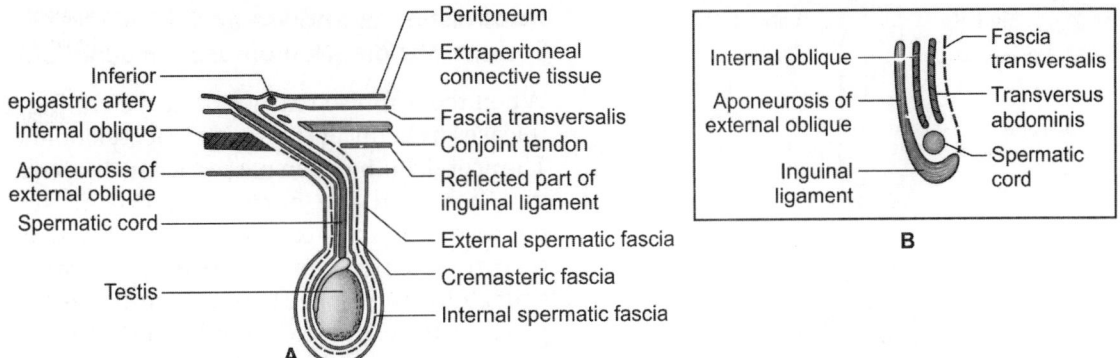

Figs 7.28A and B: Inguinal canaló(A) walls and contents and (B) anterior wall of inguinal canal

- Axillary artery with its branches
- Axillary lymph nodes.

Cubital fossa: It is present in the upper part of forearm below the elbow joint (Fig. 7.27).

It contains:

- Median nerve
- Termination of brachial artery
- Beginning of ulnar and radial arteries
- Tendon of biceps brachii
- Radial nerve with its two terminal branches.

Inguinal canal: It is an intermuscular canal, 3.5 cms. long, just above the inguinal ligament. There are two openings of this canal. These

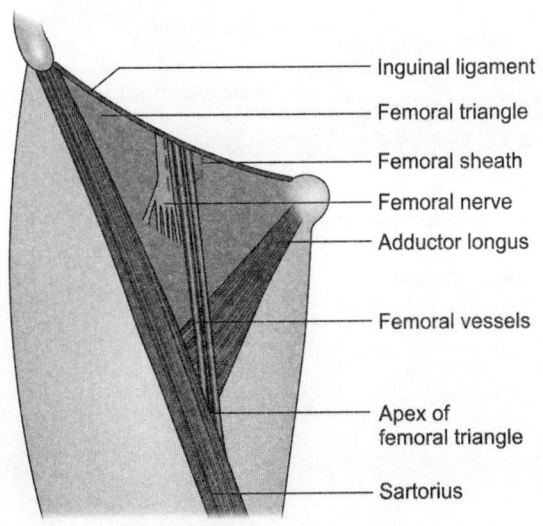

Fig. 7.29: Femoral triangle

are deep and superficial inguinal rings. It also has an anterior and posterior wall, with roof and floor. This is a site of inguinal hernia (Figs 7.28A and B).

Femoral triangle: It is triangular depression in the upper and medial side of thigh. It is bounded by inguinal ligament, sartorius and adductor longus muscle (Fig. 7.29).

Its contents are:

- Femoral artery and its branches
- Femoral vein
- Great saphenous vein
- Femoral nerve
- Inguinal lymph nodes.

Subsartorial/adductor canal: This canal is the continuation of femoral triangle beyond its apex. It ends at the opening of adductor magnus muscle.

Its contents are:

- Femoral vessels
- Nerve to vastus medialis
- Saphenous nerve.

Popliteal fossa: This fossa lies at the back of knee joint. It is diamond shaped and is bounded by muscles on all four sides (Fig. 7.30).

Its contents are:

- Popliteal vessels
- Tibial nerve
- Common peroneal nerve
- Lymph nodes.

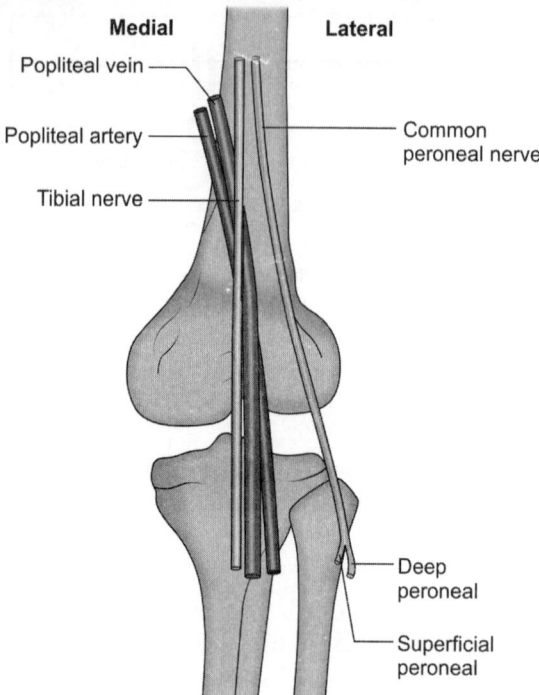

Medial   **Lateral**

Popliteal vein

Popliteal artery — Common peroneal nerve

Tibial nerve

Deep peroneal

Superficial peroneal

Fig. 7.30: Contents of popliteal fossa

Transmission of Impulse from Nerve to Skeletal Muscle (Neuromuscular Junction)

When the impulse reaches th nerve ending it releases a chemical transmitter, acetylcholine. The acetylcholine then passes across the small gap between the nerve and the muscle membrane (gap is called synaptic cleft) and it binds with the receptors, nicotinic acetylcholine receptors present on the postsynaptic muscle membrane which at this junction is specialized to form motor end plate (Fig. 7.31).

The binding of acetylcholine to its receptors on the motor end plate results in change in permeability of the muscle membrane to ions; and as a result there is impulse formation; which travels along the muscle membrane of the fiber (Sarcolemma) and produces contraction. The acetylcholine is then removed from its receptors by the action of an enzyme, acetylcholinesterase present around the motor end plate.

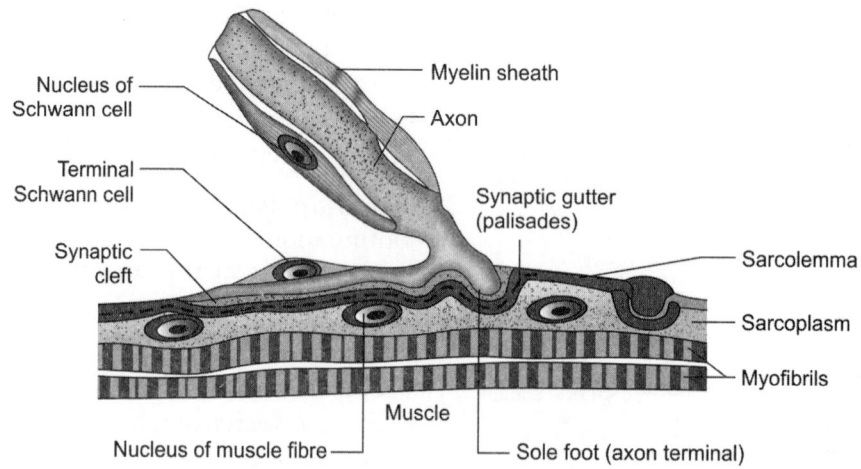

Nucleus of Schwann cell

Myelin sheath

Axon

Terminal Schwann cell

Synaptic gutter (palisades)

Synaptic cleft

Sarcolemma

Sarcoplasm

Myofibrils

Muscle

Nucleus of muscle fibre

Sole foot (axon terminal)

Fig. 7.31: Neuromuscular junction

Points to Remember

1. Cardiac muscles are least in amount, smooth are intermediate and the skeletal are maximum in amount and weight.
2. Sartorius is the longest muscle with parallel fibres.
3. Gluteus maximus is the largest muscle.
4. Richest nerve supply is to extraocular muscles as these have small motor units. One nerve fibre supplies 5–10 muscle fibres.
5. Muscles used for intramuscular injections are deltoid, gluteus medius and vastus lateralis.

MCQs

1. **Connective tissue sheath around each muscle fibre of skeletal muscle is:**
   (a) Epimysium
   (b) Perimysium
   (c) Endomysium
   (d) Sarcolemma

2. **All the following are characteristics of cardiac muscle *except*:**
   (a) Striations
   (b) Multinucleated
   (c) Intercalated disc
   (d) Involuntary

3. **Which fibres of deltoid are multipennate?**
   (a) Clavicular
   (b) Acromial
   (c) Spine of scapula
   (d) All the fibres

4. **A "motor unit" is:**
   (a) Spinal segment with all the muscles it supplies
   (b) A gamma neurons with all the muscle spindles it innervates
   (c) An alpha motor neuron with all the muscle fibres it innervates
   (d) A nerve with all the muscles it innervates

Ans! 1 c   2 b   3 b   4 c

Central Nervous System

Nervous system is the master system of the human body which controls all other systems (except endocrine glands) so as to bring homeostasis in the body. It detects and responds to changes inside and outside the body. The ability of the nervous system to maintain balance in various body functions is because of its properties of:

a. **Excitability:** Ability to receive and respond to external stimuli

b. **Conductivity:** Ability to transmit messages to and from coordinating centres.

For descriptive purposes, nervous system is divided into:

1. **Central nervous system (CNS):** Consisting of brain and spinal cord.

2. **Peripheral nervous system (PNS):** Consisting of all the nerves outside the brain and spinal cord, i.e. 12 pairs of cranial nerves and 31 pairs of spinal nerves.

The PNS has two functional parts: (1) sensory division and (2) motor division. The motor division is involved in activities that are:

* *Voluntary/somatic:* Controls movement of voluntary muscles.

* *Involuntary/autonomic:* Controls functioning of smooth and cardiac muscles and glands. It is divided into sympathetic (excitatory) and parasympathetic (inhibitory) divisions.

NEURONS

The neurons are anatomical and functional units of nervous system. Neurons are the electrically excitable cells. They initiate, receive, conduct and transmit information.

Neurons detect and transmit stimuli by means of electrochemical messages. Since the neurons are highly specialised these cannot reproduce.

The main parts of a neuron are the cell body and its cytoplasmic processes—dendrites and axon.

A typical neuron contains one **axon** and many **dendrites** extending from the cell body. The single axon conducts impulses away from the cell body. The axon may be very short or quite long up to 1 metre. A typical axon has terminal boutons (synaptic knobs). It is wrapped in a white fatty segmented sheath, the myelin sheath. The myelin sheath is produced by **Schwann cells,** which are separated by gaps called **nodes of Ranvier.**

Dendrites are multiple, short, thick diffusely branching processes that receive impulses reaching the neuron from other cells.

The neurons communicate with one another using electrical signals known as **action potential or nerve impulse.** The plasma membrane of excitable cells show a **resting membrane potential,** an electrical voltage difference across the membrane. Action potential occurs because the plasma membrane of neurons has many different ion channels that open or close in response to specific stimuli.

To communicate information from one part of the body to another, nerve impulses must travel from where they arise. This mode of travel is called **propagation/conduction.** Transmission of nerve impulse is due to movement of ions across the plasma membrane.

Transmission of Nerve Impulse

The information in the form of electrochemical impulses is transmitted in the nervous system through a succession of neurons lined up one after the other. Neurons may be stimulated by touch, pressure, heat, cold or external/internal chemicals like histamine. The meeting place or the junction between two neurons is called a **synapse** (Figs 8.1A and B).

It is formed between synaptic knob of an axon (presynaptic end) and a dendrite fibre of next neuron (postsynaptic end). The space between the two is **synaptic cleft.** In the ends of synaptic knob, there are spherical vesicles containing a chemical, the **neurotransmitter,** which is released into synaptic cleft. Neurotransmitter is released in response to an action potential and diffuses across the synaptic cleft. They act on the specific receptors on the postsynaptic end, to act as chemical stimulus for the generation of an impulse in the next neuron. Usually, neurotransmitters have an excitatory effect but sometimes they are inhibitory. The neurotransmitter is soon destroyed by enzymes.

Excitatory neurotransmitters are acetylcholine, norepinephrine, dopamine, etc. and inhibitory neurotransmitter is glycine.

Neuromuscular junction is meeting place between synaptic knobs of an axon and postsynaptic membrane of muscle fibre known as **motor end plate**. Acetylcholine is released from vesicles in synaptic knobs in response to a stimulus, which diffuses across the gap and binds to receptors at motor end plate. An action potential is generated at motor end plate which is conducted along the muscle fibre and cause muscle contraction.

PARTS AND FUNCTIONS OF CNS (BRAIN AND SPINAL CORD) BRAIN

The brain is the part of the central nervous system that lies within the skull. Its largest part is the **cerebrum,** consisting of right and left halves of **cerebral hemispheres.**

Extending down from the undersurface of the brain is the **brainstem** to which 3rd to 12th cranial nerves are attached. Situated at the back of brainstem is the little brain or **cerebellum** (Fig. 8.2).

Brain and spinal cord are most delicate and precious tissue, as neurons cannot regenerate. So, they are kept protected in three membranes, the **meninges.** From outside inwards they are—the dura mater, arachnoid mater and the pia mater, including the cerebrospinal fluid lying in the subarachnoid space (space between arachnoid and pia mater). All these are further protected by the bony skull and vertebrae (Fig. 8.3).

Cerebral Hemispheres

On the surface of each hemisphere is 3–4 mm thick **cerebral cortex**. It chiefly consists of

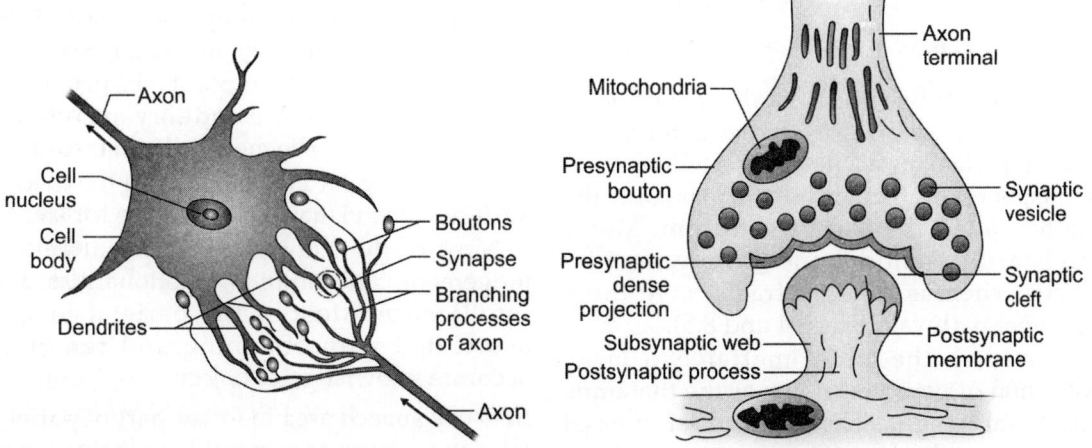

Figs 8.1A and B: Synapse (A) low power magnification and (B) high power magnification

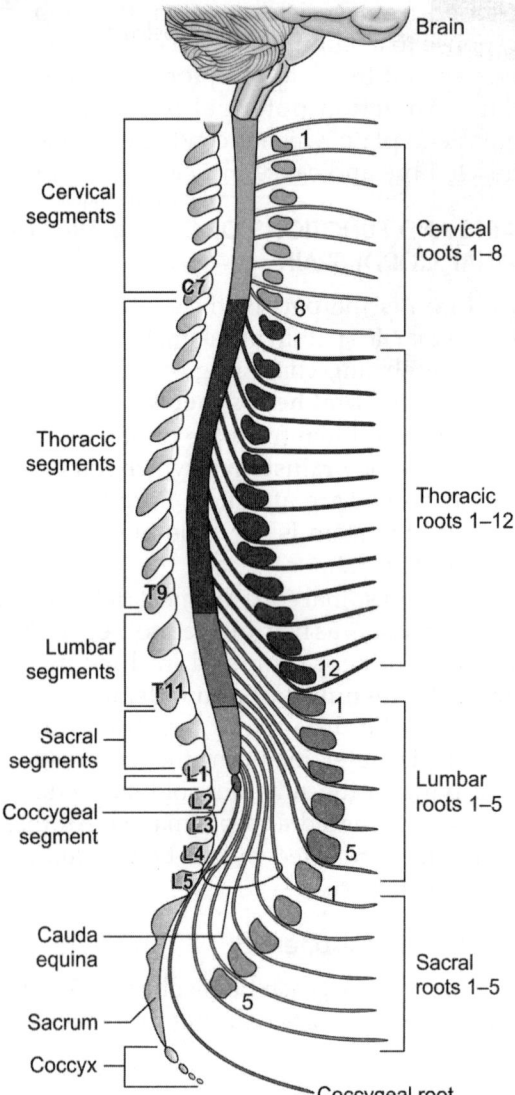

Fig. 8.2: Basic set-up of nervous system

Labels on figure: Brain; Cervical segments; Cervical roots 1–8; Thoracic segments; Thoracic roots 1–12; Lumbar segments; Sacral segments; Coccygeal segment; Cauda equina; Sacrum; Coccyx; Lumbar roots 1–5; Sacral roots 1–5; Coccygeal root; C7; T9; T11; L1; L2; L3; L4; L5

Cerebral Cortex

The surface area of cerebral cortex is increased by the presence of **sulci** and **gyri**. Each hemisphere presents following lobes and surfaces:

1. Frontal lobe, anteriorly (Fig. 8.6)
2. Occipital lobe, posteriorly
3. Temporal lobe, laterally
4. Parietal lobe, superiorly
5. Medial surface, medially
6. Superolateral surface, laterally and superiorly
7. Orbital and tentorial surface, inferiorly.

One of the most important sulci is the **central sulcus** between frontal and parietal lobes. The gyrus in front of central sulcus is the **precentral gyrus** or **motor area**, which controls the voluntary activities of opposite side of the body. Body is represented upside down in this area. Size of areas of cerebral cortex representing different parts of body are proportional to the complexity of the movement of body part. Area for thumb, hand, lips, tongue and larynx are large relative to their size. Anterior to motor area is **premotor area** which deals with learned motor activities of complex nature done in a particular sequence. In the lower part of this area just above lateral sulcus is **motor speech area**, which controls the movements necessary for speech (Fig. 8.7).

The gyrus behind central sulcus is the **postcentral gyrus** or **sensory area** and receives the sensations from the opposite half of the body. Representation is same as in motor area. On the upper part of temporal lobe just below the lateral sulcus is the **auditory area**. In the temporal lobe also lie the smell and **taste area**.

In the occipital lobe, mainly on the medial surface is the **visual area** or centre for sight.

Most of the frontal lobe is for attention, judgement, concentration, emotional state and intelligence. Most of the parietal lobe is associated with obtaining and retaining accurate knowledge of objects.

Sensory speech area in lower part of parietal lobe and adjacent temporal lobe is concerned with perception of spoken word.

neuronal cell bodies. It is also called **grey matter**. Beneath the grey matter is the **white matter** made of nerve fibres. The two cerebral hemispheres are connected by a mass of white matter called the **corpus callosum**. Motor tracts are pyramidal and extrapyramidal tracts, whereas sensory tracts have three neuronal pathway (Figs 8.4 and 8.5).

Buried in the white matter is a large collection of neurons known as the **thalamus** and **basal ganglia**. The main nuclei of basal ganglia are the lentiform nucleus and the caudate nucleus.

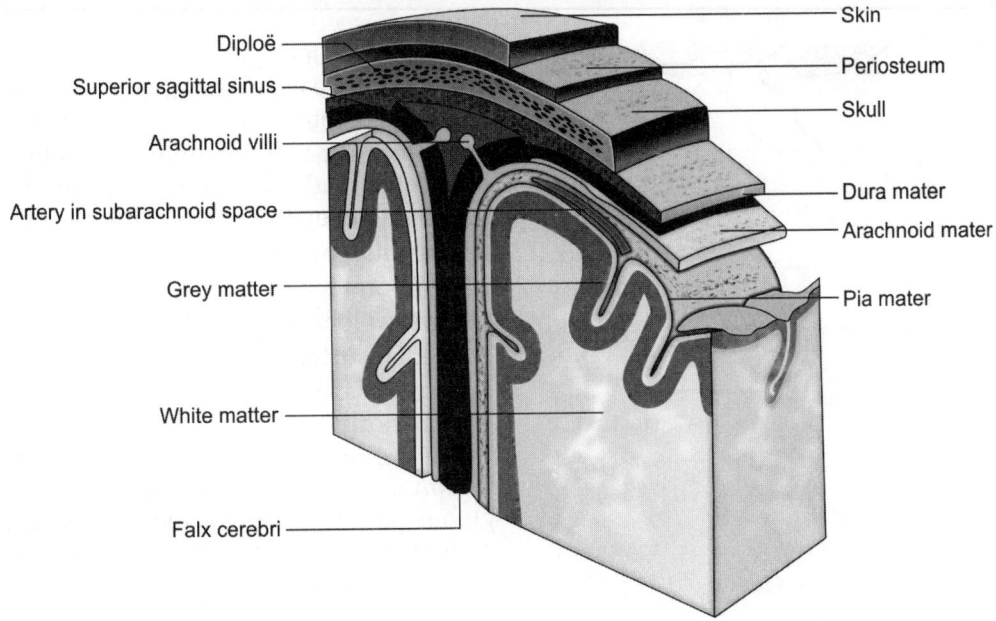

Fig. 8.3: Protective membranes of CNS

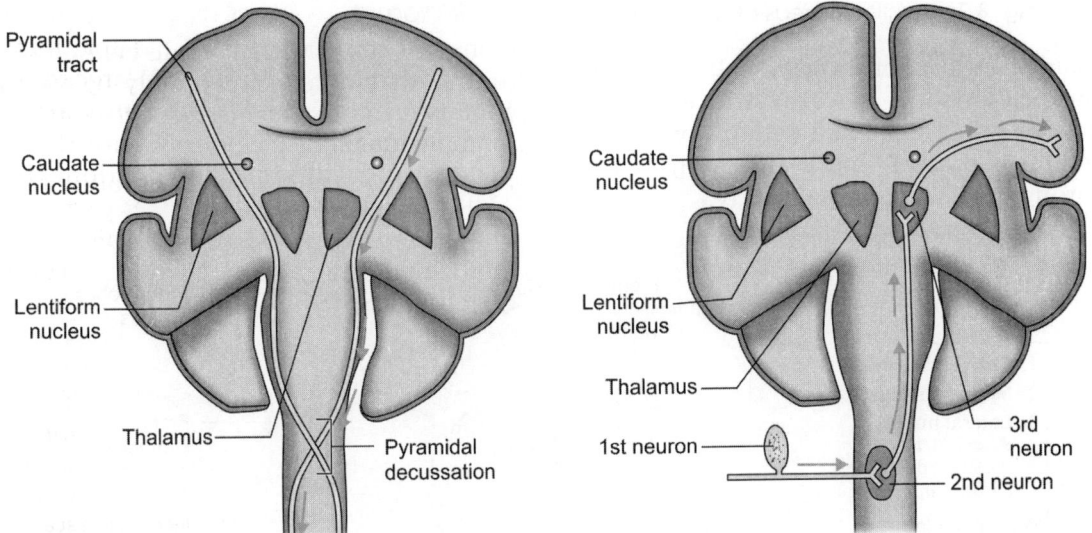

Fig. 8.4: Descending pyramidal tracts

Fig. 8.5: General pattern of sensory tracts

Thalamus

Thalamus consists of paired oval masses of grey matter organised into nuclei with interspersed tracts of white matter within cerebral hemispheres. It is a very important relay station for the afferent or sensory impulses. It is also connected with basal ganglia, cerebellum and reticular formation (Fig. 8.8). Sensory information from different organs is transmitted to thalamus before redistribution to the cerebrum. It also helps in control of autonomic activities and

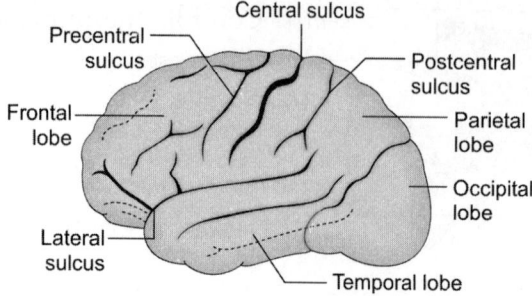

Fig. 8.6: Lobes and important sulci of cerebrum

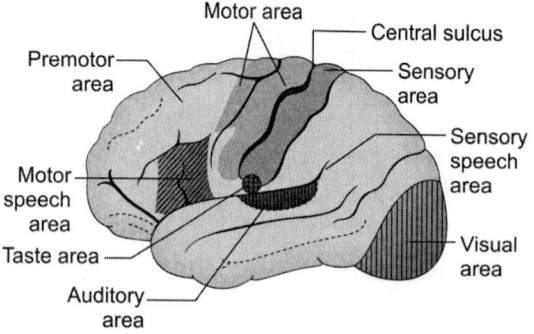

Fig. 8.7: Functional areas of cerebrum

maintenance of consciousness. It coordinates motor, sensory, visceral and emotional activities. It is connected with vision through lateral geniculate body and with hearing through medial geniculate body.

Internal Capsule

The area of white matter between the thalamus and caudate nucleus medially and the lentiform nucleus laterally is one of the most important area of the body, known as the **internal capsule**. Its parts are anterior limb, genu, posterior limb, sublentiform part and retrolentiform part. Passing through this small area are numerous sensory and motor fibres and fibres to the cranial nerve nuclei. Damage to blood supply of internal capsule causes **stroke** (Fig. 8.9).

Basal Ganglia

These are three masses of grey matter deep within each cerebral hemisphere. They are globus pallidus, with putmen together called as lentiform nucleus and caudate nucleus. These are connected with one another and cerebral cortex and thalamus. Basal ganglia function to regulate initiation and termination of movements. Basal ganglia also play a role in memory, attention and planning.

Hypothalamus

It consists of group of nerve cells below and in front of thalamus, immediately below the pituitary gland. It is connected to the pituitary gland. Its functions include:

1. Control of release of hormones from pituitary gland

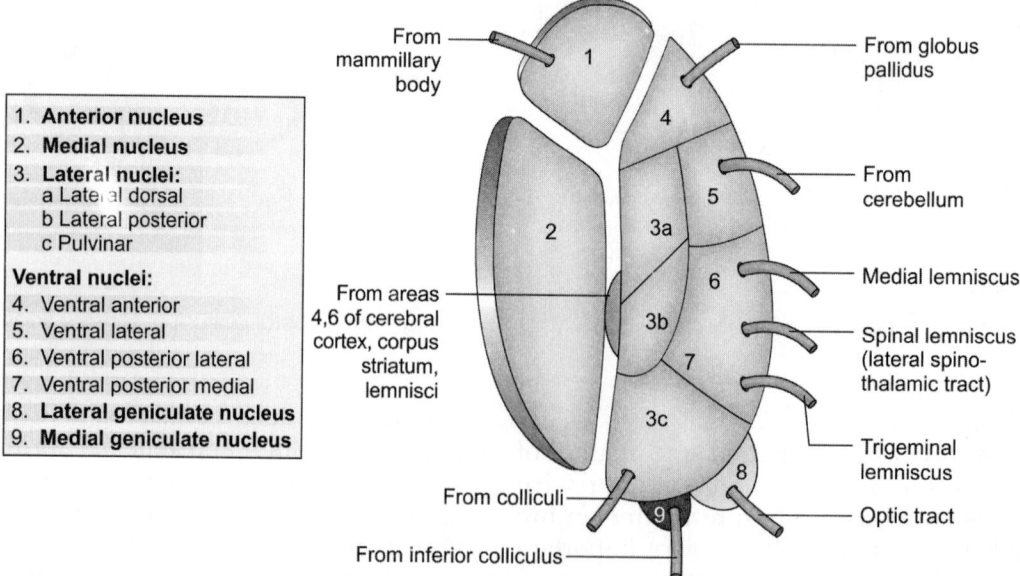

1. **Anterior nucleus**
2. **Medial nucleus**
3. **Lateral nuclei:**
   a Lateral dorsal
   b Lateral posterior
   c Pulvinar

Ventral nuclei:
4. Ventral anterior
5. Ventral lateral
6. Ventral posterior lateral
7. Ventral posterior medial
8. **Lateral geniculate nucleus**
9. **Medial geniculate nucleus**

Fig. 8.8: Nuclei of thalamus

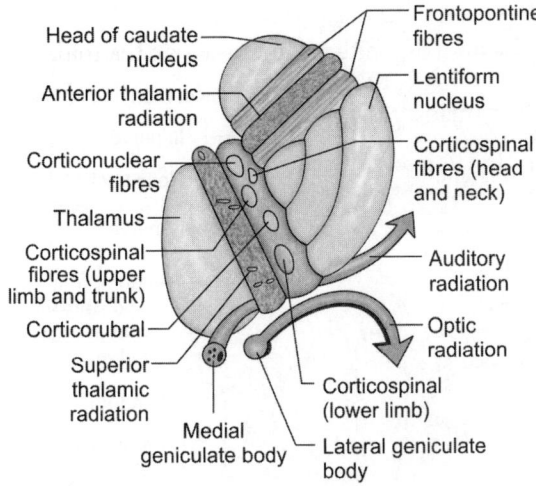

Head of caudate nucleus

Anterior thalamic radiation

Corticonuclear fibres

Thalamus

Corticospinal fibres (upper limb and trunk)

Corticorubral

Superior thalamic radiation

Medial geniculate body

Frontopontine fibres

Lentiform nucleus

Corticospinal fibres (head and neck)

Auditory radiation

Optic radiation

Corticospinal (lower limb)

Lateral geniculate body

Fig. 8.9: Internal capsule *(For colour Fig. see Plate 2)*

2. Control of the autonomic nervous system
3. Control of body temperature
4. Regulation of eating and drinking
5. Regulation of emotional and behavioural pattern
6. Regulation of biological clocks, e.g. regulates patterns of sleep and helps to maintain waking state.

Brainstem

The brainstem is the part of the brain that connects cerebrum above to the spinal cord below. It is comprised of three parts, i.e. **midbrain, pons and medulla oblongata.** In these parts, tracts and nuclei are present. The **pons** is situated in front of cerebellum, below the midbrain and above the medulla oblongata.

In pons cell bodies (grey matter) lies deeply and the nerve fibres (white matter) lie on the surface.

Medulla oblongata extends from pons above and is continuous with the spinal cord below. The **vital centres** like cardiac centre, respiratory centre, vasomotor centre and reflex centres of vomiting, coughing, sneezing and swallowing are present in medulla oblongata. The medulla oblongata has several special features:

1. *Cardiac centre:* Controls the rate and force of contraction of heart by sympathetic and parasympathetic fibres originating in the medulla and supplying the heart.

2. *Respiratory centre:* Controls the rate and depth of respiration.

3. *Vasomotor centre:* Controls the diameter of blood vessels, especially small arteries and arterioles through autonomic nervous system.

4. *Reflex centres:* When stimulated by irritating substances in stomach or respiratory tract cause reflex actions of vomiting, coughing and sneezing to expel the irritant.

5. *Crossing (decussation) of pyramids:* In medulla, motor nerves descending from the motor area of cerebrum to spinal cord in corticospinal tract cross from one side to the other. These tracts control the skeletal/voluntary muscles. By crossing over of the tracts to the opposite side, the right cerebral hemisphere controls the activity of left side and vice versa.

6. *Sensory decussation:* Sensory nerves going up from spinal cord to the cerebrum cross from one side to the other in the medulla.

In brainstem, there is **reticular formation** (collection of neurons and fibres). Neurons within reticular formation have both ascending (sensory) and descending (motor) functions. It receives afferent from cerebral cortex. This part of reticular formation is called **reticular activating system** (RAS). Reticular formation is concerned with regulation of skeletal muscle tone (state of slight degree of contraction in normal resting muscles. RAS maintains consciousness and is active during awakening from sleep. Thus, activity of this system keeps one alert. RAS gets suppressed by general anaesthetics.

Cranial Nerve Nuclei

Nuclei of 3rd to 12th cranial nerves are attached to parts of the brainstem.

• Those of 3rd and 4th are in midbrain.
• Those of 5th, 6th, 7th and part of 8th are in pons.
• Those of part of 8th, 9th, 10th, 11th and 12th are in the medulla oblongata. The fibres of these nerves are attached to the brainstem in order from before backwards (Figs 8.10A and B).

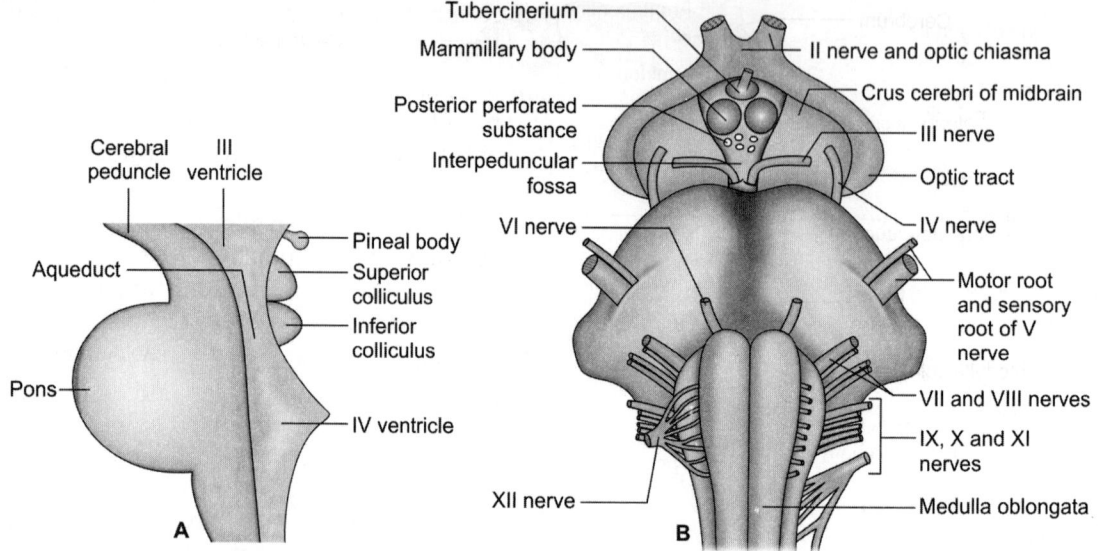

Figs 8.10A and B: (A) section of brain showing part of midbrain, pons and medulla oblongata and (B) attachment of cranial nerves to the brain

Cerebellum

The ovoid-shaped cerebellum sticks out from the back of brainstem (Fig. 8.2). It is comprised of two cerebellar hemispheres connected by a vermis.

Cerebellum is connected by three collection of nerve fibres called the **peduncles** to the midbrain, pons and medulla oblongata.

Superior cerebellar peduncle connects midbrain with cerebellum. **Middle cerebellar peduncle** connects pons with cerebellum. **Inferior cerebellar peduncle** connects medulla oblongata with cerebellum.

Cerebellum has grey matter, i.e. neuronal bodies on the surface; and white matter, i.e. fibres inside. To accommodate more neurons in a small area, the grey matter is thrown into **folia.** Within the white matter are further collections of neurons in the form of **nuclei,** the most important being the dentate nucleus.

Functions: Cerebellum is concerned with coordination of voluntary muscular activity, helping the movements to be smooth and controlled. It also controls the tone of muscles, posture and equilibrium of the body.

Diseases of the cerebellum result in clumsy uncoordinated muscular movement, stag-gering gait and inability to carry out smooth, steady and precise movements.

Ventricles of the Brain and the Cerebrospinal Fluid (CSF)

The cerebrum and brainstem contain cavities called the **ventricles.** All of them contain CSF for providing the nourishment to the neurons and take back the products of metabolism.

Each cerebral hemisphere contains a large **lateral ventricle** with anterior horn in frontal lobe, body in parietal lobe, inferior horn in temporal lobe and posterior horn in occipital lobe (Fig. 8.11).

The lateral ventricle communicates with the **third ventricle** (lying between two adjacent thalami) through **interventricular foramen.**

Cavity of midbrain is **aqueduct** while cavity of pons, medulla and cerebellum is **fourth ventricle.** The third ventricle communicates with aqueduct, which is connected to 4th ventricle. There are three openings in roof of 4th ventricle from where CSF escapes in the **subarachnoid space** (space between arachnoid mater and pia mater) and into the central canal of the spinal cord.

Cerebrospinal fluid is formed by bunches of capillaries called the **choroid plexuses** into

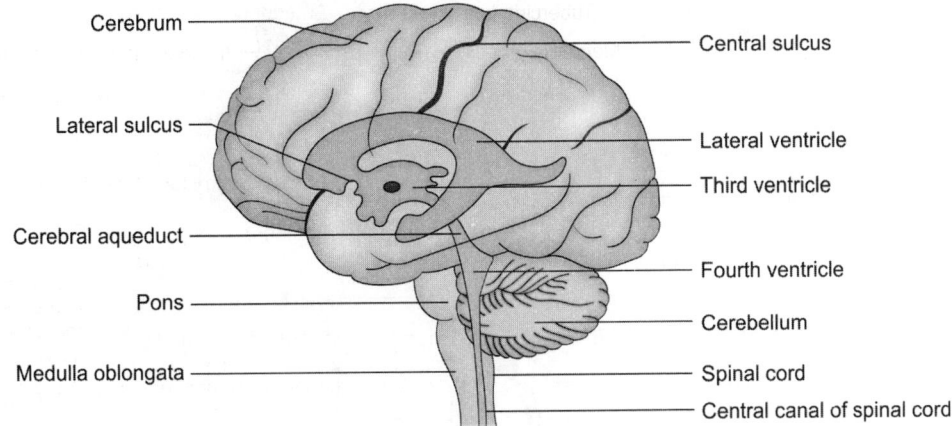

Fig. 8.11: Ventricular system

the ventricles. It circulates through lateral ventricle → III ventricle → aqueduct → IV ventricle → 3 openings → subarachnoid space and is absorbed into the superior sagittal venous sinus (Fig. 8.12).

CSF passes back into blood through tiny diverticula of arachnoid mater, called **arachnoid villi,** that project into venous sinuses.

Daily approximately about 500 mL of CSF is secreted. The amount of CSF around the brain and spinal cord is constant at 120 mL. It means that CSF absorption keeps pace with secretion.

CSF is a clear, slightly alkaline fluid with a specific gravity of 1.005. It is composed of water (98.5%) and solids (1.5%). The solids are both inorganic and organic constituent. Functions of CSF are support and protection to the brain and spinal cord; acts as a cushion and shock absorber between brain and cranial bones; and interchange of nutrients and waste products between CSF and nerve cells.

Blood Supply

Three cerebral arteries: (1) anterior, (2) middle and (3) posterior cerebral arteries supply each cerebral hemisphere. The anterior and middle cerebral arteries are branches of internal carotid, while posterior cerebral is the branch of basilar artery. The two vertebral arteries join to form the basilar artery. These three arteries of each side with a few more arteries form the **circle of Willis** at the base of brain (Fig. 8.13).

Anterior cerebral supplies mainly the medial surface of brain, middle cerebral the superolateral surface and posterior cerebral mainly the tentorial surface.

Small striate branches of the middle cerebral supply the internal capsule. Branches of the basilar artery supply parts of brainstem.

Veins do not accompany the arteries and do not have corresponding names also.

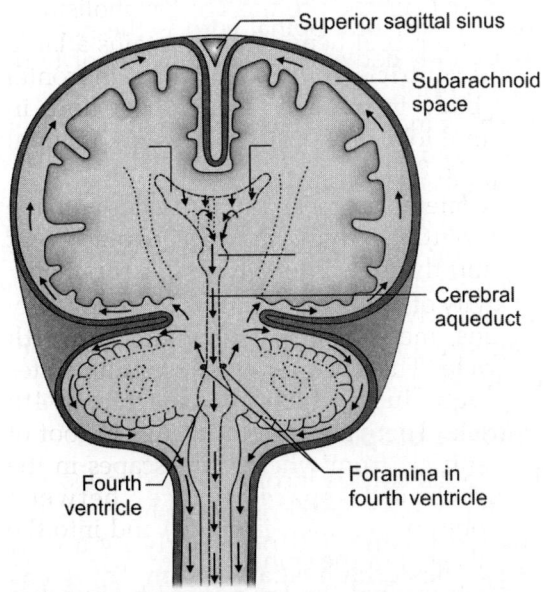

Fig. 8.12: Circulation of cerebrospinal fluid

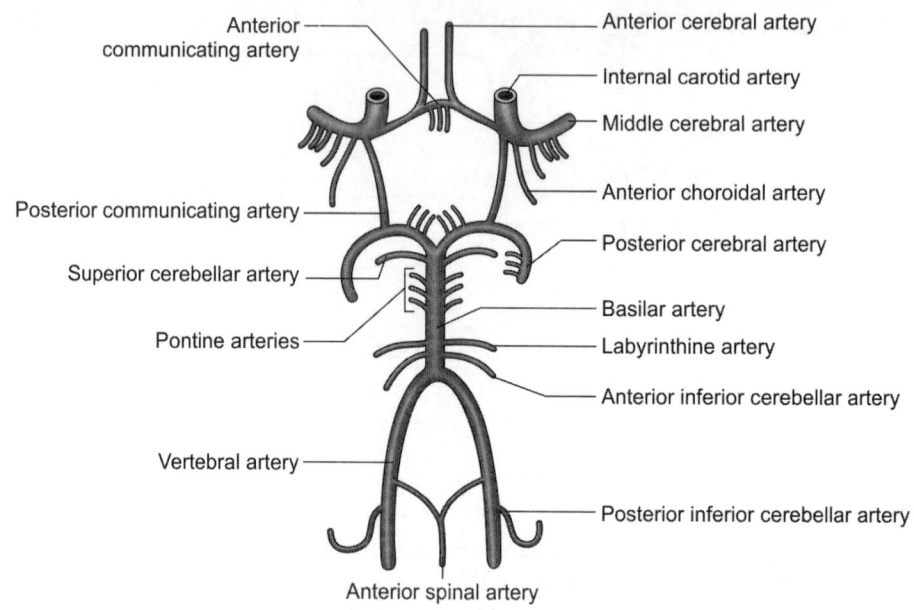

Fig. 8.13: Circle of Willis

Interior of brain is drained by **great cerebral vein,** which ends in the straight sinus, which usually becomes the left transverse sinus to continue as sigmoid sinus and finally as internal jugular vein. The superior sagittal sinus drains the superior part of brain and continues as right transverse sinus and then as right sigmoid sinus (*see* Fig. 4.27).

Inferior sagittal sinus lies deep within the brain and passes backward to form straight sinus, which runs backwards and downwards to become left transverse sinus.

Transverse sinuses begin in the occipital region. These run forward and medially and become continuous with sigmoid sinus. Each sigmoid sinus continues as internal jugular vein. Behind the clavicle internal jugular vein unites with the subclavian vein to form brachiocephalic vein.

The brain receives about 750 mL of blood per minute. Autoregulation keeps the blood flow to the brain constant across a wide range of arterial blood pressure.

The arteries of the brain can be affected by haemorrhage, i.e. bleeding or thrombosis; i.e. blockage of the artery. If the central arteries supplying internal capsule burst or get blocked, 'cerebral stroke' occurs. The opposite half of the body gets paralysed.

SPINAL CORD

The spinal cord is the continuation of medulla oblongata. It starts at level of first cervical vertebra, lies in the vertebral canal and in the adult ends at the lower border of first lumbar vertebra. Spinal cord is the nervous tissue link between brain and rest of body (Fig. 8.14).

The spinal cord is surrounded by pia mater, arachnoid mater and dura mater, the three meninges and the CSF.

Lumbar puncture in the adult is done by inserting a needle between lumbar 3 and 4 vertebral spines in the subarachnoid space to withdraw 1–2 mL of cerebrospinal fluid for diagnosis of certain diseases. It is also used for giving spinal anaesthesia.

Structure of Spinal Cord

The spinal cord is incompletely divided into two equal parts, anteriorly by a short, shallow **median fissure** and posteriorly by a deep narrow **posterior median septum.** Transverse section of spinal cord shows slightly darker, grey matter (neuronal bodies) in the form of

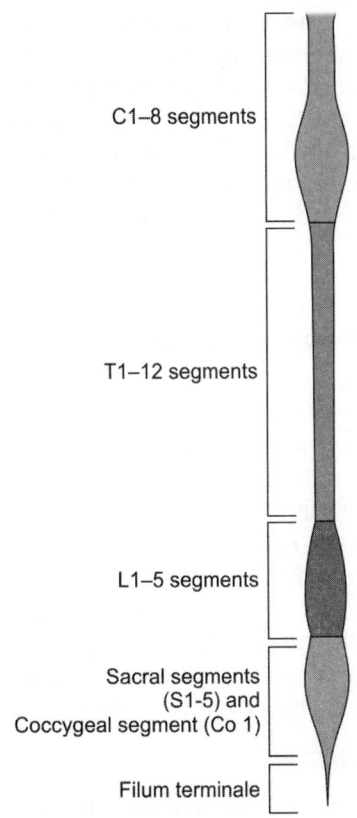

C1–8 segments

T1–12 segments

L1–5 segments

Sacral segments
(S1-5) and
Coccygeal segment (Co 1)

Filum terminale

Fig. 8.14: Parts of spinal cord

'H-shaped region', with central canal in the centre. All around it is the white matter composed of nerve fibres.

The grey matter presents **horns**—ventral/anterior, dorsal/posterior and lateral (Fig. 8.15).

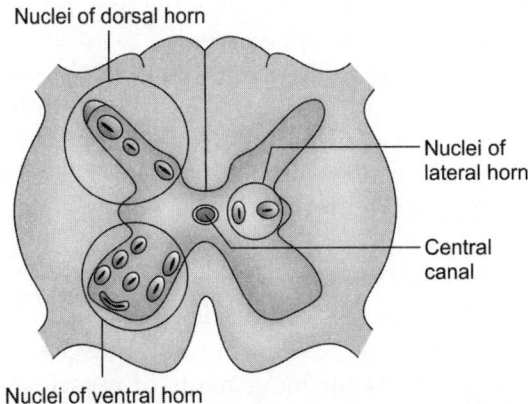

Nuclei of dorsal horn

Nuclei of
lateral horn

Central
canal

Nuclei of ventral horn

Fig. 8.15: Cross section of spinal cord

1. *Ventral horn cells* contain motor neurons, whose fibres run out in the spinal nerves to innervate various skeletal muscles. The virus of poliomyelitis affects and destroys anterior horn cells resulting in paralysis of the skeletal muscles.

2. *Lateral horn* is smaller and is present in some segments of spinal cord. It contains autonomic motor nerve cells for the innervation of cardiac muscle, smooth muscles and certain glands. It is present from 1st thoracic to 2nd lumbar segments for sympathetic activity and in sacral 2nd, 3rd, 4th segments for parasympathetic activity.

3. *The posterior horn* contains cells that are sensory/afferent in function. They receive impulses from the periphery of the body and transmit them upwards to the brain.

Grey matter also has **connector neurons** that link sensory and motor neurons at same or different levels.

White matter of spinal cord is arranged in three **columns/tracts**, i.e. anterior, posterior and lateral. These tracts are formed by motor nerve fibres descending from the brain, sensory nerve fibres ascending to the brain and fibres of connector neurons. Sensory and motor tracts of the spinal cord are continuous with sensory and motor tracts in the brain.

Spinal segment is a part or segment of spinal cord to which a pair of dorsal and a pair of ventral nerve roots are attached to form the spinal nerve on each side.

There are 31 spinal segments and 31 spinal nerves, one segment for a pair (right and left) of a spinal nerve. There are 8 cervical, 12 thoracic, 5 lumbar, 5 sacral and 1 coccygeal segments. Thus, there are 8 cervical nerves (vertebrae are 7); 12 thoracic nerves (vertebrae are 12); 5 lumbar nerves (vertebrae are 5); 5 sacral nerves (5 vertebrae are fused); 1 coccygeal nerve (4 vertebrae are fused) (Fig. 8.16).

The segments of spinal cord do not correspond to the vertebrae. Segments are higher than the vertebrae as spinal cord ends at lower border of L1 vertebra.

1. All cervical nerves arise between C1 and C7 vertebrae.

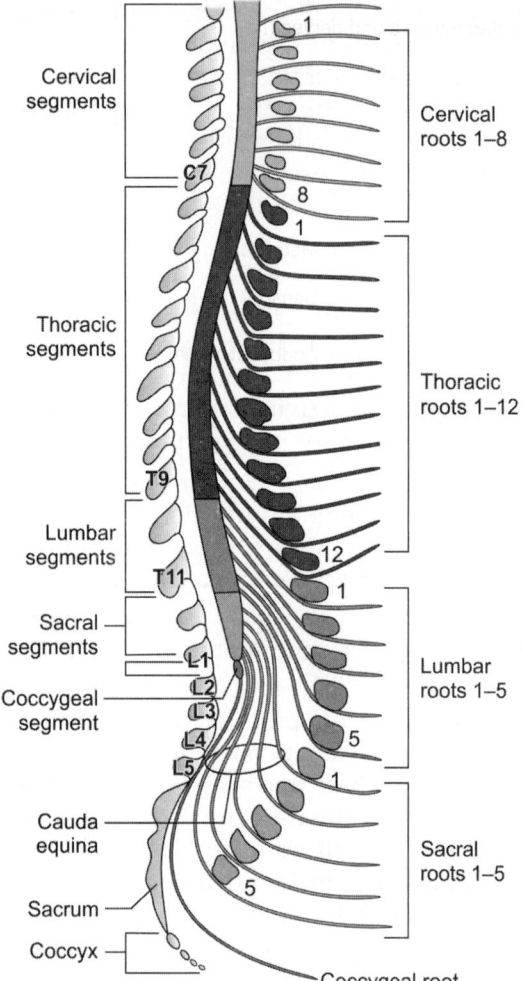

Cervical segments

C7

Thoracic segments

T9

Lumbar segments

T11

Sacral segments

L1
L2
L3
L4
L5

Coccygeal segment

Cauda equina

Sacrum

Coccyx

Cervical roots 1–8

Thoracic roots 1–12

Lumbar roots 1–5

Sacral roots 1–5

Coccygeal root

Fig. 8.16: Spinal nerves and various nerve plexuses

2. All thoracic nerves arise between T1 and T9 vertebrae.
3. All lumbar nerves arise between T10 and T11 vertebrae.
4. All sacral and coccygeal nerves arise between T12 and L1 vertebrae.

Function of spinal cord is propagation of nerve impulse by white matter tracts and integration of information in grey matter. Spinal cord gives passage to various tracts carrying different type of sensations from periphery till brain. The **spinothalamic tracts** convey impulses for pain, temperature, touch and pressure. The **posterior column** carries impulses for sense of position and movement of muscles, tendons and joints and vibration

sensation. The voluntary muscular movements of skeletal muscles are controlled by cerebral cortex via corticospinal and corticobulbar tracts. By **descending tracts** from brain stem, and cerebellum there is control of muscle tone, maintenance of posture and balance and coordination of muscle movement.

Spinal cord also acts as a reflex pathway.

PARTS AND FUNCTIONS OF PNS

The PNS consists of all the other nervous tissue outside the brain and spinal cord. Its chief components are 12 pairs of cranial nerves, 31 pairs of spinal nerves and autonomic nervous system.

Most of the nerves of PNS are composed of **motor nerve fibres** carrying impulses from brain through spinal cord to effector organs, e.g. smooth and skeletal muscles, and glands, and **sensory nerve fibres** carrying impulses from sensory end organs to the brain.

CRANIAL NERVES

The 12 pairs of cranial nerves are numbered and named in order from before backwards. They are numbered in Roman numerals. The cranial nerves originate from nuclei in the inferior surface of brain. I and II are attached to the cerebral cortex and III to XII are attached to the brainstem.

Note the following points: There are five special sensations, smell, sight, hearing, taste and touch. Their nerves are:

1. For smell, I or olfactory nerve (Fig. 8.17)
2. For sight, II or optic nerve
3. For hearing, VIII or vestibulocochlear nerve
4. For taste, VII, IX and X or facial, glossopharyngeal and vagus. These nerves have other functions also
5. For touch, V or trigeminal.

The motor cranial nerves are:
1. III, IV, VI for movements of eyes
2. V for muscles of mastication
3. VII for movements of facial muscles
4. IX, X, XI for movements of muscles of soft palate, pharynx and larynx
5. XII for movements of muscles of tongue.

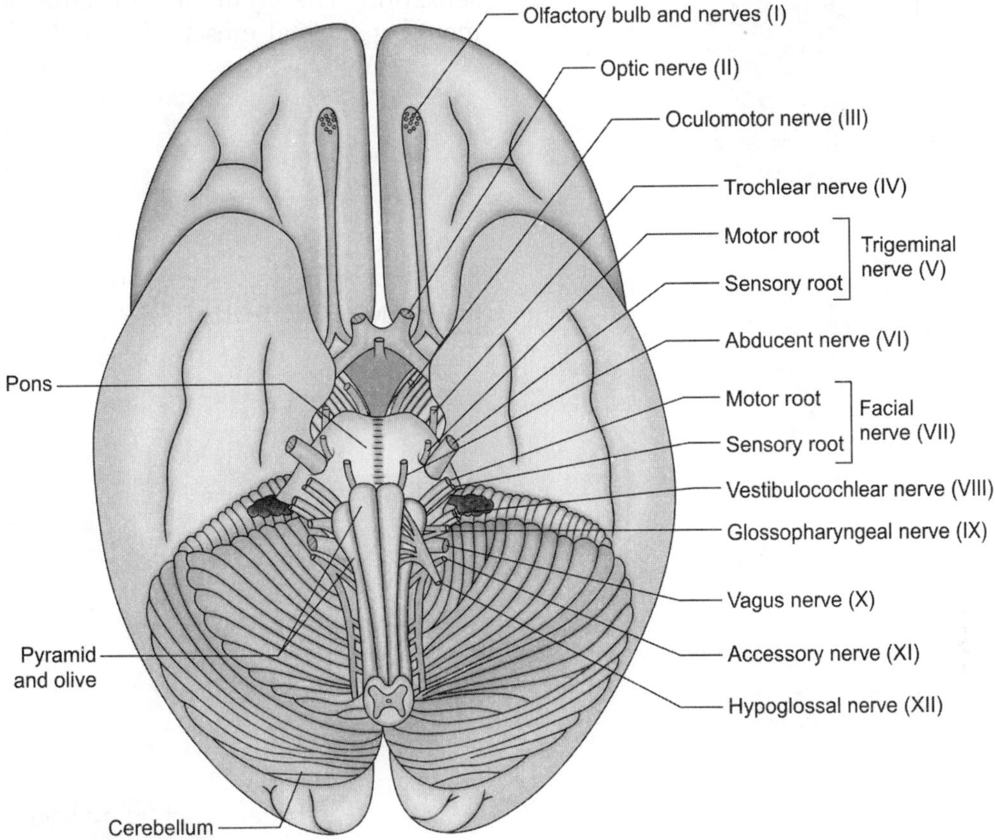

Olfactory bulb and nerves (I)

Optic nerve (II)

Oculomotor nerve (III)

Trochlear nerve (IV)

Motor root ⎤
            ⎬ Trigeminal
Sensory root ⎦ nerve (V)

Abducent nerve (VI)

Motor root ⎤
            ⎬ Facial
Sensory root ⎦ nerve (VII)

Vestibulocochlear nerve (VIII)

Glossopharyngeal nerve (IX)

Vagus nerve (X)

Accessory nerve (XI)

Hypoglossal nerve (XII)

Pons

Pyramid and olive

Cerebellum

Fig. 8.17: Attachments of cranial nerves

Also remember:

1. *I (olfactory) nerve:* Purely sensory for sense of smell (Fig. 8.18).

2. *II (optic) nerve:* Sensory for sense of sight. The nerves which move the muscles of eyeball in response to light are supplied

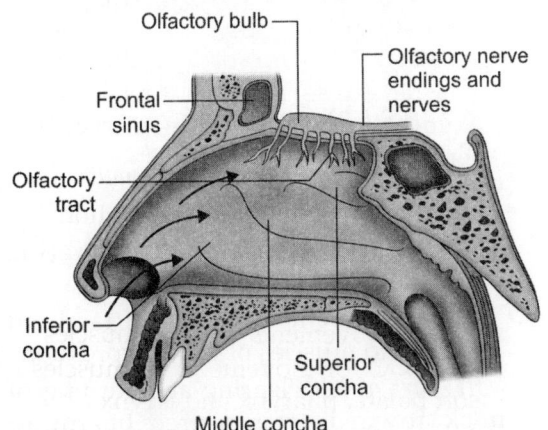

Olfactory bulb

Olfactory nerve endings and nerves

Frontal sinus

Olfactory tract

Inferior concha

Superior concha

Middle concha

Fig. 8.18: Olfactory nerve

by III, IV, VI. So, 4 cranial nerves are dedicated to eyes only (Fig. 8.19).

3. *III (oculomotor) nerve:* Supplies superior, inferior and media rectus and inferior oblique extraocular muscles for moving the eyeball; ciliary muscles of eye for focusing of light rays by changing the shape of the lens; circular muscle fibres of iris to regulate the size of the pupil; part of levator palpebrae muscle which raises the upper eyelid (Fig. 8.20).

4. *IV (trochlear) nerve:* Supplies superior oblique muscle of eye for moving the eyeball (Fig. 8.20).

5. *V (trigeminal) nerve:* Sensory to most of the face, eyes and forehead, and motor to muscles of mastication. It is the largest of the cranial nerve (Fig. 8.21).

6. *VI (abducent) nerve:* Supplies lateral rectus muscle of eye for moving the eyeball (Fig. 8.20).

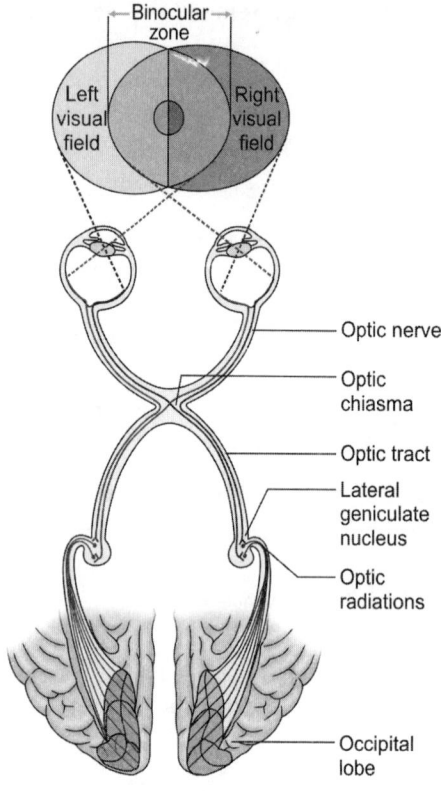

Fig. 8.19: Optic nerve

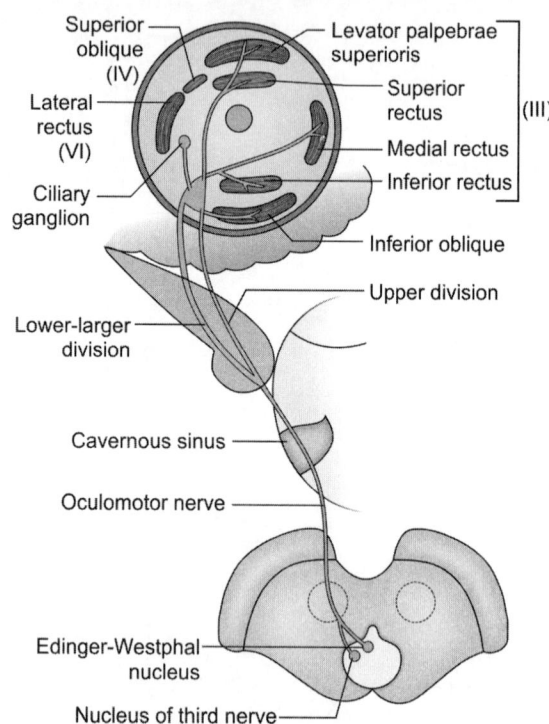

Fig. 8.20: III, IV, VI nerves

7. *VII (facial) nerve:* Motor to muscles of facial expression and sensory fibres supply the taste buds in anterior 2/3rd of the tongue for taste perception (*see* Fig. 7.9).

8. *VIII (auditory) nerve:* Sensory for maintaining the balance of body and posture, and for hearing (Fig. 8.22).

9. *IX (glossopharyngeal), X (vagus), part of XI nerve (accessory):* Motor to muscles of soft palate, pharynx, larynx. Vagus gives secretomotor fibres to stomach, small intestine and part of large intestine. Vagus nerve also has sensory fibres which convey impulses from lining membranes of same structures to the brain. IX cranial nerve also conveys sensory impulses to cerebral cortex from posterior 1/3rd of tongue, pharynx and tonsils (Fig. 8.23 and Table 8.1).

10. *Part of XI nerve:* Motor to sternocleidomastoid and trapezius muscles (*see* Fig. 7.13).

11. *XII (hypoglossal) nerve:* Supplies muscles of the tongue for movement of tongue (Fig. 8.17).

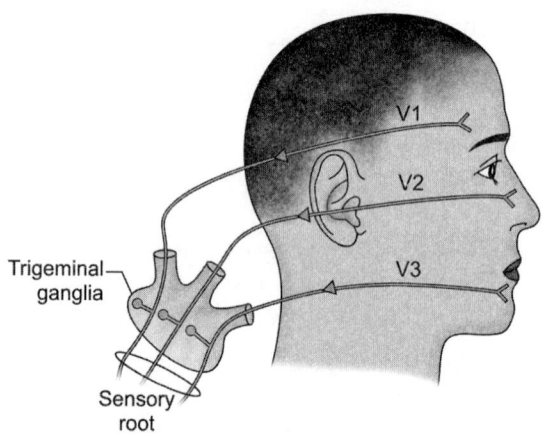

Fig. 8.21: Trigeminal nerve

These nerves can be paired functionally:

- *I and X:* Smell and gastric secretion.
- *II, III, IV, VI:* Afferent from retina and efferent to muscles of eyeball.
- *V, VII:* Afferent from skin of face and efferent to muscles of facial expression.
- *VIII, part of XI:* Hearing and turning of neck towards the source of sound (Fig. 8.17).

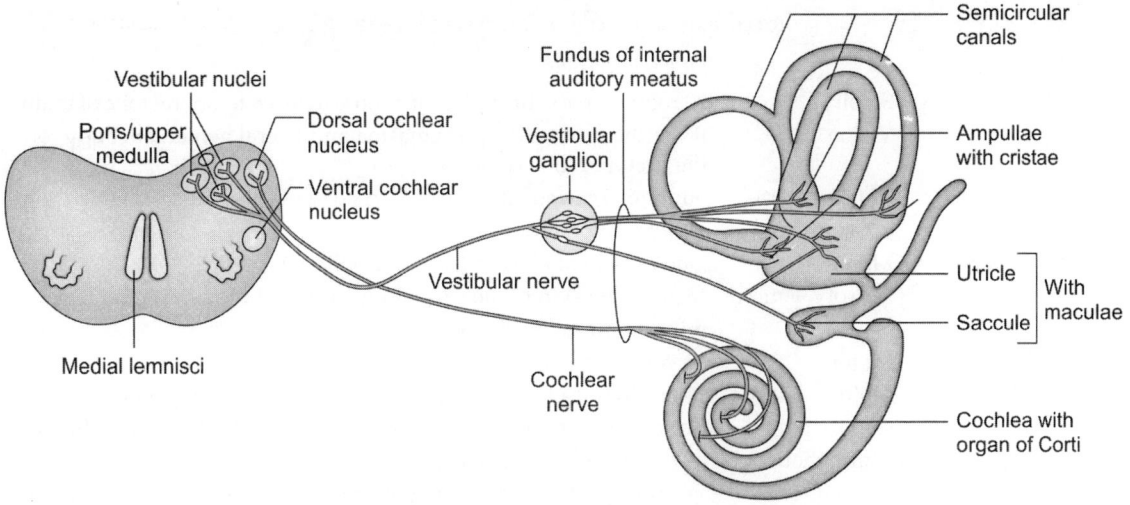

Fig. 8.22: Vestibulococclear nerve

- *VII, IX, X, part of XI, XII:* Taste and movement of tozngue, soft palate, pharynx for swallowing.

SPINAL NERVES

There are 31 pairs of spinal nerves attached to the spinal cord. Each spinal nerve is attached to spinal cord by posterior root and an anterior root (Fig. 8.24).

Dorsal (posterior) root is attached close to dorsal horn of spinal cord and is characterised by the presence of a spinal or dorsal root ganglion. Sensory nerve fibres pass through dorsal root ganglion before entering the spinal cord.

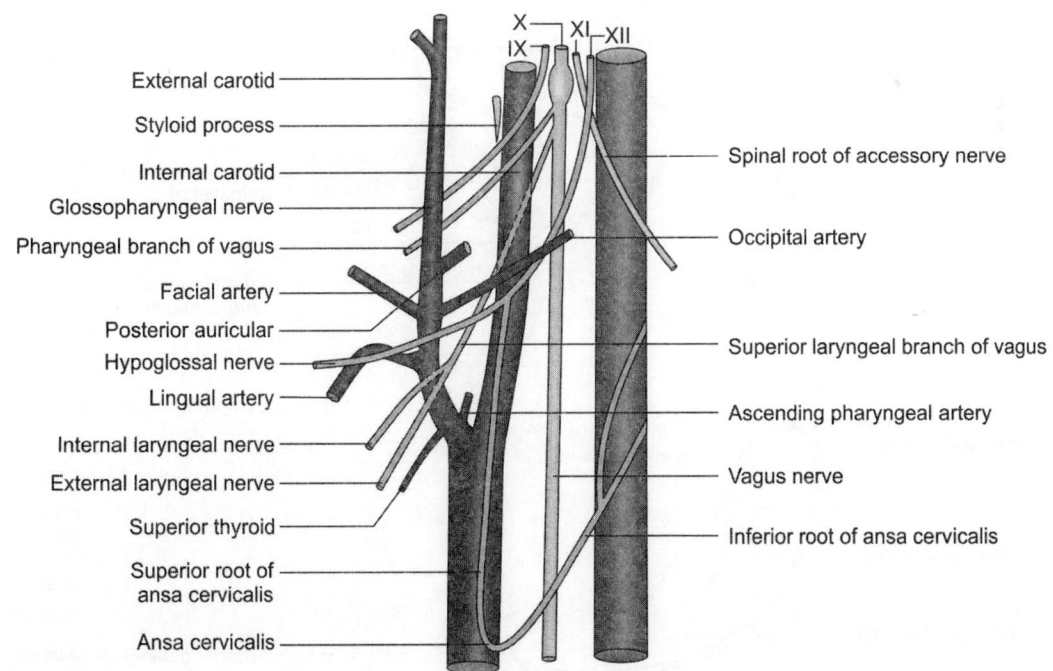

Fig. 8.23: IX, X, XI and XII nerves

Table 8.1: Summary of the cranial nerves

Nerve		Function Details
I Olfactory	Smell	20 rootlets, pass through roof of nose to reach temporal lobe of brain.
II Optic	Vision	From the retina via optic chiasma and lateral geniculate body to the occipital lobe of brain
III Oculomotor	Motor + para-sympathetic	Supplies 5 extraocular muscles. Also two sets of muscles which help in accommodation
IV Trochlear	Motor	One muscle of eyeball (superior oblique)
V Trigeminal	Sensory + motor	Most of the skin of face, nasal mucous membrane, conjunctiva; motor to muscles of mastication
VI Abducent	Motor	Motor to one muscle of eye (lateral rectus)
VII Facial	Motor + special sense + para-sympathetic	Motor to muscles of the face those around eyes and mouth; taste from anterior two-thirds of tongue; secretomotor to submandibular, lacrimal, nasal glands, etc.
VIII Vestibulo-cochlear	Hearing and balance	Vestibular part for balancing the body and maintenance of posture; cochlear part for hearing, appreciated in temporal lobe
IX Glosso-pharyngeal	Special sense + motor + para-sympathetic	Taste from posterior one-third of tongue, motor to one muscle of pharynx and secretory to parotid gland
X Vagus + cranial root of XI (accessory)	Motor + special sense+ para-sympathetic	Taste from posterior most part of tongue, motor to muscles of soft palate, pharynx, larynx, stomach and intestines and secretory to glands of respiratory and most part of digestive system
XI Spinal root of XI	Motor	Motor to two important muscles of neck, i.e. sternocleidomastoid and trapezius
XII Hypoglossal	Motor	To seven out of eight muscles of tongue

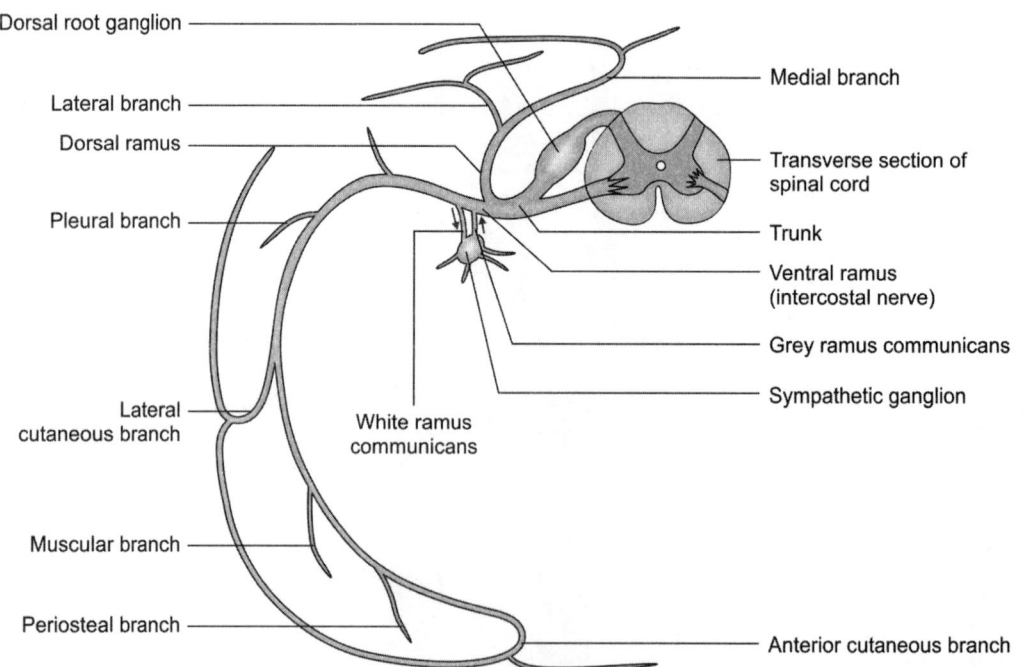

Fig. 8.24: Spinal nerve

Ventral (anterior) root is attached close to the ventral or anterior horn of spinal cord. It consists of motor nerve fibres and in the thoracic and upper lumbar regions, sympathetic nerve fibres.

Two roots unite at the respective intervertebral foramen and at once divide into a ventral or **anterior ramus** and a dorsal or **posterior ramus.**

The **dorsal ramus** is smaller, and supplies skin and muscles of the back near the midline. It is less important. The larger **ventral ramus** is highly important. These supply most of the muscles of the body and the skin overlying the muscles. The anterior rami unite and divide and reunite and redivide to form **nerve plexuses.** The importance is that one muscle gets supply from more than one segment, and injury to one segment will not paralyse the muscle.

Various nerve plexuses are:

1. *Cervical:* Formed by cervical 1st, 2nd, 3rd and 4th nerves.

2. *Brachial:* Formed by cervical 5th, 6th, 7th, 8th and 1st thoracic nerve.

3. *Lumbar:* Formed by lumbar 1st, 2nd, 3rd and part of 4th nerve.

4. *Sacral:* Formed by part of lumbar 4th, 5th and sacral 1st, 2nd, 3rd nerves.

In thoracic region, anterior rami do not form plexuses. CI nerve supplies small muscles at upper most part of back of neck.

Cervical Plexus

It is formed by ventral rami of cervical 1st, 2nd, 3rd and 4th nerves. Supplies muscles of front of neck, covering trachea and thyroid gland. It also supplies skin of front of neck. Most important branch is **phrenic nerve,** which is the sole motor supply of the muscle, diaphragm—the chief muscle of respiration.

Brachial Plexus

Is formed by ventral rami of cervical 5th, 6th, 7th, 8th and thoracic 1st nerves (Fig. 8.25). These nerves also receive sympathetic fibres.

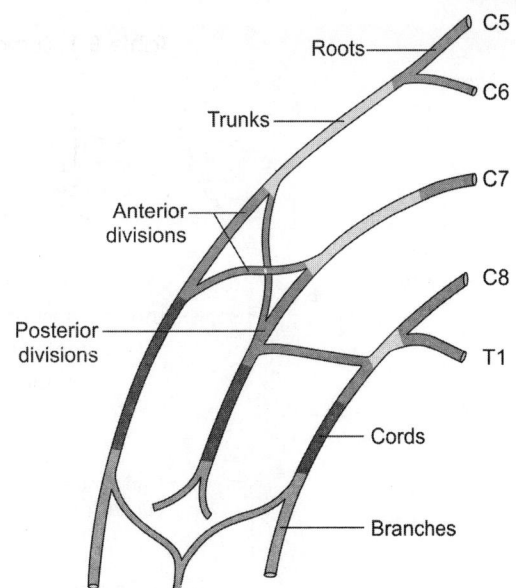

Fig. 8.25: Formation of brachial plexus with its main branches

Main branches of this plexus are axillary, radial, median, ulnar and musculocutaneous.

Axillary nerve (C5–6) supplies deltoid muscle and skin overlying lower half of the muscle and shoulder joint.

Radial nerve (C5–8, T1) supplies all the muscles on the back of arm and forearm and supinator muscle (Fig. 8.26). Since, these muscles are mainly extensors of the elbow, wrist and joints in the hand, the radial nerve is the nerve of extensor compartments in the upper limb.

Musculocutaneous nerve (C5–7) supplies both heads of biceps brachii, coracobrachialis and brachialis muscles including skin of the lateral side of the forearm (Fig. 8.27).

Median nerve (C5–8, T1) supplies muscles that flex the digits and pronate the forearm and enable the hand to grip between thumb and fingers, and skin on the lateral side of the palm (Fig. 8.28). It also supplies muscles which produce eminence on the lateral side of upper palm (thenar eminence). It is called 'labourer's nerve', and eye of the hand.

Ulnar nerve (C7, 8, T1) supplies the small muscles of the hand that are responsible for

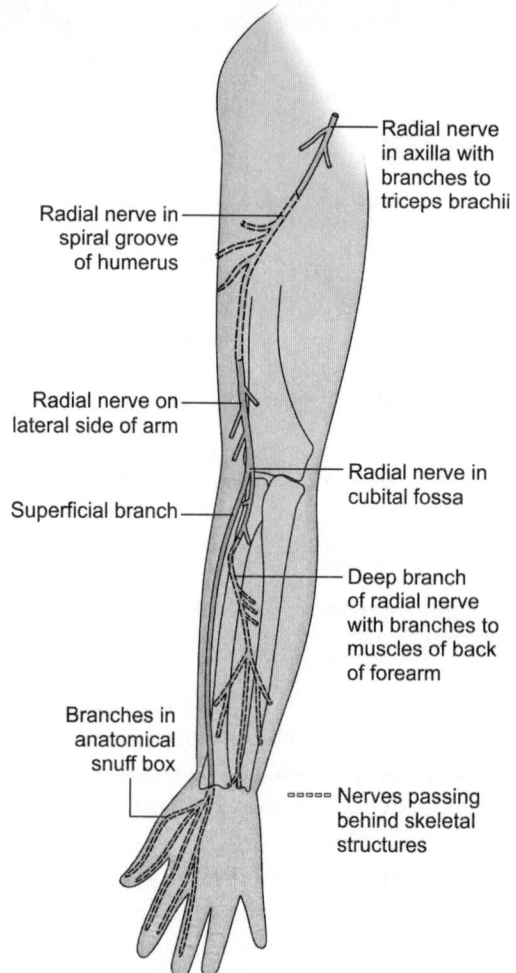

Fig. 8.26: Distribution of radial nerve

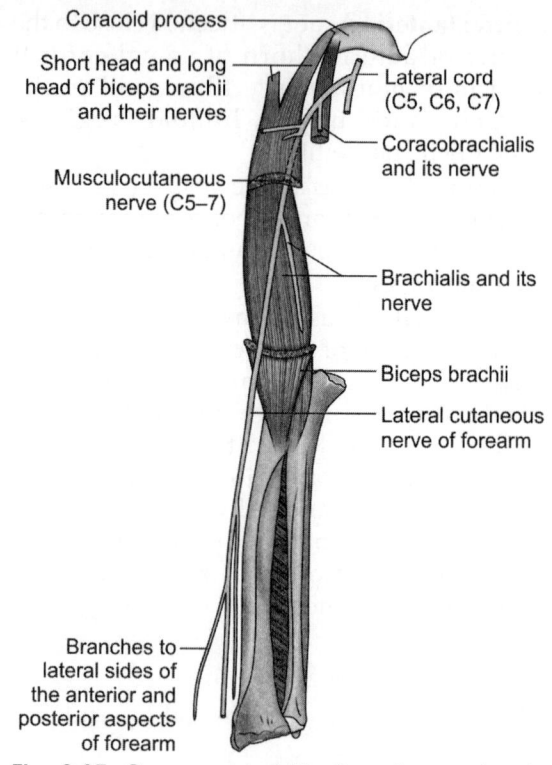

Fig. 8.27: Course and distribution of musculocutaneous nerve

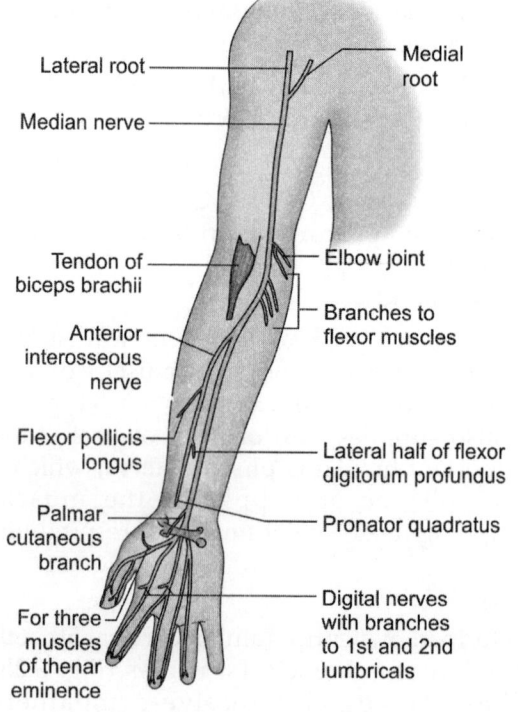

Fig. 8.28: Course and branches of median nerve

fine movements of the fingers, and skin on the ulnar side of the hand. It is called 'musician's nerve' (Fig. 8.29).

Lumbar and Sacral Plexuses

These two plexuses supply the lower limb. The large branches of lumbar plexus are the femoral and obturator nerves (Fig. 8.30).

The sacral plexus, apart from supplying the pelvic structures (part of autonomic nervous system) gives origin to the thickest nerve of the body—the sciatic nerve.

Femoral nerve (L2–4) supplies the largest muscle of front of thigh, the quadriceps femoris, the extensor of the knee joint. It supplies skin of front and medial side of thigh

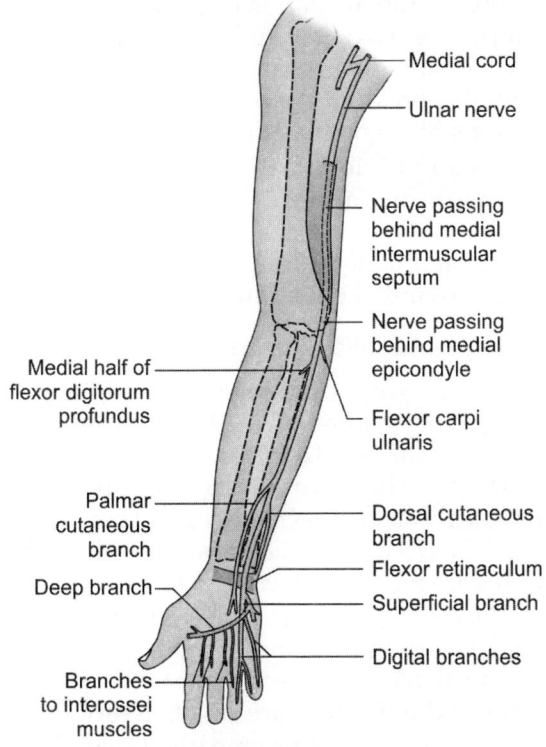

Medial cord

Ulnar nerve

Nerve passing behind medial intermuscular septum

Nerve passing behind medial epicondyle

Medial half of flexor digitorum profundus

Flexor carpi ulnaris

Palmar cutaneous branch

Dorsal cutaneous branch

Flexor retinaculum

Deep branch

Superficial branch

Digital branches

Branches to interossei muscles

Fig. 8.29: Course and branches of ulnar nerve

and by its saphenous branch supplies medial side of big toe and medial side of dorsum of foot (Fig. 8.31).

Obturator nerve (L2–4) supplies muscles on the medial side of thigh, the adductors and the skin of the medial aspect of the thigh.

Lateral cutaneous nerve of thigh is the branch of lumbar plexus and supplies skin of lateral aspect of thigh.

Superior gluteal nerve supplies gluteus medius and gluteus minimus muscles.

Inferior gluteal nerve supplies only gluteus maximus.

Sciatic nerve (L4, 5, S1–3) is the thickest and largest nerve of the body and supplies hamstring muscles, the flexors of knee joint and extensors of hip joint. In the middle of back of thigh, it divides into tibial and common peroneal nerves.

Tibial nerve supplies all the muscles of back of leg, i.e. calf region. By its two branches, the medial and lateral plantar nerves, it also supplies all the small intrinsic muscles of sole of the foot. It also supplies skin of posterior aspect of leg, sole of the foot and toes.

Common peroneal nerve supplies muscles of lateral compartment of leg, which cause eversion of foot and muscles of anterior compartment of leg, which cause dorsiflexion of foot. It also supplies skin of anterior aspect of leg, dorsum of the foot and toes.

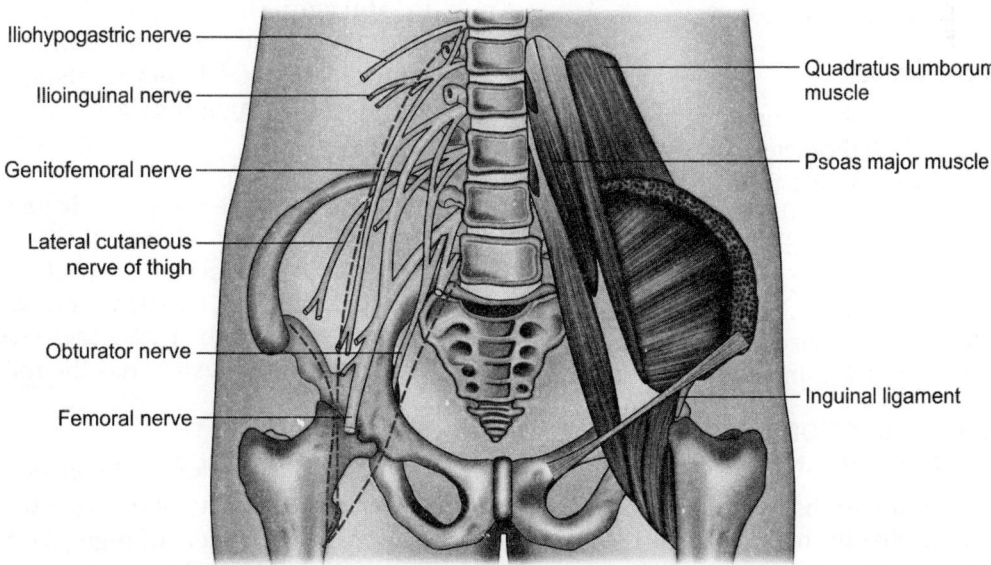

Iliohypogastric nerve

Ilioinguinal nerve

Genitofemoral nerve

Lateral cutaneous nerve of thigh

Obturator nerve

Femoral nerve

Quadratus lumborum muscle

Psoas major muscle

Inguinal ligament

Fig. 8.30: Formation and branches of lumbar plexus

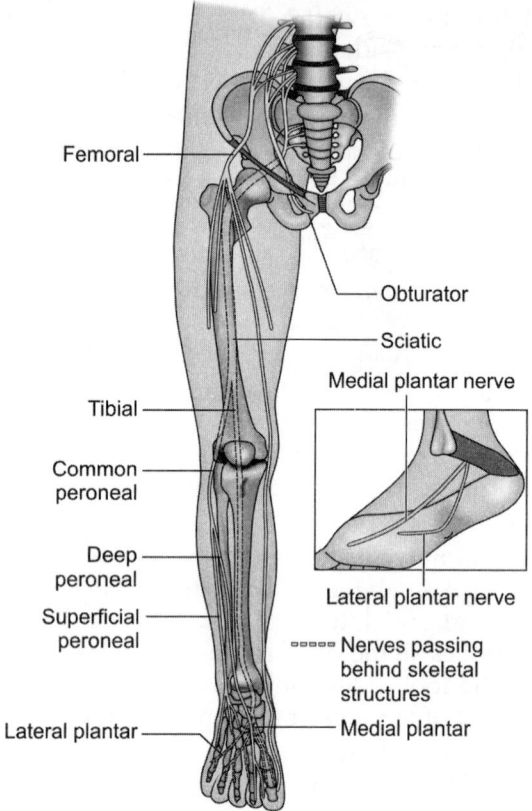

Femoral

Obturator

Sciatic

Medial plantar nerve

Tibial

Common peroneal

Deep peroneal

Lateral plantar nerve

Superficial peroneal

▫▫▫▫ Nerves passing behind skeletal structures

Lateral plantar

Medial plantar

Fig. 8.31: Nerves of lower limb

Coccygeal plexus: Small plexus formed by part of S4, S5 and coccygeal nerve. Its branches supply levator ani and coccygeus muscles and skin in the area of coccyx.

Thoracic Nerves

The ventral rami of thoracic nerves from 2nd thoracic to 12th thoracic do not form plexuses, and remain single forming the intercostal nerves that supply the muscles of thoracic wall. The 7th to 12th intercostal nerves in addition to supplying muscles of thoracic wall also supply the muscles of anterolateral wall of abdomen. These also supply skin of thoracic and anterior abdominal wall (Fig. 8.24).

PARTS AND FUNCTIONS OF AUTONOMIC NERVOUS SYSTEM (ANS)

ANS is not under the control of the will. This system supplies the muscles of the heart, other smooth muscle and glands. Autonomic pathways are interrupted by synapses in ganglia before the target organ is reached. So there are two groups of neurons, the preganglionic neuron in brain and spinal cord with its fibres and the postganglionic neuron with its fibres outside the CNS.

ANS is divided into two parts: (1) the sympathetic and (2) parasympathetic. The two act opposite to each other. On sympathetic stimulation heart rate increases while on parasympathetic stimulation it is lowered.

Parasympathetic System

The parasympathetic system has its preganglionic cell bodies in the brainstem and sacral part of spinal cord, so it has **craniosacral outflow.** The cranial nerves containing preganglionic parasympathetic fibres are III, VII, IX and X and the sacral nerves with similar fibres are S2, 3, 4 nerves (Fig. 8.32).

These preganglionic fibres terminate in the ganglia very close to the organ they supply or in the wall of the viscera itself. So, the postganglionic fibres are small or very small.

There are four parasympathetic ganglia in head and neck close to the organs supplied by them. The **cranial outflow** is as follows:

1. Parasympathetic fibres of III nerve relay in **ciliary ganglia** to supply ciliaris muscle and sphincter pupillae of eye.
2. Parasympathetic fibres of VII nerve relay in **pterygopalatine ganglia** to supply lacrimal, palatal and nasal glands.
3. Some fibres of VII nerve also relay in **submandibular ganglia** to supply the submandibular and sublingual salivary glands.
4. Fibres of IX nerve relay in **otic ganglia** to supply the parotid gland.
5. Fibres of X nerve relay in the wall of organs, i.e. heart, stomach, small intestine and part of large intestine to supply these viscera.

Parasympathetic system has the following effects:

On digestive tract:
1. Increases the secretion of the glands.
2. Increases the motility of the digestive tract.
3. Relaxes the sphincters of digestive tract.
4. Rate of digestion and absorption of food is increased.

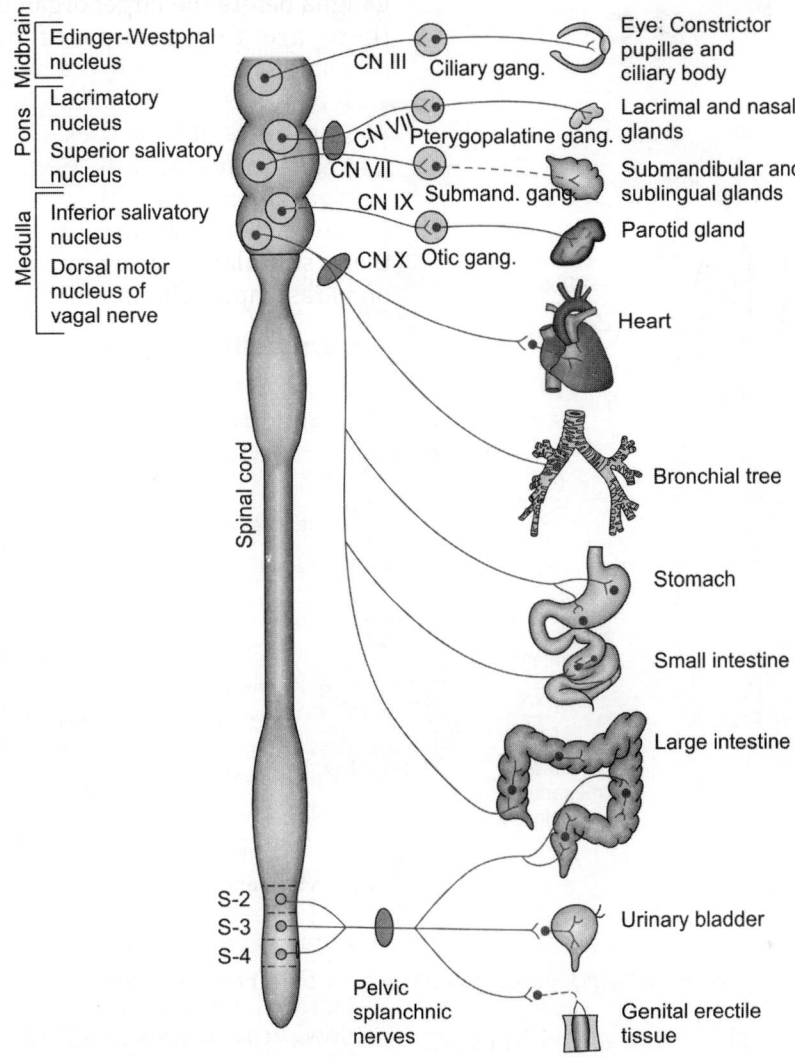

Fig. 8.32: Parasympathetic division of autonomic nervous system

Effect on heart: Decreases the heart rate and force of contraction.

Effect on respiratory system: Produces constriction of bronchi.

Effect on urinary tract: Relaxation of internal urethral sphincter and contraction of muscle of bladder wall resulting in micturition.

Effect on eye: Cause narrowing of pupil due to contraction of circular muscle fibres of iris.

Sacral outflow: The fibres that leave central nervous system through sacral 2, 3, 4 nerves leave the ventral rami of these nerves soon after they exit from ventral sacral foramina, and form a group of nerves called **pelvic splanchnic nerves.** These nerves provide parasympathetic innervation to distal part of the digestive tract and to the pelvic viscera.

Parasympathetic fibres carry pain impulses from pelvic viscera.

Sympathetic System

The preganglionic cell bodies are present in the lateral horn of the spinal cord between thoracic 1st to 12th and lumbar 1st and 2nd segments (Fig. 8.33).

The sympathetic system also comprises of two sympathetic trunks one on each side of the vertebral column. It extends from cervical to coccygeal region. It contains ganglia with

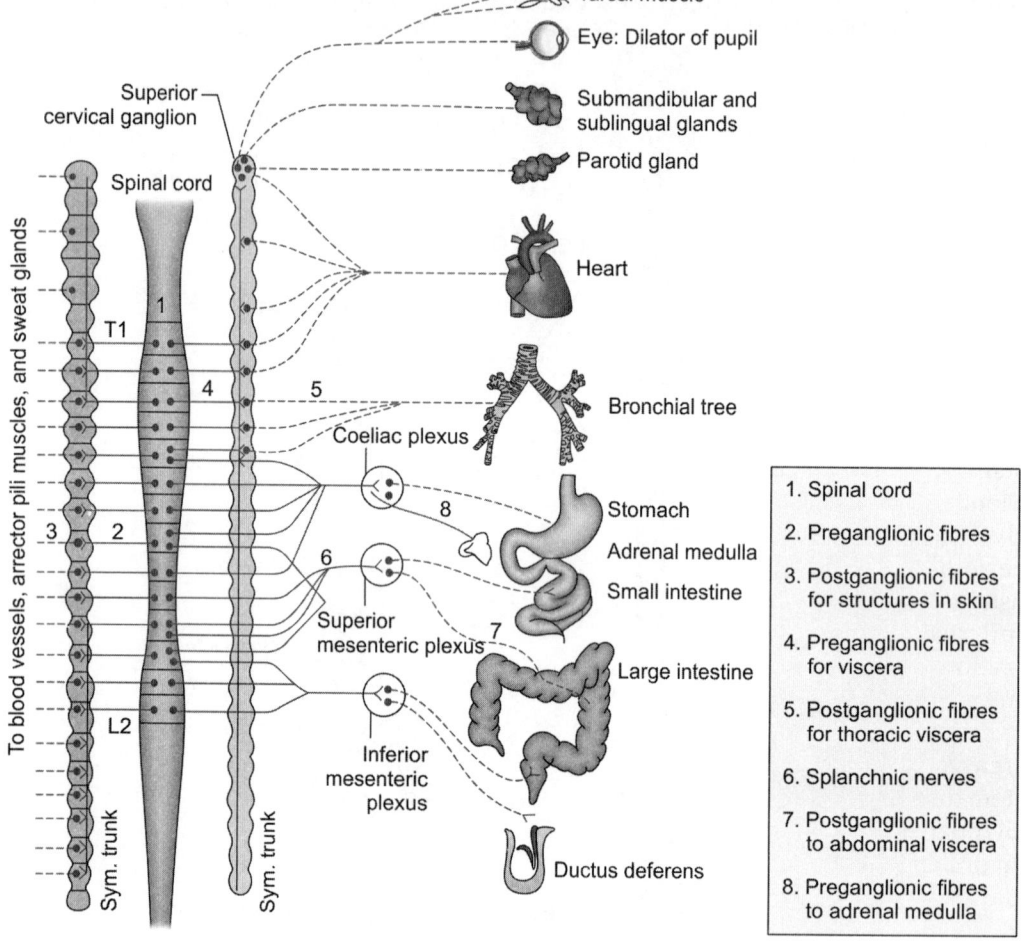

Fig. 8.33: Sympathetic division of autonomic nervous system

Legend box:
1. Spinal cord
2. Preganglionic fibres
3. Postganglionic fibres for structures in skin
4. Preganglionic fibres for viscera
5. Postganglionic fibres for thoracic viscera
6. Splanchnic nerves
7. Postganglionic fibres to abdominal viscera
8. Preganglionic fibres to adrenal medulla

neurons—3 cervical, 12 thoracic, 5 lumbar, 5 sacral and 1 coccygeal ganglia where the two trunks fuse with each other. The ganglia are attached to each other by nerve fibres.

There are **collateral ganglia,** e.g. coeliac ganglion, which give postganglionic off shoots along all the branches of the abdominal aorta and preganglionic to the adrenal gland.

The preganglionic fibres from neurons of lateral horn, reach sympathetic ganglion along white ramus communicans. Then, it may take following pathway:

1. Make synaptic connections with neurons in the ganglion of sympathetic chain at same level, i.e. thoracic spinal nerves, and pass along spinal nerves via grey ramus communicans to the arterioles of skin,

blood vessels of sweat glands and arrector pili muscles. These fibres have sudomotor (↑sweat), vasomotor (↓lumen of arterioles) and pilomotor (cause straightening of hair) function.

2. Some preganglionic fibres from T1–T2 segments pass upwards and synapse with neurons in superior, middle and inferior cervical ganglia to supply branches to 1–8 cervical nerves and also along blood vessels.

3. Some preganglionic fibres from T1 to L2 pass downwards into lumbar and sacral ganglia. These fibres relay and travel along lumbar and sacral spinal nerves and also along blood vessels of lower limb.

4. Some postganglionic fibres T2–5 sympathetic ganglia give fibres to supply heart

and lungs. Sympathetic fibres cause ↑heart rate, ↑blood pressure and ↑force of contraction of heart. It is bronchodilator for the lungs. That is why adrenaline like drugs are given for asthma.

5. Some preganglionic fibres from T5 to 12 segments pass into abdomen to reach coeliac ganglion. These fibres relay here and their postganglionic fibres travel along all the branches of abdominal aorta.

6. Some preganglionic fibres from coeliac ganglia pass to medulla of suprarenal gland.

The preganglionic fibres in sympathetic system are small and postganglionic fibres are longer.

Sympathetic system in digestive tract ↓ peristalsis, ↓ the secretion of juices. It constricts the sphincters resulting in inhibition of micturition and defaecation. It causes secretion of adrenaline and noradrenaline from adrenal medulla. It causes increased conversion of glycogen to glucose in liver and increases the metabolic rate. Sympathetic system also dilates the pupil.

Sympathetic system is the system for fright, fight or flight to prepare the body for stressful situations whereas parasympathetic is for peace, normal heart rate, digestive activities, etc. Both systems work together for the normal functioning of body.

The transmitter between the preganglionic fibres and the postganglionic neurons is acetylcholine in both sympathetic and parasympathetic system.

The transmitter at the target organs of parasympathetic system is also acetylcholine while at the target organs of sympathetic system, it is adrenaline/noradrenaline.

REFLEX ACTION AND REFLEX ARC

A **reflex** is a fast, predictable sequence of involuntary actions, e.g. muscle contraction or glandular secretion, which occurs in response to certain changes in environment. Automatic contraction of muscles is controlled by spinal cord. The immediate motor action to a painful sensory stimulus is called reflex response (Fig. 8.34).

It arises due to coordinated action of sensory receptor, sensory neuron, connector/association/integrating neuron, motor neuron and effector. Reflex arc or circuit is the functional unit of reflex response. Reflex responses occur automatically without any brain involvement to protect the body.

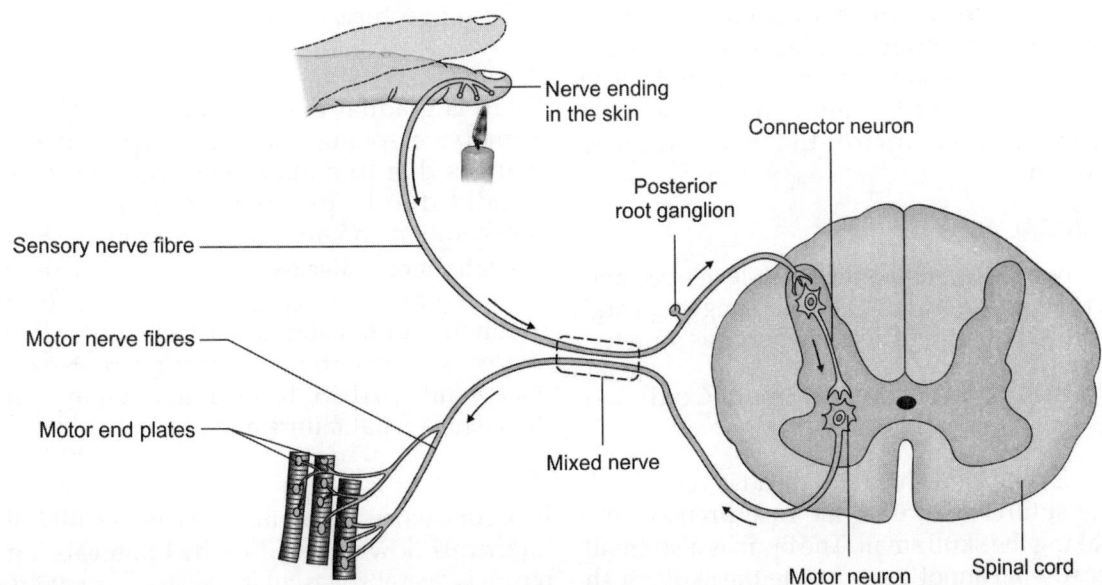

Fig. 8.34: Reflex arc

Spinal nerves which have both motor and sensory portions mediate deep tendon reflexes and superficial reflexes. Deep tendon reflexes are the involuntary contractions of a muscle after its stretching caused by a hammer.

The superficial reflexes are withdrawal reflexes elicited by tactile or noxious stimulation of the mucous membrane or cornea or skin.

A simple reflex like knee jerk reflex requires an afferent or sensory neuron, and an efferent or motor neuron. This reflex occurs as follows:

1. Sensory receptor detects the mechanical stimulus produced by the hammer striking the patellar tendon of quadriceps femoris muscle.
2. The sensory neuron carries the impulse via a spinal nerve to the dorsal root, from where it enters the spinal cord.
3. The sensory neuron synapses with the motor neuron in the anterior horn. The motor neuron carries the impulse along its axon via a spinal nerve to a particular muscle.
4. The motor neuron transmits the impulse to muscle fibres through the stimulation of motor end plate. As a result the muscle contracts and the leg extends.

ELECTROENCEPHALOGRAM (EEG)

The EEG records the background electrical activity of the brain by means of electrodes placed on the scalp or on or in the brain. The activity recorded is mainly that of the most superficial layers of the cortical grey substance.

CLINICAL ASPECTS

The nervous system is the most developed and very sensitive system. Various congenital and acquired diseases affect the nervous system.

Diseases of the Brain and Spinal Cord

Microcephaly

In this condition, the child's head is very small. The sutures of skull bone fuse prematurely making the skull small. The brain is also small because it cannot grow inside the skull. Such children are usually mentally retarded.

Increased Intracranial Pressure

The cranial cavity encloses brain, CSF, cerebral blood vessels and blood within the rigid cavity. An increase in the volume of any these raises the intracranial pressure (ICP). Rise in ICP is associated with a reduction in blood flow leading to hypoxia and neuronal damage. Rise in ICP also leads to hypertension and bradycardia. Rise in ICP also leads to herniation (displacement of part of brain from its usual compartment) of any part of brain.

Hydrocephalus

There is blockage to the flow of CSF leading to dilatation of ventricles leading to increased ICP. It leads to destruction of neural tissue.

Cerebral Oedema

It results from excessive accumulation of fluid in brain cells and/or in interstitial space leading to increased ICP. It is due to injury, haemorrhage, infections, ischaemia, hypoxia or tumours.

Parkinson's Disease

It results from gradual degeneration of dopamine releasing neurons in extra-pyramidal system. Clinical features are due to lack of control and coordination of muscle movement. It results in muscle tremors, expressionless face, stiff shuffling gait and stooping posture.

Dementia

There is gradual impairment of short-term memory, reasoning, thinking with personality changes due to mental deterioration. It is usually due to progressive, irreversible degeneration and atrophy of cerebral cortex.

Alzheimer's disease (presenile dementia) is the commonest type of dementia. It is commoner in females and affects those over 60 years. Dementia also occurs in stroke, encephalitis, AIDS, head injury, vitamin B deficiency, renal failure and alcohol abuse.

Stroke

It occurs when a vascular disease suddenly interrupts flow of blood to the brain causing hypoxia (cerebrovascular disease). It occurs due to cerebral infarction (85%) and spontaneous intracranial haemorrhage (15%). Cerebral infarction results from either thrombosis (due to atheroma) or embolism or haemorrhage (due to uncontrolled hypertension) of a cerebral artery. It may lead to paralysis of a limb or one side of body and disturbances of speech and vision.

Head Injury

The brain may be injured by a blow to the head or movement of the brain during sudden acceleration or deceleration of the head. It causes intracranial haemorrhage increasing the ICP leading to damage to the brain. It may be:

1. *Extradural haemorrhage:* There is collection of blood between inner table of skull and dura mater.
2. *Subdural haemorrhage:* There is collection of blood between layers of dura mater. It occurs from veins in dura mater.
3. *Intracerebral haemorrhage:* There are diffuse or localised haemorrhage inside the brain.

Epilepsy

It is usually idiopathic but may develop after head injury. It is characterised by seizures (fits), i.e. short, recurrent attacks of motor, sensory or psychological malfunction. The attacks are initiated by abnormal electrical discharge from neurons in the brain.

It can be treated by antiepileptic drugs.

Meningitis

The inflammation of meninges of brain is called meningitis. This occurs by blood borne infection or in injury to skull bones causing leakage of CSF. It can occur due to bacterial or viral agents. The bacterial meningitis is a serious condition and leads to high mortality while the viral meningitis is a relatively mild infection followed by complete recovery.

Clinical features of bacterial meningitis are severe headache, neck stiffness, fever and skin rash.

Encephalitis

There is infection of brain tissue. It may be because of viral or bacterial infection. There is infection of neurons and neuroglia, followed by necrosis and gliosis. As destroyed neurons (nerve cells) are not replaced, loss of function occurs, depending on the site and extent of brain damage.

Herpes Zoster

Herpes zoster virus causes **zoster** (shingles) in adults and **chickenpox** in children. Susceptible children after infection develop chickenpox. The viruses in them may remain dormant in posterior root ganglia in spinal nerves, which become active years later causing zoster. In zoster, painful vesicles develop along the course of the nerve with **hyperaesthesia** (hypersensitivity to touch). Infection is usually unilateral and is along the intercostal nerves or ophthalmic division of trigeminal nerve **(trigeminal neuralgia).**

Poliomyelitis

It is caused by poliovirus. Infection spreads by food contaminated by infected faecal matter. From alimentary tract virus spreads to the anterior horn cells of the spinal cord by blood. Usually, infection is asymptomatic or causes mild febrile illness. In less than 1% irreversible damage to anterior horn cells causes muscle paralysis. In severe cases, death may occur due to respiratory paralysis.

Poliomyelitis has been prevented by vaccination. India has eradicated poliomyelitis.

Rabies

It is a fatal disease caused by a virus that reaches the CNS via the axons. It is usually caused by bite of a rabied dog. Virus multiplies in salivary glands and are present in large number in saliva. They enter the body by bite of animal and travel to brain along the nerves. Clinical features are excitement, aggressiveness, hydrophobia, convulsions/ seizures, muscle spasm followed by paralysis and death.

Aphasia

It is the inability to use or comprehend words. It results from injury to language areas of the cerebral cortex.

Multiple Sclerosis

It results from progressive destruction of myelin sheath of neurons in CNS. It is the most common in females and in whites. The myelin sheath is replaced by irregularly distributed hardened scars or plaques (scleroses) in white matter of brain and spinal cord. It interferes with propagation of nerve impulses.

Clinical features are relapsing-remitting and include weakness in skeletal muscles, abnormal sensations, double vision or lack of coordination and movement.

Cerebral Palsy

It is a motor disorder that causes loss of muscle control and coordination. It is caused by damage to the motor areas of the brain during fetal life, birth or infancy.

Spinal Cord Injury

The spinal cord may be damaged by trauma, tumours or herniated intervertebral discs. Depending on the location and extent of spinal cord damage, paralysis may occur.

1. *Monoplegia* is paralysis of one limb only.
2. *Diplegia* is paralysis of both upper limbs or both lower limbs.
3. *Paraplegia* is paralysis of both lower limbs.
4. *Quadriplegia* is paralysis of all *four limbs*.
5. *Hemiplegia* is paralysis of upper limb, trunk and lower limb on one side of the body.

Injury to the cord results in loss of sensations and voluntary movements below the level of injury. **Spinal shock** is immediate response to spinal cord injury characterized by temporary loss of reflex function. It may last from several minutes to several months, after which reflex activity gradually returns.

Spina Bifida

It is a congenital malformation of neural canal and spinal cord. It is most commonly seen in lumbosacral region. The neural arches of the vertebrae are absent and the dura mater is abnormal. In severe cases, spinal cord is displaced backwards, the skin is deficient with leakage of CSR. There may be paralysis of both lower limbs with incontinence (loss of sphincter control) of urine and faeces, and mental retardation.

Motor Neuron Disease

There is progressive degeneration of motor neurons in cerebral cortex, brainstem and spinal cord anterior horn cells. Seen in men between 60 and 70 years of age. It leads to weakness of muscles of hand, followed by muscles of the arm and shoulder girdle. The legs are affected later.

Prolapsed Intervertebral Disc

The bodies of vertebrae are separated by **intervertebral discs,** consisting of an outer rim of cartilage, **annulus fibrosus** and a central core of soft gelatinous material, **nucleus pulposus.**

Prolapse of disc is herniation of nucleus pulposus causing annulus fibrosus and posterior longitudinal ligament to protrude into the neural canal.

It is most common in the lumbar region, followed by cervical region. It is the most common cause of compression of spinal cord and/or nerve roots. It usually occurs suddenly in young adults during strenuous exercise (Fig. 8.35).

Tumours

Tumours mostly arise from the neuroglial cells as these are capable of dividing. Neurons do not form tumour as these have lost the power of division due to their high evolution.

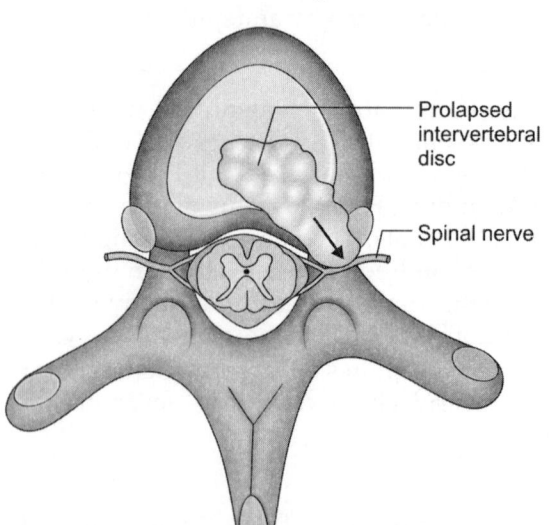

Fig. 8.35: Prolapsed intervertebral disc

Diseases of Peripheral Nerves

Neuropathies

This is a group of diseases of peripheral nerves not associated with inflammation. It can be polyneuropathy (several neurons are affected) or mononeuropathy (single neuron is affected).

Polyneuropathy occurs in metabolic or toxic disorders, e.g. diabetes mellitus; folic acid, vitamin B_{12} or thiamine deficiency; toxicity due to lead, arsenic, mercury.

Mononeuropathy is usually due to pressure which causes ischemia.

1. *Erb's paralysis:* The small area where C5 and C6 ventral nerve roots join to form upper trunk which divides into a ventral and dorsal division. Two branches arise from here. In damage to this area, there is paralysis of many muscles of upper limb. The position of limb is adducted at shoulder joint, extended at elbow joint, pronated forearm with flexed fingers **(policeman taking a tip).**

2. *Axillary nerve paralysis:* The deltoid muscle is paralysed. The patient cannot abduct the shoulder joint between 20° and 90°. Rounded contour of shoulder is lost.

3. *Median nerve paralysis:* This is usually involved in **'carpal tunnel syndrome'.** There is atrophy of muscles of thenar eminence **(ape-like hand),** loss of sensation over lateral 3½ digits, clawing of index and middle fingers.

4. *Radial nerve paralysis:* Paralysis of this nerve in axilla, radial groove or upper arm results in paralysis or weakness of extension of elbow with **'wrist drop'.**

5. *Ulnar nerve paralysis:* Since ulnar nerve supplies 15 intrinsic muscles of the hand, there is **clawing** of the fingers, especially ring and little fingers, loss of hypothenar eminence and atrophy of muscles of the palm.

6. *Common peroneal nerve paralysis:* The most common nerve which gets paralysed in lower limb is the common peroneal nerve. Injury to this nerve causes inability to dorsiflex the foot, resulting in **'foot drop'.**

Guillain-Barré Syndrome

There is acute, progressive, bilateral ascending paralysis beginning in lower limbs and spreading to arms, trunk and cranial nerves. It usually occurs 1–3 weeks after an upper respiratory tract infection. There is widespread demyelination of nerves.

Bell's Palsy

It results from compression of facial nerve causing paralysis of facial muscles with drooping and loss of facial expression on affected side. Compression of facial nerve occurs at stylomastoid foramen. Recovery is usually complete within a few months.

Points to Remember

1. Neuron is the unit of nervous tissue.
2. Astrocytes form part of "blood–brain barrier."
3. Cervical (spinal) nerves are 8 while cervical vertebrae are 7 only.
4. Limbs are mostly supplied by ventral primary rami of the spinal nerves.
5. Plexuses are cervical, brachial, lumbosacral and coccygeal.
6. Sympathetic nervous system is thoracolumbar outflow.
7. Parasymphathetic nervous system is craniosacral outflow.
8. Sympathetic nerves are mostly responsible for the referred pain.

MCQs

1. **Number of spinal nerves in cervical region is:**
   (a) 7 nerves
   (b) 8 nerves
   (c) 6 nerves
   (d) 9 nerves

2. **Bipolar neurons are present in:**
   (a) Spiral ganglia
   (b) Vestibular ganglia
   (c) Olfactory cells
   (d) Neurons in posterior horn of spinal cord

3. **Reflex arc is made up of all parts *except*:**
   (a) Receptors, e.g. skin
   (b) Afferent neuron
   (c) Efferent neuron
   (d) Gland

4. **Thoracolumbar outflow arises from lateral horns of one of the following segments of spinal cord:**
   (a) $T_1 - L_2$ segments
   (b) $T_1 - L_1$ segments
   (c) $T_1 - L_1$ segments
   (d) $T_1 - S_1$ segments

5. **Parasympathetic outflow does not arise from which of following nerves:**
   (a) III nerve
   (b) VII nerve
   (c) XII nerve
   (d) $S_2–S_4$ nerves

6. **Referred pain of myocardial ischaemia is mostly felt at:**
   (a) Precordium aspect of left upper limb
   (b) Lateral aspect of left upper limb
   (c) Right shoulder region
   (d) Left shoulder region

Ans! 1 b   2 d   3 d   4 a   5 c.   6 a

Sensory Organs

The sensory organs of taste (tongue), smell (nose), hearing (ear), sight (eye) and touch (skin) have specialised receptors present outside the brain. These sense receptors are in close vicinity of brain and are governed by cranial nerves. Special senses work in harmony with each other and also with various muscles and glands.

TONGUE

It is a voluntary muscular organ situated in the oral cavity. It has following functions:

1. Helps in speech
2. Helps in swallowing
3. Contains **taste buds** which make us aware of various tastes. The multitude of eating shops like Pizza Huts, etc. are to please the taste buds. Stomach has none at all.

Musculature of tongue is comprised of intrinsic muscles (lying within tongue) and extrinsic muscles (one attachment is outside the tongue and other within it). Most of these are supplied by XII or hypoglossal nerve.

The sensation of taste is carried by branch of VII (facial) from most of the anterior two-thirds; by branch of IX (glossopharyngeal) from vallate papillae and posterior one-third of tongue; by branch of X (vagus) from posterior most part of tongue.

General sensation from anterior two-thirds is carried by lingual branch of V3 (mandibular branch of trigeminal nerve); from posterior one-third by IX; from posterior most part by X.

There are three types of papillae according to their shape.

1. *Filiform,* which make the dorsal surface of tongue rough.
2. *Fungiform* seen on the sides, contain few taste buds.
3. *Vallate* present in posterior part of anterior two-thirds of tongue. Contain maximum taste buds (Figs 9.1A and B).

The basic tastes are sweet, salt, sour and bitter (Fig. 9.2).

1. **Sweet:** Mainly on tip of tongue

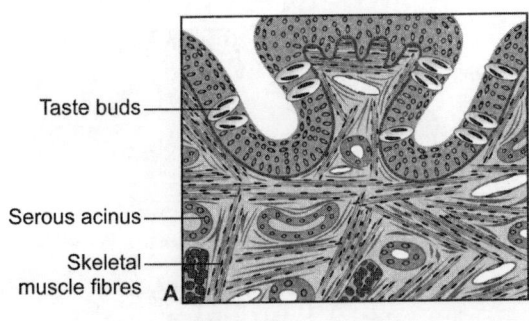
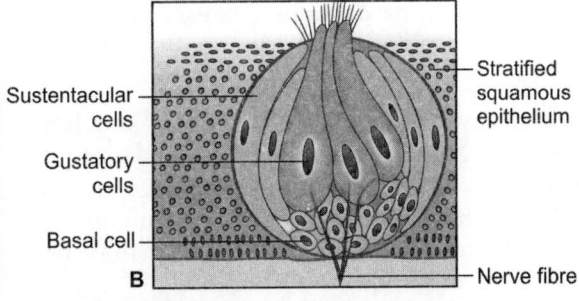

Figs 9.1A and B: Circumvallate papilla of tongue. Taste buds contain receptors on papillae of tongue. These are stimulated by chemicals that enter the pores dissolved in saliva

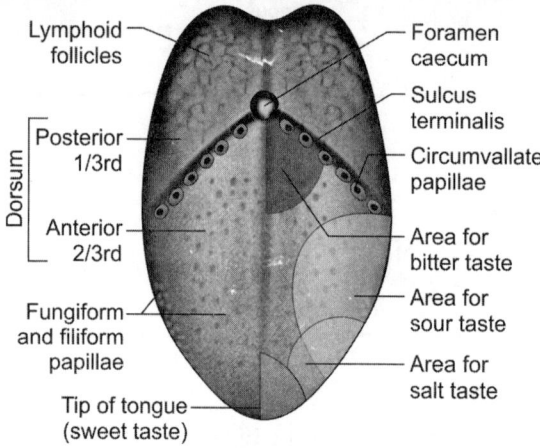

Fig. 9.2: Tongue with areas for taste

2. **Sour:** Mainly on edges of tongue
3. **Salt:** Mainly on dorsum anteriorly
4. **Bitter:** Mainly at back of tongue.

Arterial supply of tongue is by lingual artery branch of external carotid artery.

Veins unite to form lingual vein which drains into internal jugular vein.

Lymph drains to submandibular and deep cervical nodes. Lymph vessels cross within tongue from one side to the other.

Cancer of the tongue may involve lymph nodes of both sides. Cancer is common in people who keep betel nuts with lime for hours in their mouth.

NOSE

The nose is for breathing and the upper part of its lining contains olfactory nerve cells for smell. The nose consists of external nose and nasal cavity. The **external nose** is made of only two bones, the nasal bones, the rest is cartilage. The two openings on the face are the **anterior nares.**

Nasal cavity is divided into right and left halves by a median **nasal septum.** The septum is formed by thin bones and cartilage and is covered by mucoperiosteum or mucoperichondrium. At times, the septum may be deviated to one side.

Nasal cavity opens at the back into the nasopharynx through the posterior nares.

The lateral wall of nasal cavity shows three projections: (1) superior, (2) middle and (3) inferior **conchae** to increase the surface area. Below each concha is the respective **meatus.**

The paranasal air sinuses open into these meatuses. These are sphenoidal, ethmoidal, frontal and maxillary. These sinuses make the skull lighter, give resonance to the voice and humidify the inspired air (Fig. 9.3).

The main **artery** of the nasal cavity is sphenopalatine artery, the continuation of maxillary artery. Veins drain into maxillary vein.

Lymph drains into pharyngeal and deep cervical nodes.

The nerve supply to nasal cavity is of two types, **general sensation** like pain, touch, temperature carried by branches of V1 (ophthalmic) and V2 (maxillary) divisions of V or trigeminal nerve. The upper most part of septum and lateral wall (1 cm) contains olfactory cells for carrying sense of smell.

The nerve rootlets pass through holes (cribriform plate) in the ethmoid bone and reach lower aspect of frontal lobe. These join the olfactory bulb, which continues into olfactory tract to end in the uncus of temporal lobe.

Sense of smell is related to sense of taste. Sense of smell is also connected to X or vagus nerve which secretes the gastric juice in relation to good smell. Human beings can distinguish 2,000 to 4,000 different odours. Highly lipid and water soluble substances produce strong odours.

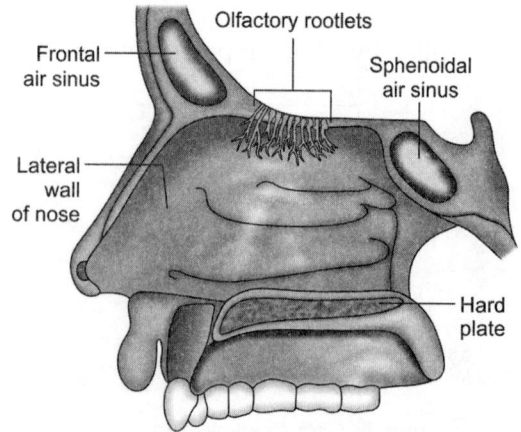

Fig. 9.3: Olfactory rootlets for sense of smell

Adaptation: It is a term used when olfactory receptors are exposed to a odour for a long time, the perception of that odour decreases and eventually ceases.

EAR

The ear is an important organ. Its functions are hearing and maintenance of the balance of body.

Ear consists of three parts: (1) external ear, (2) middle ear and (3) internal ear.

External Ear

Made up of **pinna or auricle and external auditory meatus. Auricle** projects from the side of head and is composed of elastic cartilage covered with skin. **External auditory meatus is** a 'S' shaped tube about 2.5 cm long and extends from auricle to tympanic membrane (Fig. 9.4).

Outer one-third of external auditory meatus is cartilaginous and inner two-thirds is bony. It is covered with skin, that contains numerous ceruminous glands in outer third, that secrete ear wax and has hair follicles. **Tympanic membrane** separates the external auditory meatus from middle ear. It is an oval shaped membrane placed obliquely.

Middle Ear

A box like small cavity with six walls, having a **chain of ossicles, malleus, incus and stapes** from lateral wall towards the medial wall (Fig. 9.5). The ossicles transmit the sound

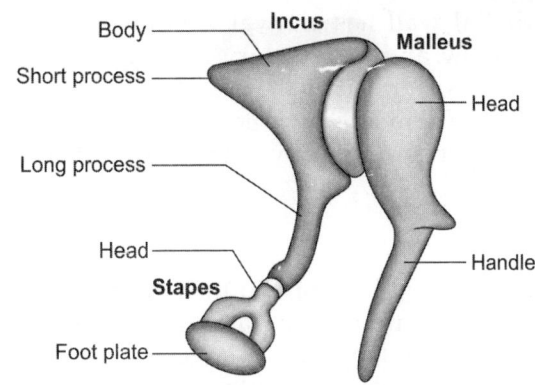

Fig. 9.5: Ossicles of middle ear

vibrations of tympanic membrane to internal ear.

Its **roof** is thin plate of bone in the middle cranial fossa.

Floor is small piece of bone near carotid canal.

Anterior wall contains auditory tube which equalises the pressure outside the ear and within the ear. It opens into the nasopharynx. Opening of auditory tube usually remains closed but opens during chewing, swallowing, yawning. Anterior wall also contains a canal for tensor tympani muscle.

Posterior wall consists of mastoid antrum, facial canal, pyramid containing stapedius muscle.

Lateral wall is formed by tympanic membrane (Fig. 9.6).

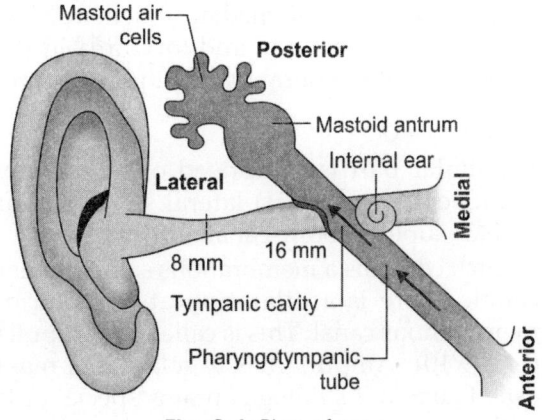

Fig. 9.4: Plan of ear

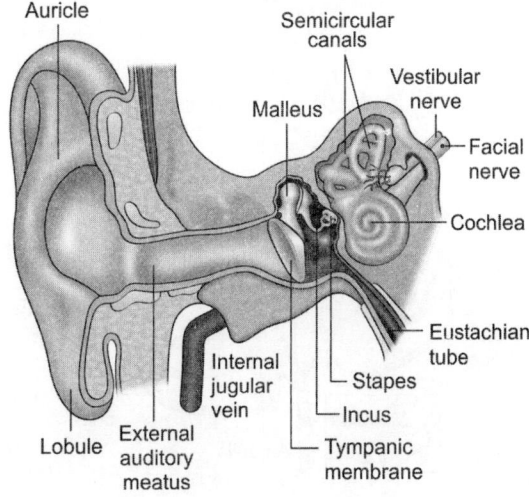

Fig. 9.6: Components of ear

Medial wall has an oval window, a round window and promontory between the two windows formed by the basal turn of cochlea. The oval window is occluded by part of stapes and round window by a fine sheet of fibrous tissues.

Internal Ear

Internal ear is a cavity in the temporal bone. It is made up of two parts, one within the other. **Bony labyrinth** is larger and encloses the membranous labyrinth of the same shape which fits into it, like a tube within a tube. Between bony and membranous labyrinth there is watery fluid called **perilymph** and within membranous labyrinth there is watery fluid called **endolymph** (Figs 9.7 and 9.8). There is no communication between spaces filled with endolymph and those filled with perilymph.

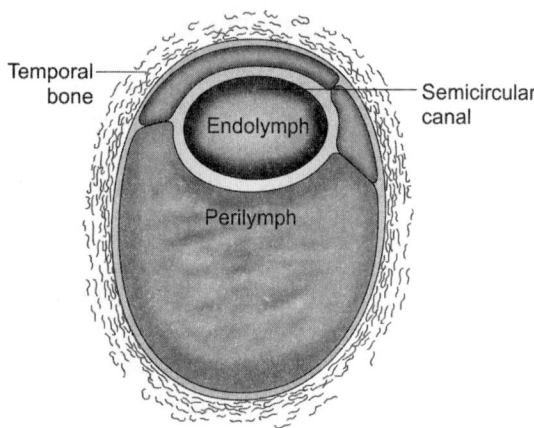

Fig. 9.7: Internal ear

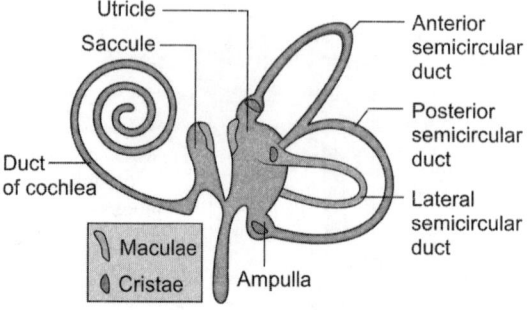

Fig. 9.8: Membranous labyrinth

Bony labyrinth consists of:

1. *Vestibule:* Expanded part nearest the middle ear. It contains oval and round windows in its lateral wall.

2. *Cochlea:* It has broad base where it is continuous with vestibule and a narrow apex.

3. *Semicircular canals:* The three tubes are arranged so that one is situated in each of the three planes of space. They are continuous with the vestibule.

Membranous labyrinth comprises of same three parts but the vestibule contains utricle and saccule.

The membranous labyrinth comprises the cochlea which functions as a hearing unit and a vestibular part which functions for proper balancing of the body and maintenance of posture of the body.

Cochlea

There is a bony cochlea like a shell which forms two and three-fourth circle. It contains perilymph and inside it is the membranous cochlea or cochlear duct.

The cochlear duct or scala media consists of basilar membrane on which phalangeal cells and rods of Corti are resting (Fig. 9.9).

The phalangeal cells support the hair cells.

Movement of perilymph through bony cochlea causes vibrations in the basilar membrane, to stimulate the hair cells.

Nerve fibres from hair cells reach the spiral ganglion from where the impulses travel along auditory (cochlear) nerve to reach cochlear nuclei. Then, through medial geniculate body the impulses reach the auditory area in the upper part of temporal lobe of the cerebrum.

Vestibular Part

Vestibular part is comprised of three bony semicircular canals: (1) lateral, (2) posterior and (3) superior bony canal.

Each contains a membranous semi-circular canal. There is a dilatation at one end of membranous canal. This is called the ampulla (Fig. 9.10). Ampulla has a gelatinous mass called cupola. Its lining contains special cells with nerve endings. Any deformation of these

Plate 1

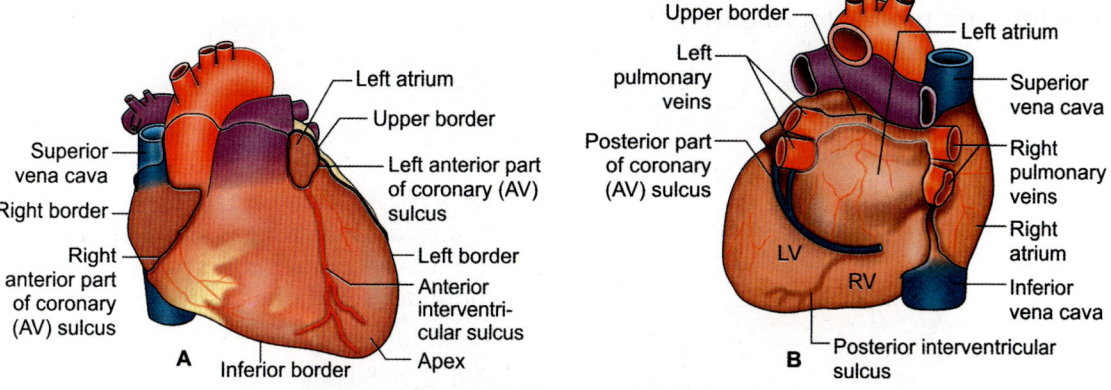

Figs 4.15A and B: Gross features: (A) sternocostal surface and (B) base of heart

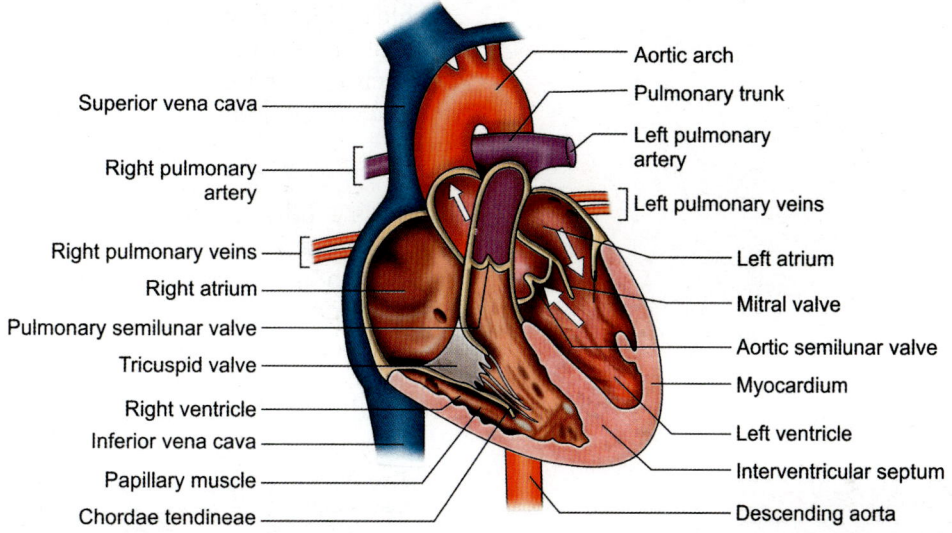

Fig. 4.16: Interior of the heart

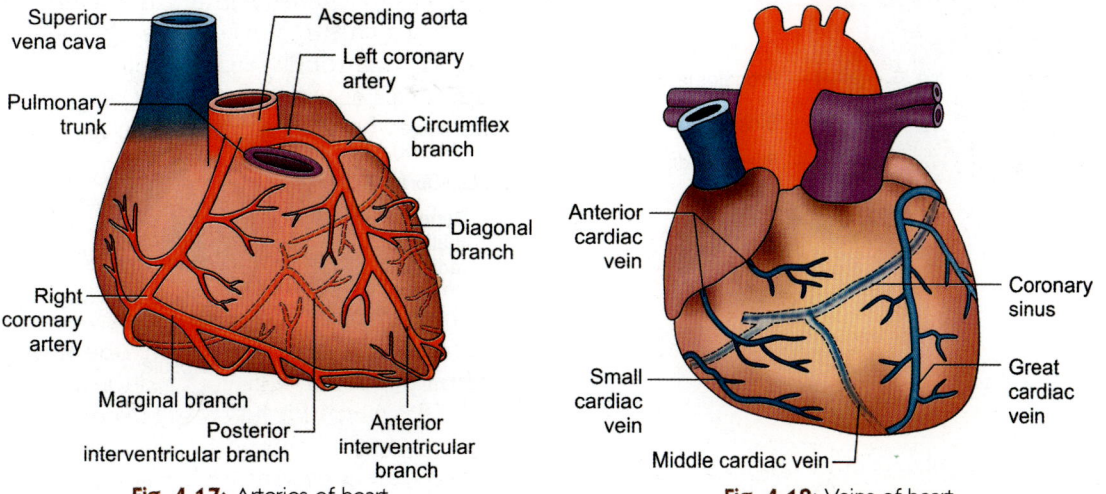

Fig. 4.17: Arteries of heart

Fig. 4.18: Veins of heart

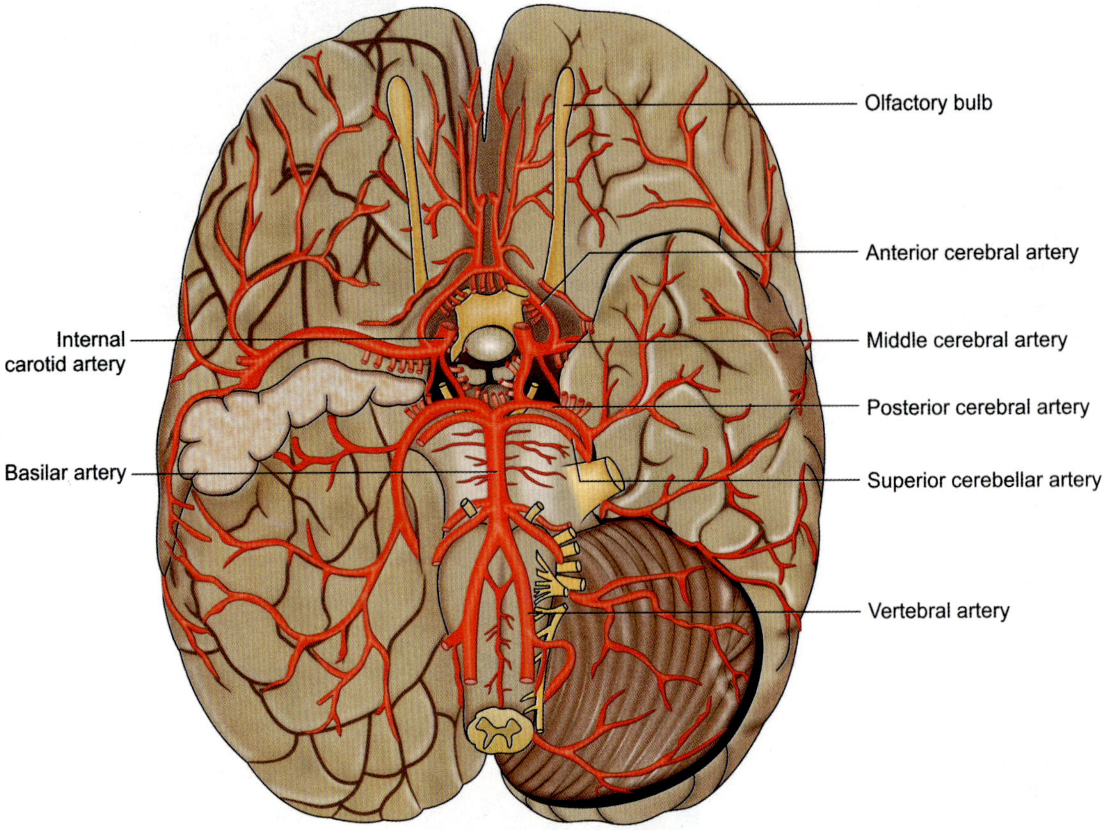

Plate 2

Olfactory bulb

Anterior cerebral artery

Internal
carotid artery

Middle cerebral artery

Posterior cerebral artery

Basilar artery

Superior cerebellar artery

Vertebral artery

Fig. 4.26: Arteries of brain

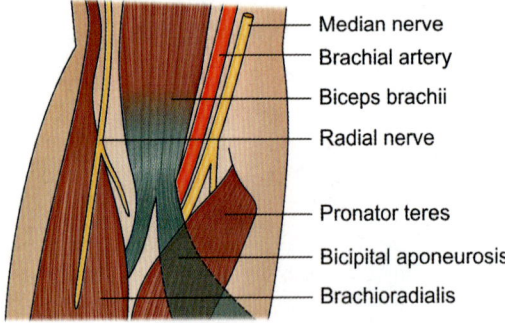

Median nerve

Brachial artery

Biceps brachii

Radial nerve

Pronator teres

Bicipital aponeurosis

Brachioradialis

Fig. 7.27: Cubital fossa

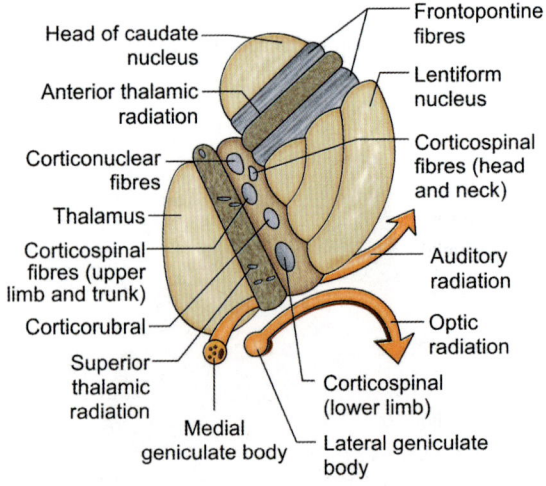

Frontopontine
fibres

Head of caudate
nucleus

Anterior thalamic
radiation

Lentiform
nucleus

Corticonuclear
fibres

Corticospinal
fibres (head
and neck)

Thalamus

Corticospinal
fibres (upper
limb and trunk)

Auditory
radiation

Corticorubral

Optic
radiation

Superior
thalamic
radiation

Corticospinal
(lower limb)

Medial
geniculate body

Lateral geniculate
body

Fig. 8.9: Internal capsule

Plate 3

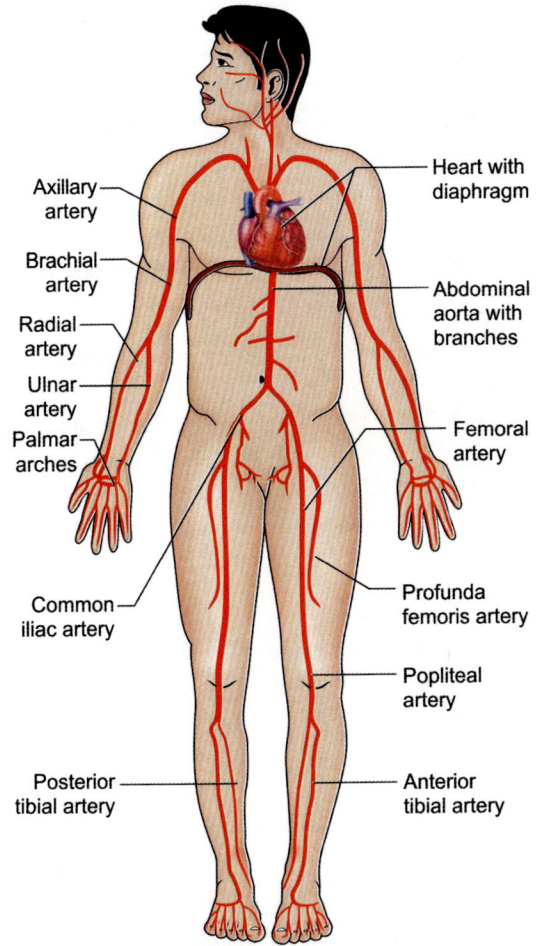

Axillary artery

Brachial artery

Radial artery

Ulnar artery

Palmar arches

Common iliac artery

Posterior tibial artery

Heart with diaphragm

Abdominal aorta with branches

Femoral artery

Profunda femoris artery

Popliteal artery

Anterior tibial artery

Fig. 14.2B: Arterial system

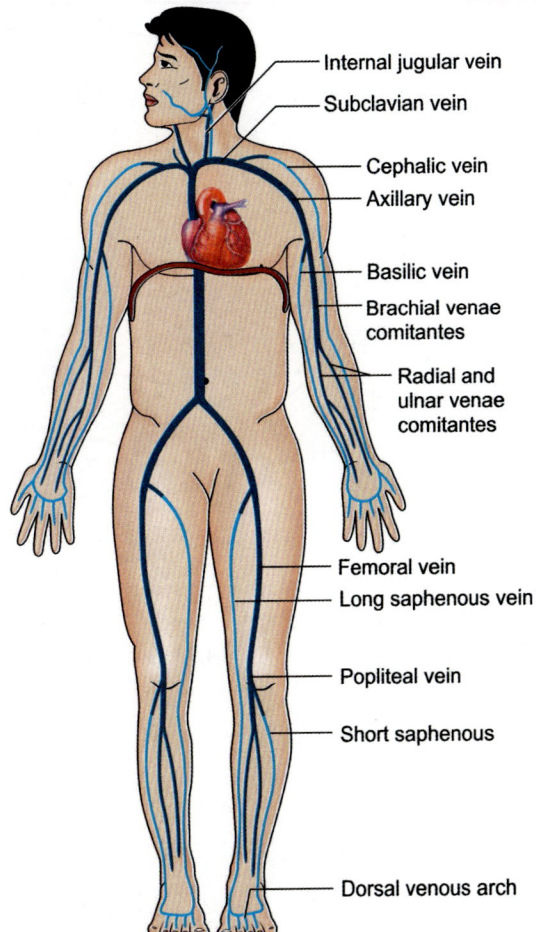

Internal jugular vein

Subclavian vein

Cephalic vein

Axillary vein

Basilic vein

Brachial venae comitantes

Radial and ulnar venae comitantes

Femoral vein

Long saphenous vein

Popliteal vein

Short saphenous

Dorsal venous arch

Fig. 14.2C: Venous system

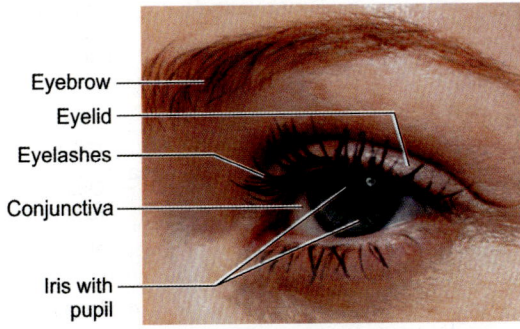

Eyebrow

Eyelid

Eyelashes

Conjunctiva

Iris with pupil

Fig. 14.7A: Parts of eye as seen from outside

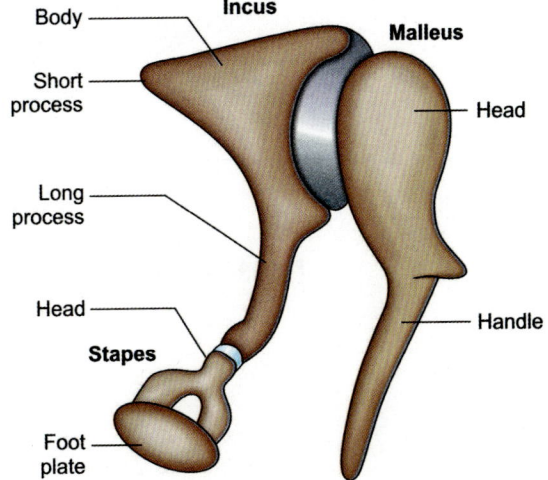

Body

Short process

Long process

Head

Stapes

Foot plate

Incus

Malleus

Head

Handle

Fig. 14.8B: Ossicles

Plate 4

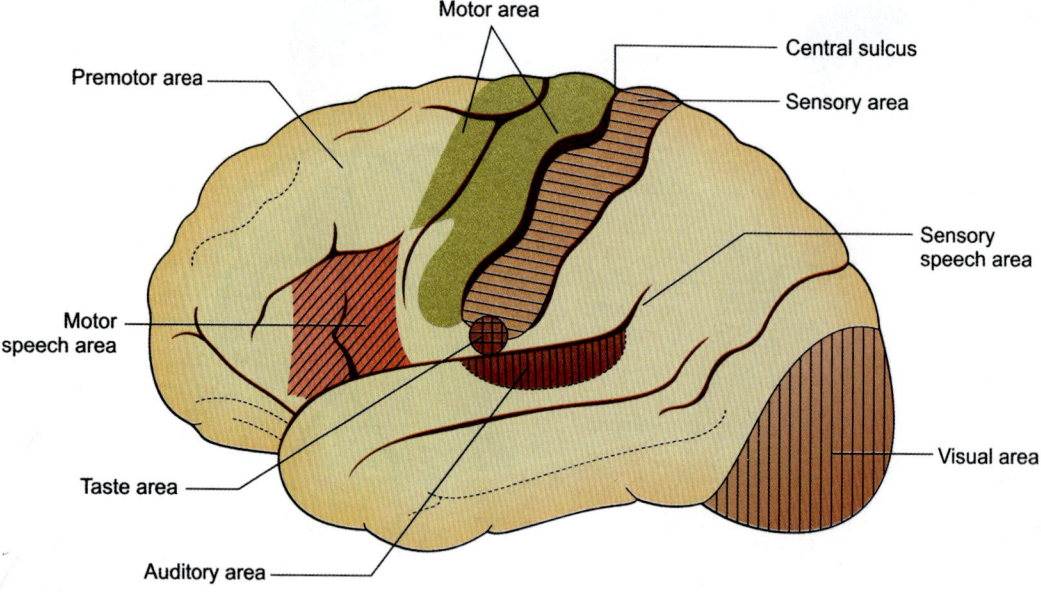

Fig. 14.9B: Superolateral surface of left cerebral hemisphere

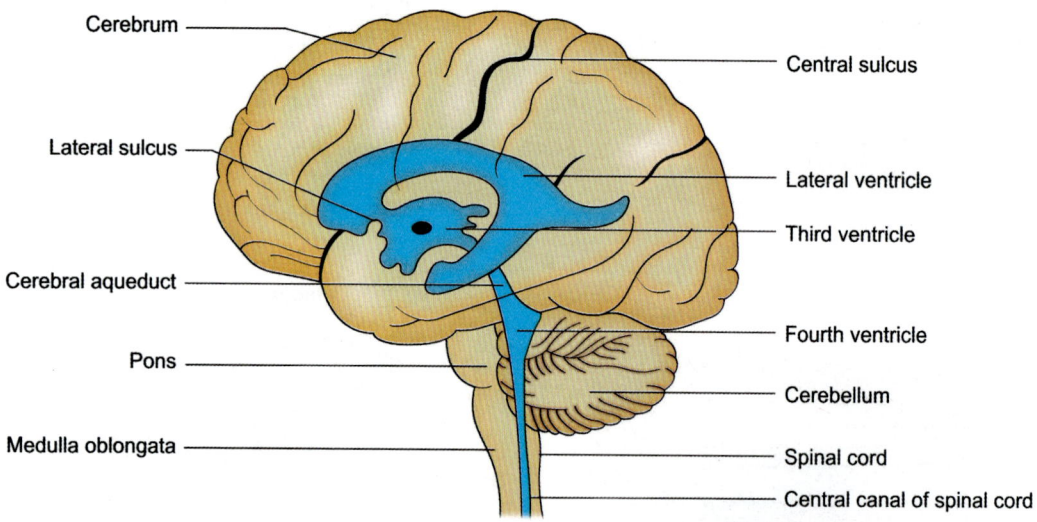

Fig. 14.9C: Ventricles of the brain with central canal of spinal cord

Plate 5

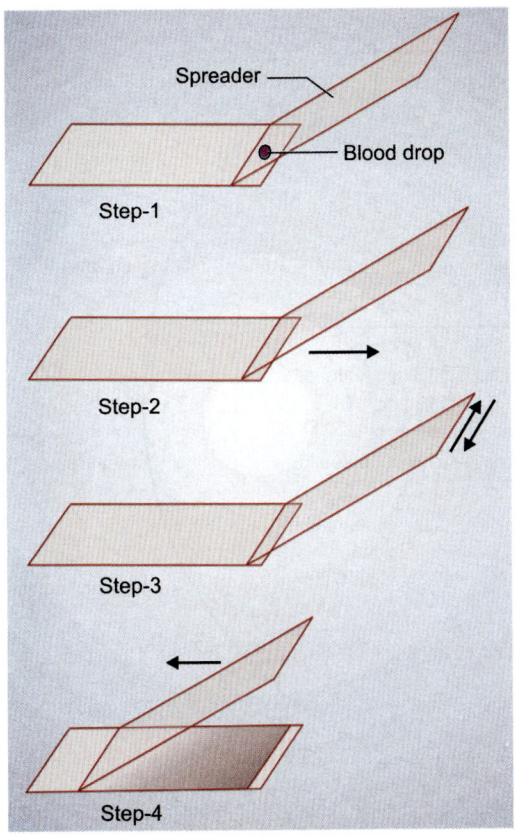

17.6: Steps of peripheral blood smear preparation

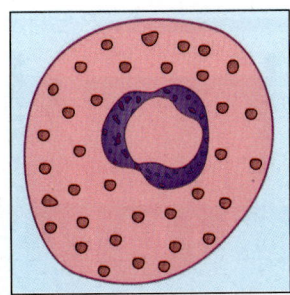

Fig. 17.8B: Neutrophil (polymorph)

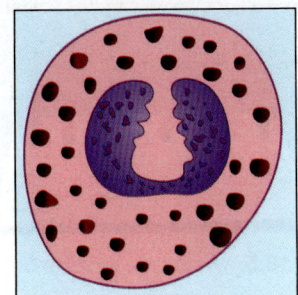

Fig. 17.9B: Eosinophil

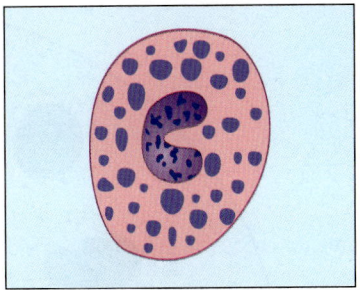

Fig. 17.10B: Basophil

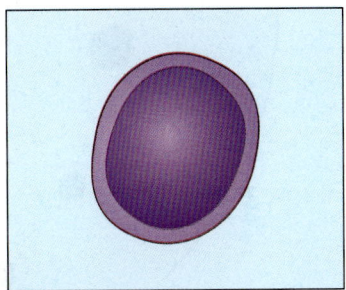

Fig. 17.11B: Small lymphocyte

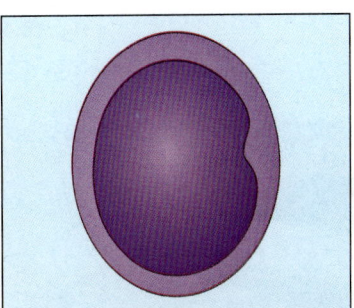

Fig. 17.12B: Large lymphocyte

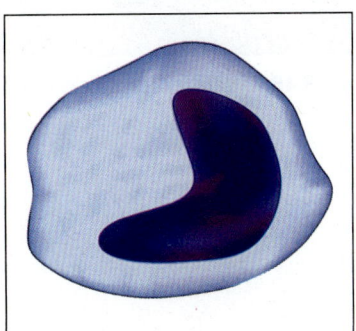

Fig. 17.13B: Monocyte

Plate 6

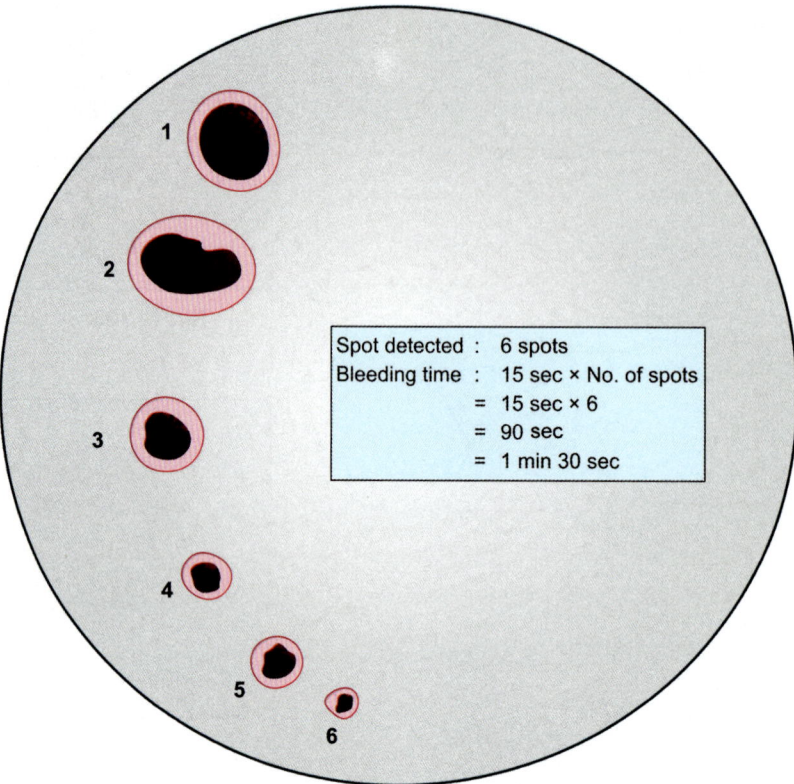

Spot detected   :   6 spots
Bleeding time   :   15 sec × No. of spots
              =   15 sec × 6
              =   90 sec
              =   1 min 30 sec

Fig. 18.4A: Determination of bleeding time

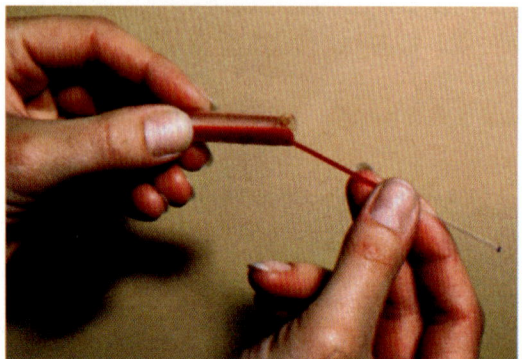

Fig. 18.4B: Determination of clotting time

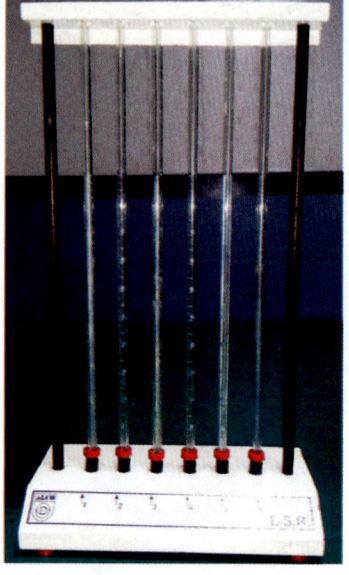

Fig. 18.5: Westergren tubes and stand

Plate 7

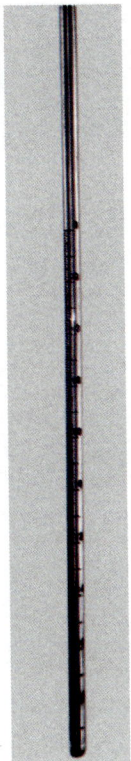

Fig. 18.6: Westergren pipette marking

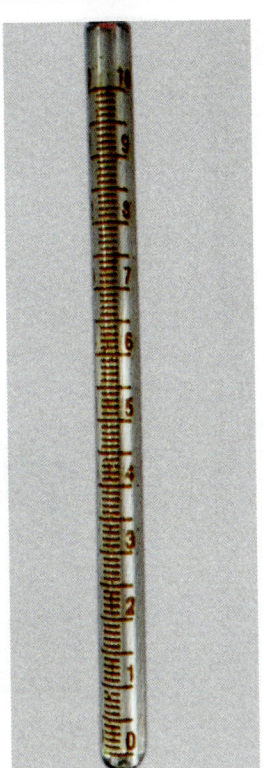

Fig. 18.8: Wintrobe tube marking 10 to 0

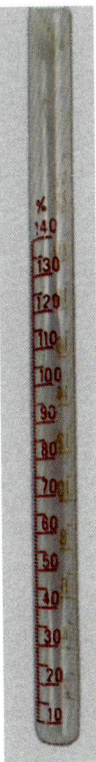

Fig. 18.11: Sahli graduated tube percentage marking

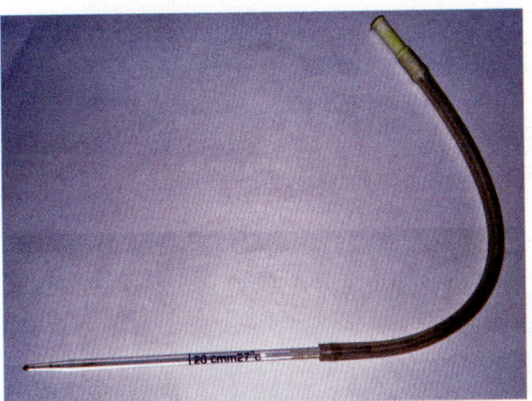

Fig. 18.12: Haemoglobin pipette

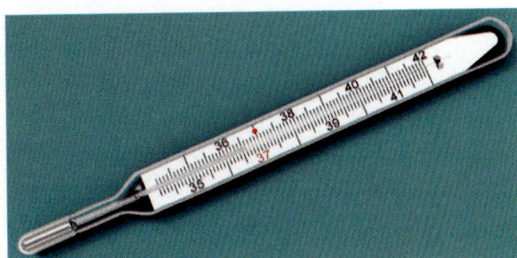

Fig. 19.1: Clinical glass thermometer for oral and axillary temperature measurement

Plate 8

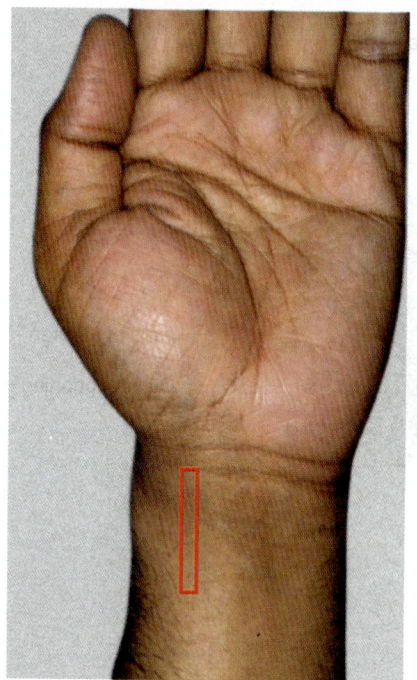

Fig. 19.2: Location of radial artery

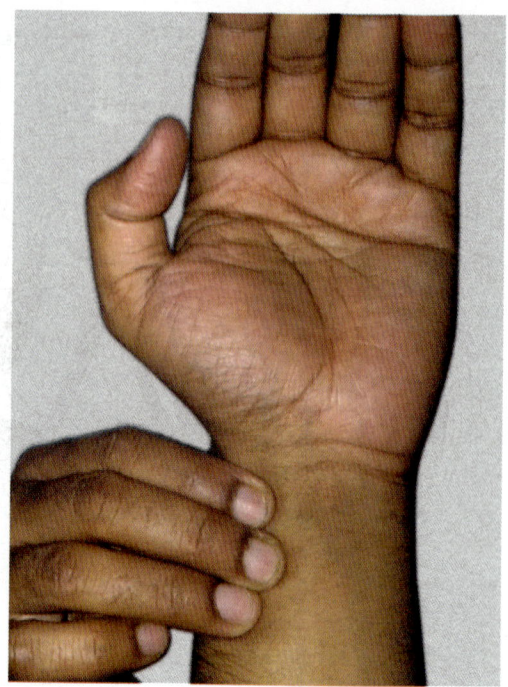

Fig. 19.3: Pulse rate measurement from radial artery

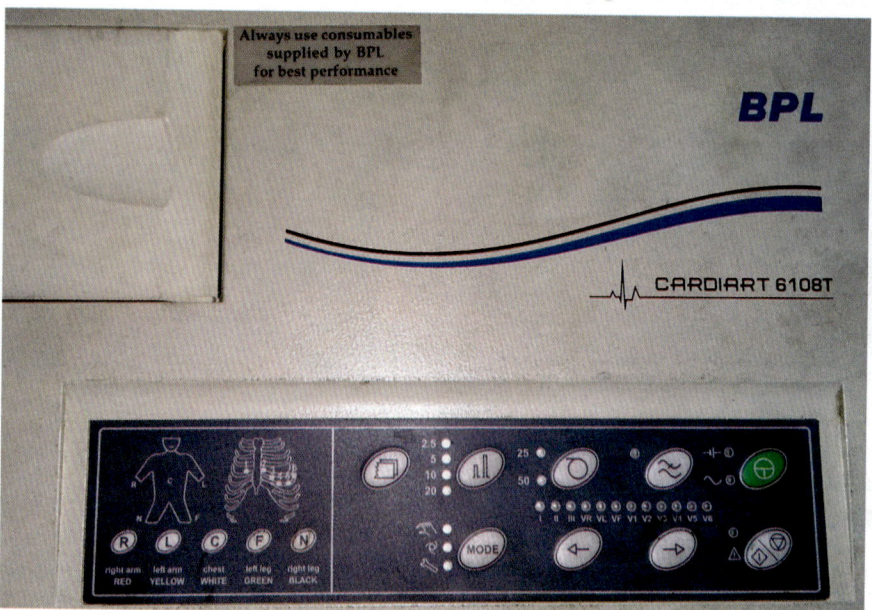

Fig. 19.7: ECG machine

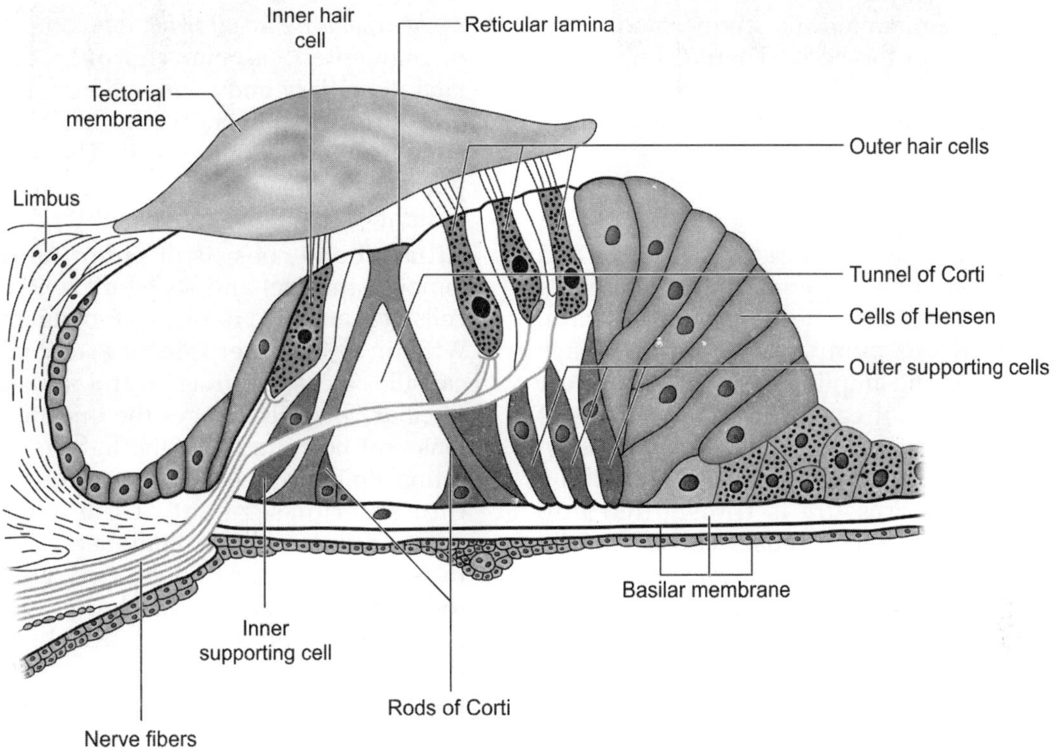

Inner hair cell

Reticular lamina

Tectorial membrane

Limbus

Outer hair cells

Tunnel of Corti

Cells of Hensen

Outer supporting cells

Basilar membrane

Inner supporting cell

Rods of Corti

Nerve fibers

Fig. 9.9: Cochlea

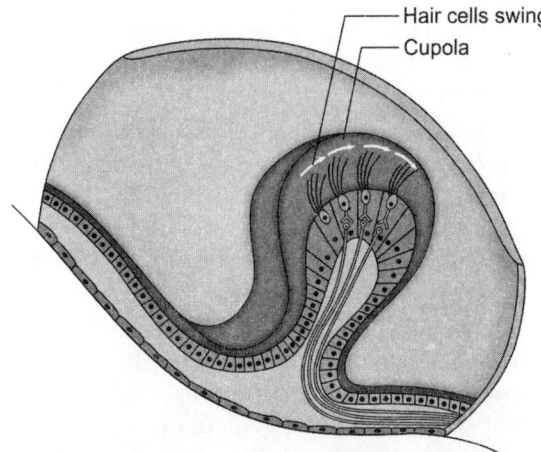

Hair cells swing

Cupola

Fig. 9.10: Ampulla of semicircular canal

cells send impulses to vestibular division of VIII nerve, to reach the vestibular nuclei. These are connected to cerebellum of brain. The semicircular canals maintain the angular equilibrium of the body.

Vestibular part is also comprised of **bony vestibule,** which contains the **utricle** con-

nected to three semicircular canals and **saccule** connected to the cochlea.

Utricle and saccule also contain end organs for providing the linear equilibrium to the body. These contain an **otolith membrane** (Fig. 9.11).

The movement of special hair cells stimulate the nerve endings and sends impulses along vestibular part of VIII nerve. Thus, the vestibular nerve, semicircular canals, utricle

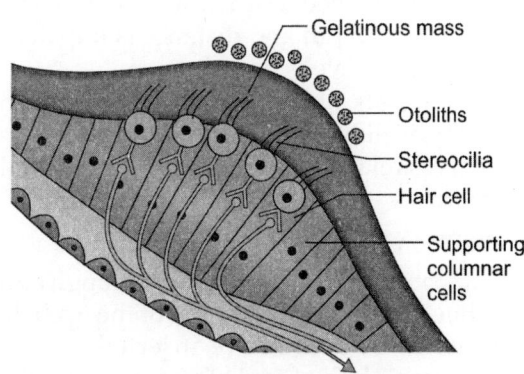

Gelatinous mass

Otoliths

Stereocilia

Hair cell

Supporting columnar cells

Fig. 9.11: Otolith membrane of utricle and saccule

and saccule maintain the angular and linear equilibrium of the body. There is one artery for internal ear. This end artery is the **labyrinthine artery,** branch of basilar artery.

Physiology of Hearing

Sound produces vibrations or sound waves in ear. The auricle concentrates the waves and direct them along external auditory meatus causing tympanic membrane to vibrate. Vibrations of tympanic membrane are transmitted and amplified through middle ear by movement of ear ossicles. Movement of foot plate of stapes in oval window sets up fluid waves in perilymph of scala vestibuli. Most of the pressure is transmitted into cochlear duct, which causes corresponding waves in endolymph. It results in vibration of basilar membrane and stimulation of auditory receptors in hair cells of spiral organ. Nerve impulses pass to the brain in the auditory branch of VIII cranial nerve.

The auditory nerve and cochlea subserve the function of hearing appreciated in the temporal lobe of brain.

EYE

Eye is the sense organ for the sense of sight. It is situated in the orbital cavity and sense of sight is carried by optic nerve.

Each eye is almost spherical in shape and has a diameter of about 2.5 cm. The space between the eye and orbital cavity is occupied by adipose tissue. Activities of both the eyes are coordinated so they function as a pair. It is possible to see with one eye but the judgement of depth and distance is impaired when only one eye is used.

Eye consists of the **eyeball** (partly seen when the eyelids are open) including muscles and nerves related to the eyeball and **lacrimal apparatus.**

Eyeball consists of following three layers:

1. *Outer most is the sclera,* which is tough and white in colour forms 5/6th of the eyeball. Muscles of eyeball are inserted into it. Anterior 1/6th of eyeball is formed by the transparent **cornea** (Fig. 9.12).

2. *Middle coat is the uveal tract.* It is comprised of pigmented vascular **choroid,** antero-laterally **ciliary body** with ciliary muscles and anteriorly curtain like iris with a circular aperture, the **pupil.** The size of pupil can change according to the amount of light entering the eye (Fig. 9.12).

Ciliary body consists of **ciliary muscle** (smooth muscle) and secretory epithelial cells. It is attached to suspensory ligament which, at its other end is attached to capsule of lens. Contraction and relaxation of ciliary muscle changes the thickness of lens and helps to focus the light rays on retina. Epithelial cells secrete aqueous fluid into anterior segment of the eye, i.e. anterior and posterior chambers. Ciliary muscles are supplied by 3rd cranial (oculomotor) nerve. Stimulation causes contraction of smooth muscle and accommodation of eye.

Iris is visible coloured part of eye, lying behind cornea in front of lens. It consists of two layers of smooth muscle fibers.

Lens is circular biconvex structure lying behind the pupil. It is enclosed in a capsule and suspended from ciliary body by suspensory ligament.

3. *The inner most layer is the photosensitive retina,* comprising of layers of numerous **rods** (for night vision) and **cones** (for day vision, colour vision and brightness of vision), bipolar cell layer and ganglionic cell layer.

Axons of ganglionic cell layer form the optic nerve (II), which courses through the optic canal, forms optic chiasma, optic tract, synapses in the lateral geniculate body to end in the occipital lobe of the cerebral cortex.

Anterior segment of eye, i.e. anterior and posterior chambers contain **aqueous humour.** It is secreted into posterior chamber by ciliary glands. It circulates in front of the lens, through pupil into the anterior chamber and return to venous circulation through **canal of Schlemm** in the angle between iris and cornea. Aqueous humour supplies nutrients and removes metabolic products from transparent

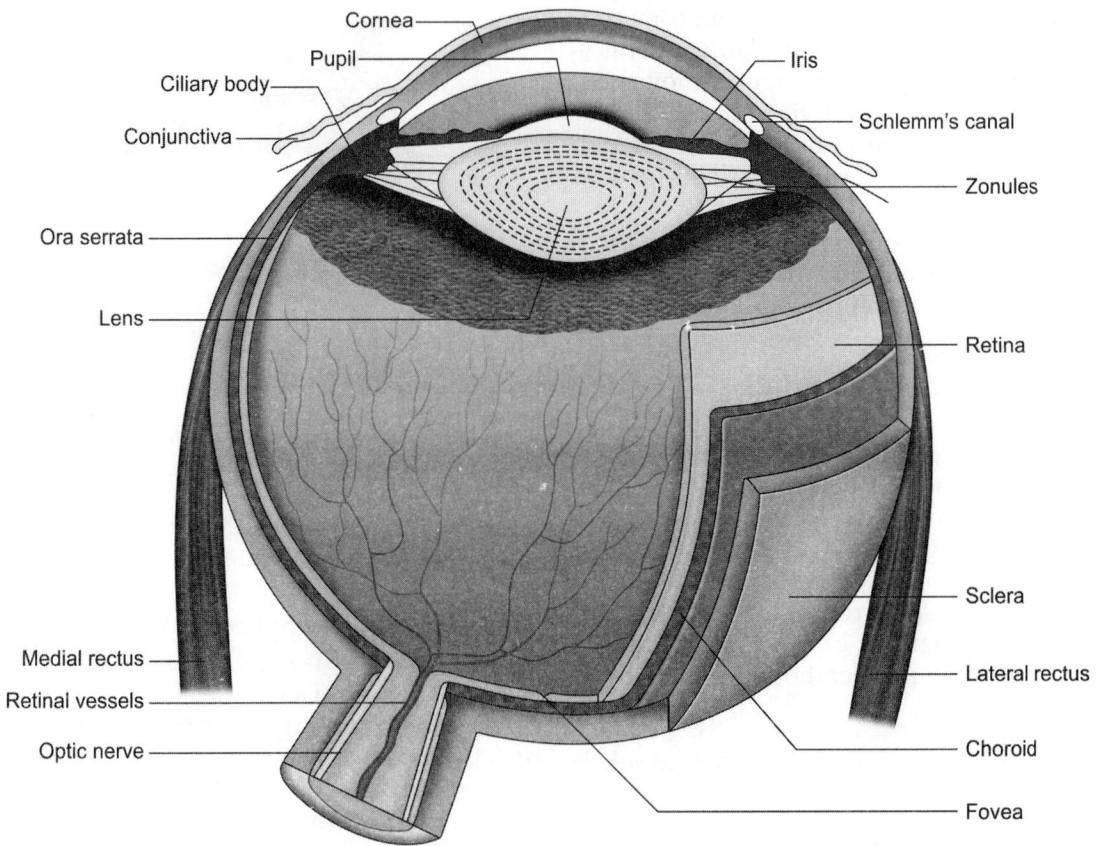

Fig. 9.12: Horizontal section of the eye

structures in front of eye that have no blood supply, i.e. cornea and lens.

Behind the lens, filling the posterior segment is **vitreous humour,** which is a transparent, soft jelly like substance. Both aqueous and vitreous humour help to maintain the shape of the eyeball because of the intraocular pressure exerted by these. Normally, the intraocular pressure is maintained between 10 mmHg and 20 mmHg.

Image Formation

The receptors for the vision are rods and cones present in the retina. To achieve clear vision, light reflected from objects within the visual field is focused on to the retina of each eye. The light rays have to pass through other layers to reach rods and cones, i.e. conjunctiva, cornea, aqueous humour, pupil of iris, lens and vitreous humour.

The process involved in production of a clear image are—refraction of light rays, changing the size of pupils and accommodation.

When light rays, pass from one medium to another medium of different density, the rays slightly bent out and it is known as **refraction.** This principle is used to focus light on the retina, lens is the only structure in eye that changes its refractive power to focus the light rays on the retina.

Pupil size influences accommodation by controlling the amount of light entering the eye. In dim light, the pupils are dilated and in bright light the pupils are constricted.

Accommodation

Accommodation is the process by which curvature of lens is increased to see an object close to the eye.

To see a near object, i.e. within 6 metres, the eye makes the following adjustments—constriction of pupils, convergence movement of eyeballs on the object viewed so that they stimulate the corresponding areas of two retina and changing the power of lens to focus the light on retina.

Distant objects, i.e. more than 6 metres away are focused on retina without convergence or change in power of lens.

Functions of Retina

Retina contains two light-sensitive nerve cells: (1) **rods** and (2) **cones.** Light rays cause chemical change in photosensitive pigments in these cells and they generate nerve impulses which are transmitted to the cerebrum via optic nerves. **Rhodopsin** is a photosensitive pigment present only in rods. It is degraded by bright light and it regenerates in darkened area. Visual pigment of cones also undergo breakdown and regeneration like in the rods.

Binocular Vision

When an object is viewed, both eyes see it slightly differently. There is an overlap in the middle but right eye sees more on the right than can be seen by the left eye and vice versa. The images from two eyes are fused in cerebral cortex so that only one image is perceived. Binocular vision is important to perceive the depth and proportion of the object.

Extraocular Muscles

The eyeball is situated in the anterior part of the bony **orbit.** In the posterior part of bony orbit are the various muscles, to move the eyeball in various directions. Their associated nerves and blood vessels.

There are seven muscles. These are:

1. *Lateral rectus, medial rectus* which move the eyeball laterally and medially (Fig. 9.13).
2. *Superior rectus* moves the centre of cornea upwards and medially while **inferior** rectus moves it downwards and medially.
3. *Superior oblique* moves centre of cornea downwards and laterally and **inferior** oblique takes it upwards and laterally.
4. *Levator palpebrae superioris* lifts the upper eyelid to open the eye.

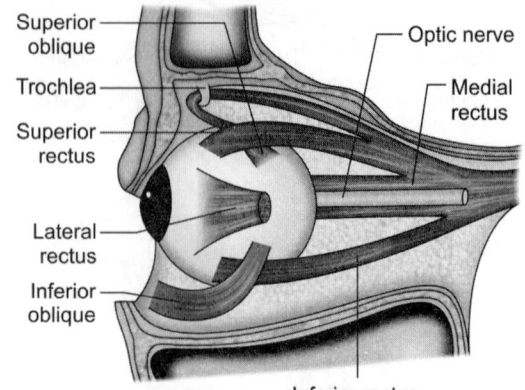

Fig. 9.13: Muscles of eyeball

Muscles of two eyes move in coordination. To look to right side, lateral rectus of right eye and medial rectus of left eye would contract.

5. *Lateral rectus* is supplied by VI nerve.
6. *Superior oblique* is supplied by IV nerve.

Rest of the muscles, i.e. medial rectus, inferior oblique, superior rectus, inferior rectus and part of levator palpebrae superioris are supplied by III nerve. Muscles which constrict the pupil and muscles which increase the curvature of lens are supplied by parasympathetic fibres through III nerve.

Blood supply is from ophthalmic artery, branch of internal carotid. The central artery of retina is the branch of ophthalmic artery for retina. It is an end artery. It does not anastomose with any other artery. If blocked, it leads to blindness in the affected eye. Venous drainage occurs into cavernous venous sinus. The retinal artery and vein are encased in optic nerve, entering the eye at the optic disc.

Lacrimal Apparatus

These are the components in relation to anterior part of eyeball which secrete lacrimal fluid for lubrication between the eyelids and the eyeball. These are the laterally situated **lacrimal gland** and its ducts which open into the conjunctival sac (Fig. 9.14).

At the medial end of the conjunctival sac are the two **lacrimal canaliculi.** They join together to open into **lacrimal sac,** which is connected by **nasolacrimal duct** to the inferior meatus of the nose.

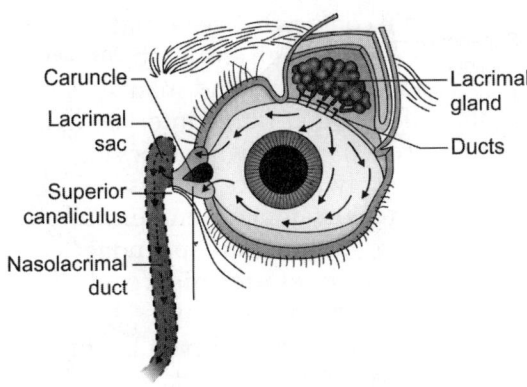

Fig. 9.14: Lacrimal apparatus

The secretions **(lacrimal fluid)** flows in the sac and is drained into the nasal cavity. If excessive amount is secreted, these are called the **tears.**

Eyelids and Eyebrows

Protecting the delicate and precious eyeball are the upper and lower **eyelids** with **eyelashes** (Fig. 9.15). Front of the eyeball and eyelids are covered by a fine transparent membrane, conjunctiva. It protects the cornea and the front of eye. The medial and lateral angles of eye where upper and lower lids come together are called medial and lateral **canthus** respectively. The eyelids can be moved by two muscles, orbicularis oculi and levator palpebrae superioris. Eyelid margin also has opening of several glands. The eyebrows prevent the sweat of forehead from entering the eyes and protect the anterior aspect of eyeball from injuries by foreign objects.

Eyes are very important to a person, as one views the external world through his/her eyes. The clinician can see retina, central artery and vein of retina through an instrument called **ophthalmoscope**, put opposite the cornea with dilated pupil.

SKIN

Skin is the outermost garment of our body. The thickness of skin varies from 0.1 to 4.0 mm depending on requirement. It is thinnest on the lips (mucocutaneous) and thickest on the soles. It is made up of two layers, the outer is the epidermis and inner is the dermis (Fig. 9.16).

Epidermis is composed of stratified (multiple layered) squamous (uppermost cells are flattened), keratinised (cells produce **keratin**, a protein which is water proof) epithelium.

The outermost layer is especially thick in palm and sole to protect the underlying structures. Epidermis has no blood vessels or

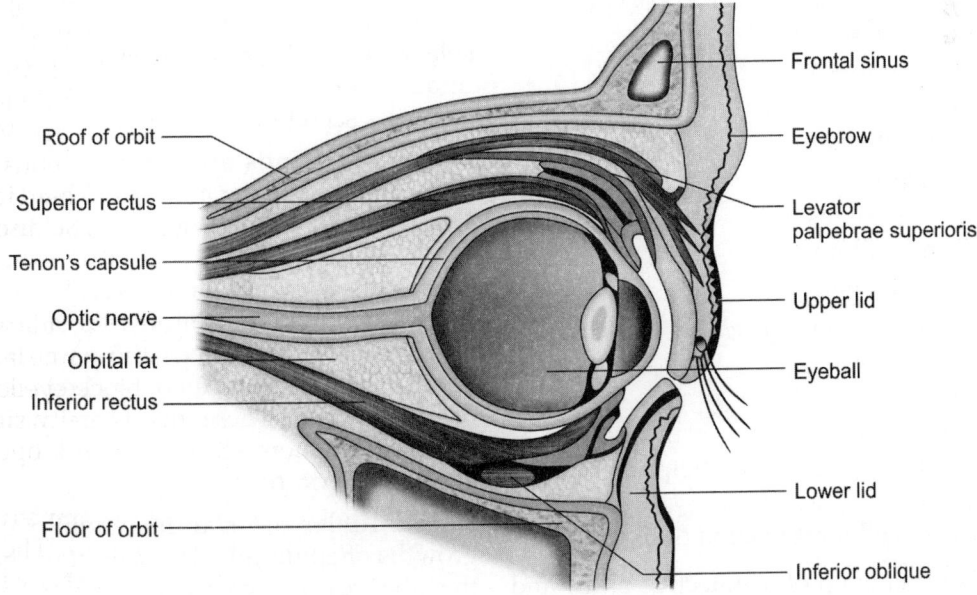

Fig. 9.15: Section of the eye and its accessory structures

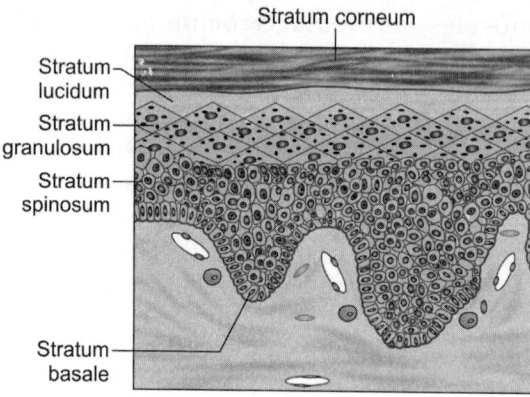

Fig. 9.16: Histological structure of skin

nerve endings. Epidermis is several layered thick. The deepest layer is **stratum germinativum.** Cells in this layer multiply to give rise to the superficial layer.

Stratum corneum is the outermost layer. It has flat, thin, non-nucleated, dead cells in which cytoplasm and its contents are converted into keratin. These cells are constantly shed off and are replaced by cells originating in the deepest layer and gradually change as they progress towards the surface. Complete replacement of epidermis takes about 40 days. There are melanocytes also in the epithelium, which secrete melanin. It protects skin from ultraviolet rays of sun. Various layers of epidermis are shown in Fig. 9.16.

The germinal layers are:
1. Stratum basale
2. Stratum spinosum.

The horny layers are:
1. Stratum granulosum
2. Stratum lucidum
3. Stratum corneum.

There are four types of cells in the epidermis. They are:

1. Keratinocytes
2. Melanocytes
3. Langerhans cells which help in immune response
4. Merkel's cell for sensation of touch.

Dermis is made up of connective tissue and shows projections, the **papillae,** which help

to make tight contacts between epidermis and dermis. Dermis is tough and elastic. It is made up of connective tissue and matrix, varying number of collagen fibres interlacing with elastic fibres. It contains phagocytes, small blood vessels, lymphatics, nerves and nerve endings for pain, touch, temperature and pressure and various skin appendages. The nourishment to epidermis reaches via diffusion from dermal blood vessels.

The direction of dermal papillae produce specialised patterns like whorls, loops, arches at the tips of fingers and in toes. This science is called dermatoglyphics.

Deeper to the dermis is areolar tissue and varying amount of adipose tissue (fat).

Appendages of Skin

These are sweat gland, sebaceous gland, hair follicle and nails.

Sweat gland is an invagination of the epidermal cells into dermis, which get modified to form sweat glands. These glands are like coiled tubes. Their ducts pierce the epidermis like a corkscrew to open on the skin surface, forming pores on the skin.

The sweat helps to lose heat and waste materials and also helps to maintain temperature and water balance of the body.

Sweat glands are maximum in palm, sole, axilla and groin. The sweat glands are under sympathetic control, its stimulation increases secretion of sweat.

Sebaceous glands are modified clusters of epidermal cells lying adjacent to hair follicle. These secrete an oily substance, **sebum,** into hair follicles. They are present in skin of all parts of body except palm and sole. They are most numerous on skin of scalp, axilla, face and groin. Sebum keeps the hair soft and pliable. **Acne** are a result of blocked secretion of these glands. These glands are maximum in scalp. If their secretions gets blocked, **sebaceous cyst** results.

Hair follicles are slanting tubular downgrowths of epidermis. The cells at the base of the tube are called **hair matrix,** which produce a type of hard keratin—the hair. At the obtuse

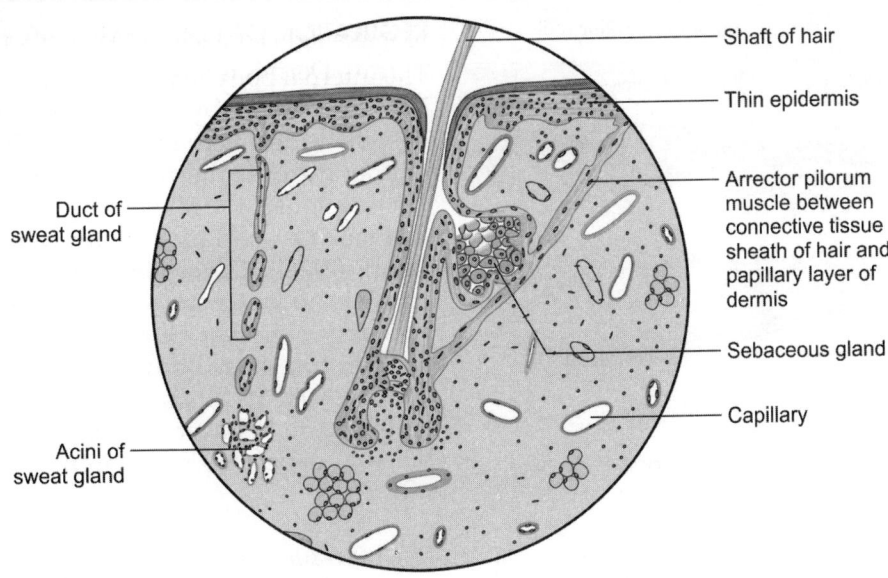

Fig. 9.17: Schematic view of the skin showing structures therein

side of the follicle are few smooth muscle fibres attached. These are the **arrector pili** muscle. Sebaceous glands are present between the muscle and the upper part of hair follicle. As the muscle contracts under the effect of sympathetic fibres, the hair shaft becomes straight to hold the air between the hair and the sebum is secreted out. Part of the hair above the skin is shaft and the remainder is root. The **shaft** of the hair consists of medulla centrally and cortex at periphery. The hair **root** is enlarged—hair bulb and is lodged in superficial portion of dermis called the hair follicle. Growth of the hair occurs at the hair bulb. The daughter cells are progressively pushed upwards and get keratinised to form cells of shaft of hair. Rate of growth of hair varies from 1.5 to 2.2 mm per week depending on the location (Fig. 9.17).

Colour of hair is due to **melanin.** With age, melanin production decreases and air is engulfed into the shaft of hair, giving it grey appearance. One can 'grey gracefully', or use various kinds of physical or chemical agents to colour them as one wants.

Nails are also composed of hard keratin, which grows from specialised epidermal area, the **nail matrix.** Nails are placed on the dorsal distal part of the fingers and toes. Its proximal part, the **root** is implanted into a groove in skin. Its exposed part is **body/nail plate** and distal border forms the **free edge.** The root of nail is overlapped a little by skin, called **nail fold** (cuticle) and has a white, crescentic part called **lunula** (Figs 9.18 and 9.19).

The nail bed appears pinkish because of underlying capillaries. Nail shows the health of the person. Nails normally grow at rate of 0.5 mm/week. Finger nails grow faster than the toe nails. These can also be coloured according to the choice of the individuals. That is how cosmetic industry flourishes.

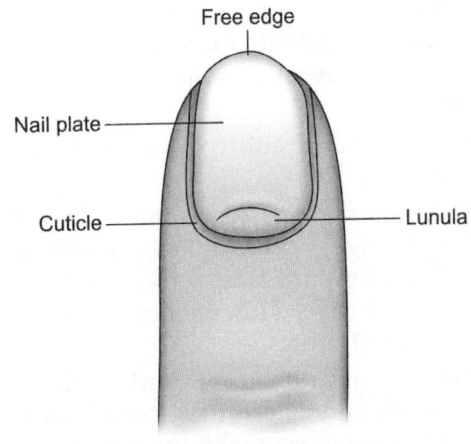

Fig. 9.18: Nail

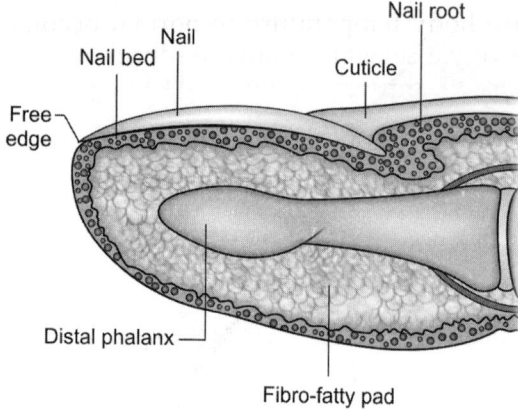

Fig. 9.19: Parts of nail

Functions of the Skin

1. Skin is a water proof covering of the body. It prevents escape of fluid from the body, prevents bacteria from entering the body.
2. Sweat helps to maintain body temperature.
3. Skin has receptors for touch, pressure, temperature or pain. These protect body from extremes of temperature and pressure.
4. Melanocytes of skin antagonise harmful effects of sun rays. Negroes are dark because in their land sun is very hot. Europeans are fair because sun is less hot, but are vulnerable to cancer of the skin.
5. Sunlight helps to synthesise vitamin D required for bone formation and maintenance.
6. It has partial ability to excrete out selective substances through sweat and sebaceous glands.
7. It has limited ability to absorb certain substances.
8. Patterns of whorls, loops and arches on the tip of fingers are used to identify individuals (the criminals) as these are fixed for the whole life. This science is known as **dermatoglyphics.**
9. Healthy skin even without make up is beautiful and reflects the inner health of the person, whereas make up tries to 'show off', which is necessary at times.

REGULATION OF BODY TEMPERATURE

The internal body temperature is maintained in a normal range by homeostatic mechanisms despite wide fluctuations in environmental temperature. If the rate of body heat production equals the rate of heat loss, the body maintains a constant core temperature near 98.6°F (37°C). **Core temperature** is temperature in body structures deep to the skin and subcutaneous layer. **Shell temperature** is the temperature near body surface in the skin and the subcutaneous layer. Normally shell temperature is lower than core temperature by 1–6°C depending on environmental temperature.

Heat Production

The production of body heat is proportional to metabolic rate. Factors affecting the metabolic rate are:

1. *Body temperature:* Higher the body temperature, higher is the metabolic rate. For each 1°C rise in core temperature metabolic rate increases by 10%.
2. *Exercise:* During strenuous exercise metabolic rate may increase up to 20 times the basal metabolic rate (BMR) due to contraction of skeletal muscles.
3. *Nervous system:* Stimulation of sympathetic division of autonomic nervous system releases norepinephrine and epinephrine, both of which increase the metabolic rate.
4. *Hormones:* Thyroid hormones are the main regulators of BMR. BMR increases as blood levels of thyroid hormones rise. Growth hormone, testosterone and insulin also increase the BMR.
5. *Ingestion of food:* Raises the metabolic rate by 10–20% due to the increase in metabolic rate due to digestion, absorption and storage of nutrients. This food induced increased heat production is maximally seen after eating a high protein diet.
6. *Metabolic rate* is also affected by sex (lower in females except during pregnancy and lactation), sleep (lower), age (higher in children).

Heat Loss

Normal body temperature is maintained only when heat is lost to the environment at the same rate as it is produced by metabolic reactions. Heat from the body can be lost by:

1. *Conduction:* It is the exchange of heat that occurs between molecules of two materials that are in direct contact with each other. At rest, about 3% of body heat is lost via conduction to solid materials in contact with body such as chair and clothing. If a body is submerged in cold or hot water, heat loss or gain via conduction is much greater because water conducts heat 20 times more effectively than air.

2. *Convection:* It is the transfer of heat by movement of a gas/liquid between areas of different temperature. Contact of air/water with human body results in heat transfer by both conduction and convection. When cool air comes in contact with body, it warms and become less dense and is carried away by convection currents created as less dense air rises. At rest, about 15% of body heat is lost to air via conduction and convection.

3. *Radiation:* It is the transfer of heat in the form of infrared rays between a warmer object and a cooler one without physical contact. About 60% heat loss occurs via radiation in a resting room at 21°C.

4. *Evaporation:* It is the conversion of liquid to a vapour. Every millilitre of water evaporates taking with it about 0.58 cal heat. At rest, about 22% heat is lost through evaporation of about 700 mL water per day (300 mL in exhaled air and 400 mL from skin surface).

Hypothalamic Thermostat

The **control centre** that regulates the temperature is the **preoptic area** in the **anterior hypothalamus.** Nerve signals from preoptic area are transmitted to the **heat losing centre and heat promoting centre** of the hypothalamus.

Thermoregulation

If core temperature declines, mechanisms that conserve heat and increase heat production to raise body temperature to normal become active via several negative feedback mechanisms. Temperature receptors in skin and hypothalamus send nerve impulses to control centres in hypothalamus, which in turn sends impulses to heat promoting centre.

These impulses also cause release of thyroid stimulating hormone (TSH). These impulses help to raise the core temperature by:

1. Constriction of blood vessels of the skin: Decreases heat loss through skin by decreasing flow of blood to skin.

2. Increased release of hormones by adrenal medulla. These hormones bring about an increase in cellular metabolism, which increases heat production.

3. Increased TSH releases increased secretion of thyroid hormones from thyroid gland, which in turn increases metabolic rate.

4. Impulses from the brain cause **shivering** (skeletal muscles contract in a repetitive cycle), increasing the metabolic rate.

All the mechanisms above result in increase in body temperature.

If the body temperature rises above normal, the hypothalamic control centre send nerve impulses which stimulate heat losing centre and inhibit heat promoting centre. Stimulation of heat losing centre causes dilatation of blood vessels in skin and excess heat is lost to the environment via radiation and conduction as an increased volume of blood flows from warmer core of body into cooler skin. Also metabolic rate decreases and shivering does not occur. Increased perspiration also leads to increased loss of heat. All these responses help to return body temperature to normal.

Hypothermia is present when core temperature is below 35°C (95°F). At core temperature below 32°C (89.6°F) compensatory mechanisms to restore body temperature fail and there is muscle rigidity, cramps and lowered blood pressure, pulse and respiratory rate, followed by mental confusion and disorientation. Death usually occurs when body temperature falls below 25°C (77°F).

Fever usually results from infection and is due to release of chemicals **(pyrogens)** from affected tissue. The pyrogens through prostaglandins act on the hypothalamic thermostat and reset it to higher temperature. The body responds by activating heat producing mechanisms, e.g. shivering and vasocons-triction, until the new higher temperature is reached. When hypothalamic thermostat is reset to normal level due to disappearance of pyrogens, heat loss mechanisms are activated, e.g. sweating and vasodilatation, until body temperature falls to the normal. Death occurs if core temperature rises above 44–46°C (112–114°F).

PHYSIOLOGY OF PAIN

In its simplest form, pain stimulates pain receptors, and this stimulus is transferred via specialised nerves to the spinal cord and from thre to the brain.

Pain Receptors

Pain receptors are present everywhere in the body, especially the skin, surfaces of the joints, wall of the arteries. It is interesting to note that th brain itself does not have any pain receptors at all and is therefore insensitive to pain.

Pain receptors are free nerve endings. There are three types of pain receptor stimuli: mechanical, thermal and chemical. A mechanical stimulus would be, for example, high pressure or stretching, and a thermal pain stimulus would be extreme heat or cold.

Compounds called prostaglandins are released with painful stimuli, and although they do not directly stimulate pain receptors, they do increase their sensitivity. Paracetamol and non-steroidal anti-inflammatory drugs (NSAIDs) decrease the effect of prostaglan-dins, that is why they work as painkillers. Paracetamol operates in the central nervous syster and the NSAIDs are peripheral-acting substances.

Pain Nerve Fibres—Fast Pain and Slow Pain

From the pain receptors, the pain stimulus is transmitted thorugh peripheral nerves to the spinal cord and from there to the brain. This happens via two different types of nerve fibre: "fast pain" and "slow pain" fibres.

Fast Pain

Fast pain, like pricking yourself with a needle or touching a burning object, is mainly related to painful stimuli of the skin, mouth and anus.

Fast pain is well-localised, meaning that a person can normally describe very accurately where exactly the pain is sharp and "cutting".

Slow Pain

Slow pain, which starts immediately after the fast pain, can only be transmitted slowly to the brain.

Comparison of slow pain and fast pain is shown in Table 9.1.

Pain Transmission in the Spinal Cord and the Brain

The peripheral nerves (nerves outside the central nervous system) carry the pain impulse to the spinal coard. In the spinal coard, fast pain and slow pain are carried up to the brain via different pathways. The impulse of the fast pain goes to specific and limited areas on the

Table 9.1: Comparison of slow pain and fast pain	
Slow pain	*Fast pain*
Transmitted by very thin nerve fibres	Transmitted by relatively thicker (and therefore faster conducting) nerve fibres
Poorly localised	Well-localised
All internal organs (except the brain)	Mainly skin, mouth, anus
Body wants to be immobile to allow healing (guarding, spasm, rigidity)	Immediate withdrawal of stimulation to avoid further damage
Pain often radiates, or is referred	Pain does not radiate
Effective relief from opioids	Little relief from opioids
Examples: Labour pain, pain starting after fast pain from an injury	Example: Pain from a surgical incision

surface of the brain (the coartex), allowing for the relatively precise localisation of the pain stimulus. The impulse from slow pain is distributed diffusely in the brain.

What can the Body do to Temper the Pain Sensation?

A very common remedy is "rubbing the pain bettter". When you get hurt, you instinctively rub the painful area, which partly relieves the pain. The reason is that rubbin or pressing stimulates certain other nerve fibres, and their input in the spinal cord receives preference over the input from the nerve fibres transmitting the pain.

When a pain stimulus reaches the brain, the brain itself sends a signal back to the spinal cord via a very complex system of nerve connections to diminish the transmission of the pain impulse that has been sent up to the brain. In a nutshell, the brain puts a "brake" on the pain impulse as it enters the spinal coard. Important molecules in this process are enkephalin and serotonin.

In the pain-processing parts of the brain there are also exists a system of natural opioids. When a pain impulse reaches the brain, these opioids are released from their storage areas and bind with receptors in the pain pathway to block the transmission nad perception of pain. Examples of these natural opioids are enkephalin, endorphin and dynorphin. The same receptors in the brain to block pain perception.

CLINICAL ASPECTS

Tongue

1. *Ulcers:* The sides of the tongue show small/big ulcers. These are mostly due to deficiency of vitamin B complex. Eating food containing chillies is very painful in such times. If the ulcer does not heal, it must be followed closely, as the chronic ulcers may change into cancer of tongue.

2. *Ageusia* is term used for absence of sense of taste. **Hypogeusia** is diminished sense of taste. **Dysgeusia** is distorted sense of taste.

Nose

The nose and nasal cavity are affected by following maladies:

1. Forceful hit on the nose may cause fracture of nasal bones. Nasal bone is the most common facial bone to be fractured.
2. The nasal septum may be deviated to one or the other side.
3. The anteroinferior area of nasal septum can bleed, if it is picked too often. It is called 'Little's area'.
4. Many paranasal sinuses open into each side of the nasal cavity. In **sinusitis,** there is mucus or watery discharge from the nose.
5. Common cold affects the nose. It is a viral infection and takes about 1 week for the person to become alright.
6. Loss of sense of smell is known **anosmia. Hyposmia** is decreased sense of smell and **dysosmia** is distorted sense of smell.

Diseases of the Ear

1. *Otitis externa:* Occurs due to infection of the external auditory meatus by a boil. It is painful, as there is very limited space.
2. *Otitis media:* This is the inflammation of the narrow middle ear cavity. Mostly, the infection reaches from the throat via the auditory tube. If not treated completely, acute otitis media may become chronic and cause meningitis, mastoiditis, labyrinthitis and other complications.
3. *Otosclerosis:* If the foot plate of stapes get fused to the oval window, the condition is called 'otosclerosis'. The sound waves cannot be transmitted to the internal ear and the person develops conductive hearing loss.
4. **Deafness:** Inability to hear properly is called deafness. It may be **conductive deafness** (due to impaired transmission of sound waves from outside to oval window) or **nerve deafness** (due to diseases of cochlea, cochlear nerve) or mixed, i.e. both conductive and nerve deafness.

Meniere's disease: Excessive accumulation of endolymph leads to increased pressure and distension within the membranous labyrinth.

Patient presents with recurrent attacks of dizziness, nausea, vomiting, ringing in the ear and gradually nerve deafness develops.

Presbycusis is gradual hearing loss associated with ageing. It is due to gradual loss of hair cells and neurons.

Diseases of the Eye

1. **Congenital:** There may be abnormalities in the eye. There may be 'congenital cataract'. This is usually due to rubella or Down's syndrome. There may be non formation of lacrimal gland, absence of nasolacrimal duct.

2. **Inflammatory diseases**
   - *Blepharitis* is inflammation of margin of the eyelid. If there is additional ulceration of margin of eyelid, there may be fibrosis of eyelid and it may not close completely.
   - *Hordeolum:* It is infection of tarsal glands of the margin of eyelid. The hordeolum or stye occur repeatedly.
   - *Conjunctivitis:* This is inflammation of the conjunctiva, due to infection or allergy.
   - *Trachoma* is a chronic inflammation of the conjunctiva caused by *Chlamydia trachomatis*. It is an important cause of preventable blindness in developing tropical countries.
   - *Corneal ulcers:* These ulcers develop due to infection of cornea following any injury even by edge of newspaper or infection.
   - *Uveitis:* It is the inflammation of the uveal tract, i.e. inflammation of iris, ciliary body or choroid.
   - *Glaucoma:* There is increased intraocular pressure due to lack of drainage of aqueous humour through the canal of schlemm. Glaucoma leads to pressure on optic nerve fibres and blindness.

3. **Cataract:** The lens gets opaque, interfering with the passage of light. The cataract causes blurring of vision and the lens needs to be removed. This is replaced by an artificial lens (intraocular lens implant).

4. **Retinal detachment:** In this condition, there is partial or complete separation of the inner nine layers of retina from the outer pigmented layer. It needs surgery for its correction.

5. **Retinitis pigmentosa:** It is a hereditary disease in which there is degeneration of retina, mainly affecting the rods. There is defective vision in the dim light **(night blindness).**

6. **Dacryocystitis:** There is inflammation of the lacrimal sac. It is associated with partial or complete blockage of the lacrimal duct.

7. **Squint:** Normally, the movements of the two eyes are synchronous, so that the same image falls on corresponding parts of the retina in both eyes. In weakness or paralysis of one muscle, the images fall on different parts of the two retina, leading to two images for the brain and **diplopia** (double vision).

8. **Myopia (near sightedness):** The image of distant objects falls in front of the retina because eyeball is too long. So, concave lens is given to diverge the image, so that these fall on the retina. Near objects are seen in focus.

9. **Hypermetropia (far sightedness):** The near image falls behind the retina because eyeball is too short. Convex lens is required to correct the defect. Distant objects are focused normally.

10. **Astigmatism:** The curvature of the part of the cornea is abnormal. The light rays are refracted to a different focus causing a blurred image. It is corrected by a cylindrical lens.

Diseases of the Skin

Skin is the outer garment and is subjected to many maladies.

1. **Albinism:** The child is born without any melanin pigment in the skin. It is usually inherited.

2. **Eczema/dermatitis:** There is redness, swelling, itching and exudation in acute cases. It may become chronic. Dermatitis may be due to allergy to soap or cosmetics.

3. **Herpes virus:** It causes chickenpox and herpes zoster.
4. **Fungal infections**
   a. *Ringworm* is a superficial fungal infection with rings of inflammation. It most commonly affects the scalp.
   b. *In 'athlete's foot'* there is fungal infection between the toes. If toes and area between toes is kept dry, it improves.
5. **Pressure sores:** The skin slowly dies over pressure sites, e.g. pressure sores on the lower back when patient is too sick to get up.
6. **Acne:** It usually occurs at puberty due to blockage of sebaceous glands in the hair follicle. Acne mostly appears on face and chest.
7. **Burns:** It is a common condition and occurs due to heat, too much cold, strong alkalis or acids, electricity, etc. If only epidermis is involved, the burn is **superficial.** But if both epidermis and dermis are affected by burns, the burn is **deep.** Severe burns result in shock, dehydration, renal failure and contractures.
8. **Tumours:**
   a. *Malignant melanoma* is due to malignant multiplication of melanocytes of the epidermis. It mostly occurs in white people. The tumour causes metastases in liver, lung, intestine and brain.
   b. *Basal cell carcinoma:* It is most common type of skin cancer occurring in face, head, neck. It is associated with long-term exposure to sunlight.
9. **Impetigo and cellulitis:** Impetigo is bacterial infection of skin caused by *Staphylococcus aureus* or *Streptococcus pyogenes.* Superficial pustules develop around the nose and mouth.
10. **Cellulitis** is spreading bacterial infection of skin.

Points to Remember

1. The basic tastes are sweet, sour, salt and bitter.
2. Anything to be smell has to be in form of vapour.
3. Only uppermost part of nasal cavity has olfactory epithelium.
4. Eyeball comprises three layers. These are—sclera with cornea; choroid, ciliary body, iris and retina.
5. Internal ear functions both for hearing and balance.
6. Fingerprints are unique to each and every person.
7. Acne occurs due to blockage of duct of the sebaceous gland.

MCQs

1. **Appendages of skin are all except:**
   (a) Hair
   (b) Nail
   (c) Sebaceous gland
   (d) Arrector pilorum muscle

2. **Full nail grows in:**
   (a) 30–60 days
   (b) 60–90 days
   (c) 90–120 days
   (d) 120–160 days

3. **Circumvallate papillae are present at:**
   (a) Tip of tongue
   (b) Lateral border of tongue
   (c) Anterior to sulcus terminates
   (d) Posterior to sulcus terminates

4. **Order of bony ossicles from lateral to medial side are:**
   (a) Malleus, stapes, incus
   (b) Stapes, incus, malleus
   (c) Malleus, incus, stapes

Ans! **1** d   **2** c   **3** c   **4** c

Digestive System

The digestive system is concerned with the ingestion and breakdown of food including its absorption.

Digestive system is responsible for maintaining a continuous supply of required elements for the, cellular metabolism in every tissue, organ and system of body.

The main components of the digestive system are the **digestive tract/alimentary canal.** The tract begins at mouth where food is taken in and ends at the anus from where the unwanted material is eliminated (Fig. 10.1).

Associated with the tracts are a number of glands which help in the digestive process. These are the salivary glands, liver, gall bladder, pancreas and intestinal glands.

The activities of the digestive system can be grouped as:

1. *Ingestion:* Taking in of food in the digestive tract.
2. *Digestion:* During this process food is broken down into smaller pieces by mastication and various enzymes secreted by glands of digestive system. Enzymes of salivary glands, gastric juice, intestinal juice, pancreatic juice, and bile aid the digestive process.
3. *Absorption:* The digested food products are absorbed from the walls of intestine to be deposited in liver.
4. *Elimination:* Substances which cannot be digested or absorbed are expelled out from anal canal as faecal matter.

LAYERS OF THE ALIMENTARY CANAL

The wall of the alimentary canal from the lower oesophagus to the anal canal has the same basic, four layered arrangement of tissue. The four layers from deep to superficial are the mucosa, submucosa muscle layer and adventitia or serosa (Fig. 10.2).

Mucosa

It is the inner lining of the digestive tract. It is composed of three layers of tissue.

1. *Mucous membrane:* Composed of epithelial cells. Its function is protection, secretion and absorption. Epithelium in mouth, pharynx, oesophagus and anal canal is nonkeratinised stratified squamous epithelium (protective in function). Stomach and intestine are lined by simple columnar epithelium (function in secretion and absorption). Cells of the epithelium are replaced every 5–7 days.

2. *Lamina propria:* Consists of areolar connective tissue containing blood and lymphatic vessels. It also contains lymphoid tissue that has protective function. It supports the epithelium and binds it to muscularis mucosa (Fig. 10.2).

3. *Muscularis mucosa:* It is a thin layer of smooth muscle. It throws, mucous membrane into folds thus increasing the surface area for digestion and absorption in stomach and small intestine.

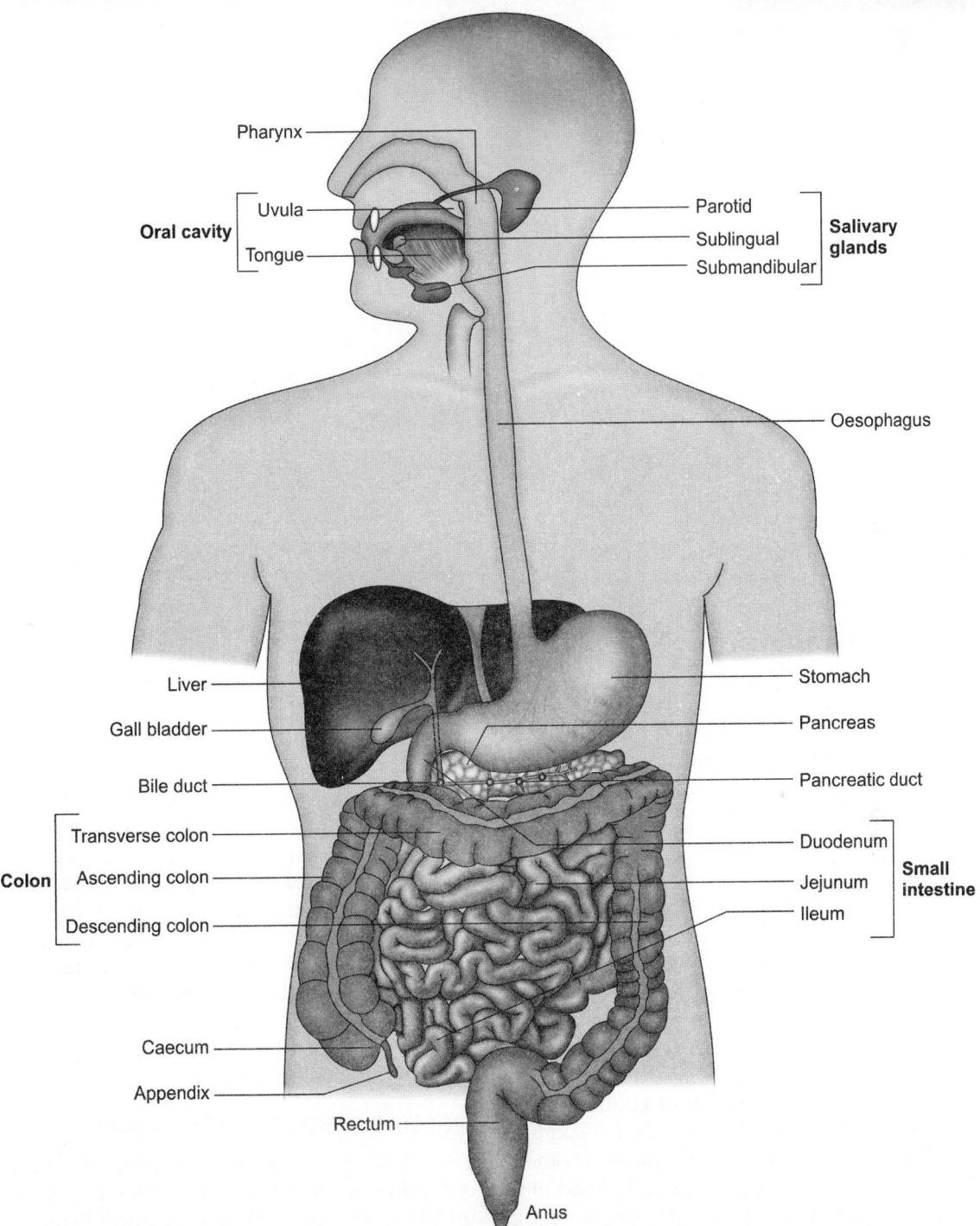

Fig. 10.1: Gastrointestinal system

Submucosa

It consist of loose areolar connective tissue. It binds mucosa to the muscle layer. It has many blood and lymphatic vessels and lymphoid tissue. It also has a network of neurons, **submucosal plexus/plexus of Meissner,**

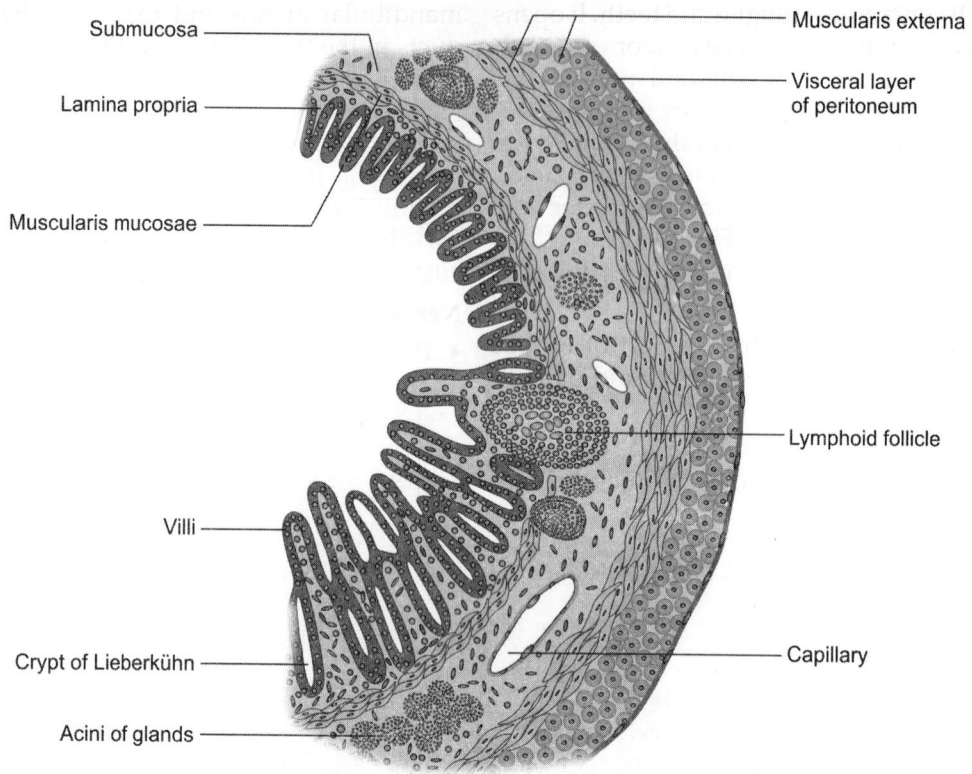

Submucosa

Lamina propria

Muscularis mucosae

Villi

Crypt of Lieberkühn

Acini of glands

Muscularis externa

Visceral layer of peritoneum

Lymphoid follicle

Capillary

Fig. 10.2: Layers of the alimentary canal

which has sympathetic and parasympathetic nerves which supply the mucosa and submucosa.

Muscle Layer

It consists of two layers of smooth muscle inner layer of circular fibres and outer layer of longitudinal fibres. Between two muscle layers a network of sympathetic and parasympathetic nerves and neurons is present, the **myenteric or Auerbach's plexus.** It controls motility of digestive tract especially the frequency and strength of contraction of the muscle layer. Contraction and relaxation of this layer **(peristalsis)** push the food content of digestive tract and also mixes the food with digestive secretions. In mouth, pharynx and upper part of oesophagus muscle layer has skeletal muscle that produces voluntary swallowing. Skeletal muscle is also present in external anal sphincter which allows control of defaecation.

Serosa

It consists of a serous membrane consisting of a areolar connective tissue and simple squamous epithelium. It covers the organs of abdomen in membrane and is known as **peritoneum.** Peritoneum consists of a closed sac and consists of two layers **parietal peritoneum,** which lines the abdominal wall and **visceral peritoneum,** which covers the organs in abdominal cavity. The space between two membranes is **peritoneal cavity** and contains serous fluid.

DIGESTIVE TRACT/ALIMENTARY CANAL

The main parts are the mouth, pharynx, oesophagus, stomach, small intestine, large intestine. The last part of large intestine is the rectum and anal canal which ends at the anus.

Mouth

Mouth is the beginning of digestive tract and is guarded by two **lips** with the **cheeks** at the sides. It contains the **tongue** and **teeth.** It opens posteriorly into the **pharynx.** Roof of mouth is formed by palate. It is divided into anterior **hard palate** which is bony part is longer and separates mouth cavity from the nasal cavity. The posterior part of the palate, the **soft palate,** is like a curtain. It is muscular, shorter and hangs down at the back (Fig. 10.3).

Floor of the mouth is formed by two mylohyoid muscles.

Vestibule of the mouth: It is part of mouth cavity inside the lips and cheeks and outside the gums and teeth.

Mouth cavity proper: This is the cavity lying within the teeth and gums all around. It contains the mobile tongue. In the midline, the floor of front of oral cavity is a fold of mucous membrane, the **frenulum** of tongue.

Salivary Glands

Three pairs of salivary glands are parotid glands, submandibular glands and sublingual glands (Fig. 10.1).

Parotid glands are situated one on each side of face just below the external acoustic meatus. Each gland has a **parotid duct,** opening into the vestibule of mouth opposite the 2nd upper molar tooth.

Submandibular glands lie one on each side of face under the angle of jaw.

The **duct of submandibular gland** opens on the side of the frenulum.

Sublingual glands lie under mucous membrane of the floor of mouth in front of sub-mandibular glands and they open by 10–12 ducts in the floor of the mouth.

Each gland is made up of several lobules made up of small acini lined with secretory cells. The secretions are poured into ductules which join to form larger ducts leading into mouth. The saliva provides the necessary fluid for chewing and swallowing and some enzymes as well.

Nerve supply is by autonomic nervous system
- Parasympathetic: Increases secretion with enzymes
- Sympathetic: Depresses secretion

Tongue

The tongue is muscular organ within the mouth cavity proper.

Functions:
- It helps in swallowing of food
- It helps in speech.

Parts:

Tongue consists of a **root** with which it is attached to the mandible and hyoid bone and is prevented from swallowing. Its **dorsal surface** is rough and divided into posterior 1/3rd and anterior 2/3rd by V-shaped **sulcus terminalis.** The **ventral surface** is smooth and a **tip** pointing anteriorly (Fig. 10.4).

The dorsum of tongue is rough as it contains 3 types of papillae.

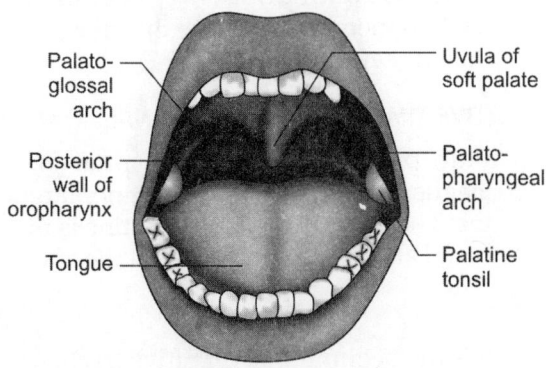

Fig. 10.3: Mouth

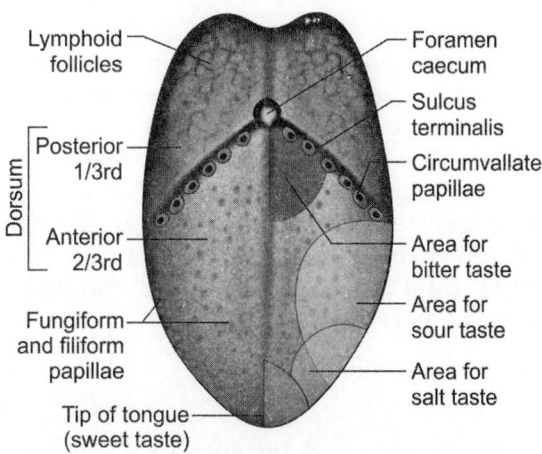

Fig. 10.4: Tongue

1. *Filiform:* Thin and pointed with no taste buds. They are present on anterior two thirds of the tongue.
2. *Fungiform:* Mushroom like structures with a few taste buds. They are present on sides and tip of tongue.
3. *Vallate papillae:* 10–12 in number lying in front of 'V' shaped sulcus. These contain maximum number of taste buds.

Different areas of tongue are demarcated for different tastes (Fig. 10.4).

Muscles: Eight voluntary muscles are present in each half of the tongue. **Intrinsic** muscle change the shape of tongue. Extrinsic muscle **moves the tongue. Genioglossus** is the most important muscle as it keeps the tongue anteriorly in position and prevents it from blocking the air pathway.

Nerve supply: Most of the muscles are supplied by hypoglossal nerve (12th cranial nerve).

Arterial is derived from lingual artery, a branch of external carotid artery. **Venous drainage** is by lingual vein which joins the internal jugular vein.

Teeth

There are no visible teeth in the newborn. Between 6 months and 3 years 20 **temporary/deciduous teeth** erupt, 5 in each quarter of the jaw

Incisor	Canine	Molar
2	1	2

These are named from before backwards as **central incisor, lateral incisor, canine, 1st molar and 2nd molar.** These fall off and are replaced by permanent teeth, between 6 and 24 years age. The **permanent teeth** are 8 in each quarter of the jaw. These are named **central incisor, lateral incisor, canine, first and second premolars, 1st molar, 2nd molar and 3rd molar** (Fig. 10.5).

Incisor	Canine	Premolar	Molar
2	1	2	3

The incisors are for cutting, canine for tearing and premolars and molars for

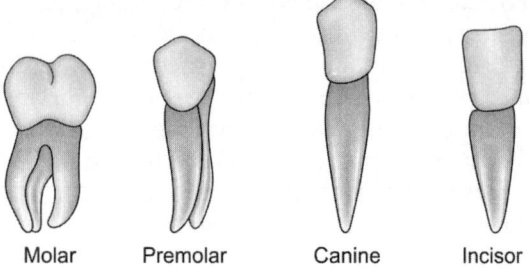

Molar   Premolar   Canine   Incisor

Fig. 10.5: Permanent teeth

grinding the food. The tooth consists of a crown, neck and a root. The principal component is the **dentine,** a hard calcified tissue (Fig. 10.6).

Crown of the tooth is best seen in the mouth and is covered by hardest calcified tissue, the **enamel. Root** is buried in the jaw and held by the **cementum** which anchors tooth to the surrounding bone. **Neck** is present at the gum margin where enamel and cementum meet. In the centre of the dentine is a **pulp cavity** with vessels and sensory nerves.

Gum or gingiva is the part of the lining of mouth, which adheres firmly to the bone of the jaw.

Nerve supply: Upper teeth are supplied by branches of maxillary division of trigeminal

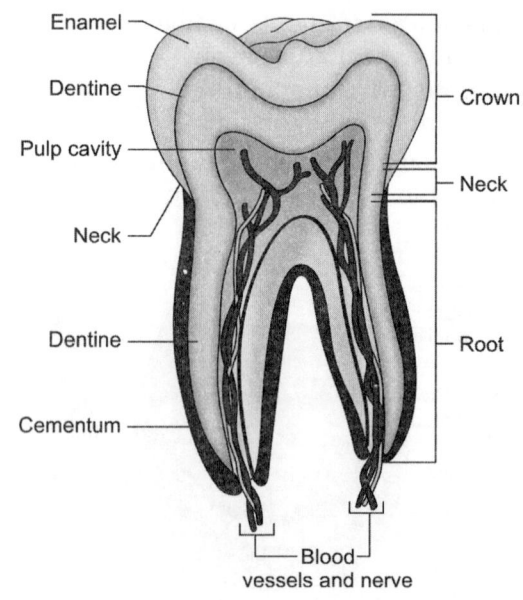

Fig. 10.6: Structure of tooth

(V cranial nerve) while lower teeth are supplied by the mandibular division of trigeminal (V cranial nerve).

Pharynx

Pharynx is a 12–14 cm long tube that extends from base of skull to level of 6th cervical vertebra. It is divided into three parts— nasopharynx, oropharynx and laryngo-pharynx (Fig. 10.7).

Nasopharynx is nasal part of pharynx and lies behind the nose above the level of soft palate. It is important in respiration. Oropharynx and laryngopharynx are passages common to respiratory and digestive systems.

The oropharynx is the part of the pharynx between the soft palate and the upper border of epiglottis at level of third cervical vertebra. **Palatoglossal arch** on each side divides the mouth from pharynx. Oropharynx includes two palatine tonsils (Fig. 10.7). During swallowing, nasal and oral parts are separated by soft palate and the uvula.

Laryngopharynx extends from oropharynx above and continues as oesophagus below, i.e. from 3rd to 6th cervical vertebra. Food passes from oral cavity into oropharynx and laryngopharynx and then to oesophagus below.

Pharynx is composed of 3 layers of tissue— mucosa, middle layer of fibrous tissue and outer layer of three constrictor muscles. These are superior, middle and inferior constrictor muscles.

Blood supply to pharynx is by facial vessels and **nerve supply** is by pharyngeal plexus (X + XI nerves).

Palatine Tonsils

These are a pair of lymphoid tissue masses lying in tonsillar bed in oropharynx between anterior palatoglossal arch and posterior palatopharyngeal arch (Fig. 10.3).

Tonsil is made of lymphoid follicles embedded in connective tissue and covered on superficial surface by stratified squamous epithelium. This epithelium dips into the underlying tissue to form **crypts,** which can trap bacteria and become site of infection. Tonsils are large till puberty but regress in adulthood. These provide immunity to the body.

Oesophagus

It is muscular tube 25 cm long. It starts at level of **6th cervical vertebra,** runs the most of its part through the thoracic cavity. At the level of **10th thoracic vertebra,** it enters the diaphragm to reach abdominal cavity, where again it has a small course, to continue with the stomach. It lies behind the trachea in upper part of its course, then it passes anterior to thoracic aorta.

Proximal one-third of oesophagus contains striated muscles and distal third smooth muscles. Oesophagus is lined by stratified squamous non-keratinised epithelium. Middle third contains a mixture of the two types of muscles.

Its function is to conduct the bolus/mass of food from the pharynx into the stomach. It is distended only during the passage of bolus, rest of the time it remains collapsed.

Arterial blood supply is by branches from thoracic aorta to the thoracic part and by branches of coeliac artery to abdominal part.

Venous drainage of thoracic part is into azygos and hemiazygos vein. Abdominal part drains into left gastric vein.

Upper end of oesophagus is guarded by **cricopharyngeal sphincter** which prevents

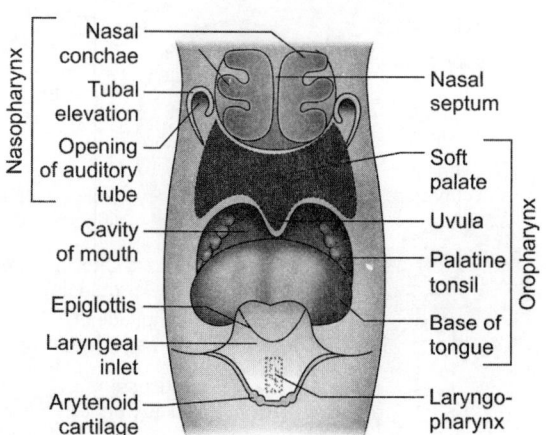

Fig. 10.7: Pharynx

Nasal conchae
Tubal elevation
Opening of auditory tube
Cavity of mouth
Epiglottis
Laryngeal inlet
Arytenoid cartilage
Nasopharynx

Nasal septum
Soft palate
Uvula
Palatine tonsil
Base of tongue
Laryngo-pharynx
Oropharynx

passage of air during inspiration and aspiration of oesophageal contents. **Lower (cardiac) oesophageal sphincter** prevents reflux of acid gastric contents into the oesophagus.

Before the abdominal viscera are learnt, let us see the subdivisions of abdominal cavity.

Subdivisions of Abdominal Cavity

Two horizontal lines are drawn, one at the level of tip of 9th costal cartilage (level of first lumbar vertebra) and other at the level of tubercle of iliac crest (level of fifth lumbar vertebra).

Two vertical lines each passing through the midclavicular and midinguinal points are drawn. The upper limit of abdomen is diaphragm and lower limit is the inguinal ligament and upper border of pubic bone.

Thus, the abdominal cavity is subdivided into 9 regions:

- Right and left **hypochondriac** with **epigastric** region in centre (Fig. 10.8).
- Right and left **lumbar** with **umbilical** region in the centre.
- Right and left **iliac** with **hypogastric** region in the centre.

Various organs of abdomen are approximately placed in these nine regions.

The viscera in the abdominal cavity are related to a serous membrane, the **peritoneum.** Some are completely enveloped like the stomach and small intestine, some are partly covered and few are only covered anteriorly.

Peritoneum helps in friction free movements of the various viscera present.

Stomach

The stomach acts as a mechanical mixer, chemical digester and temporary storehouse of food. It is the most dilated part of digestive tube. Its capacity in adults is 1–1.5 litres.

Position: Left hypochondriac and epigastric regions.

Parts: The junction of oesophagus and stomach is the cardio-oesophageal junction. The stomach consists of:

- 2 ends, the proximal **cardiac** and distal **pyloric end** (Fig. 10.9).
- 2 borders, the lesser curvature and the greater curvature.
- 2 surfaces, anterosuperior and posteroinferior surface. The latter rests on a number of organs forming the **stomach bed.**

Part of the stomach above the gastro-oesophageal junction is called the **fundus** of the stomach. The main part is the **body** and the distal part is the **pyloric part.** This part possesses a sphincter, the **pyloric sphincter** at its distal part.

Relations

Anterior: Anterior abdominal wall and left lobe of liver

Posterior: Left kidney, left suprarenal, spleen and pancreas. **These form the stomach bed.**

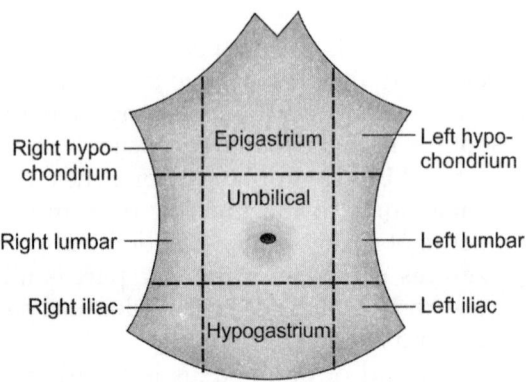

Fig. 10.8: Anterior view of abdominal regions

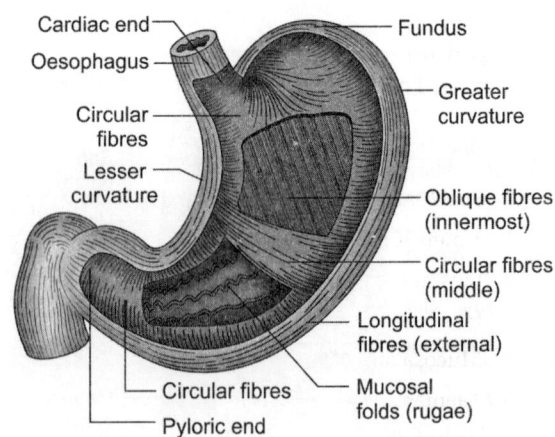

Fig. 10.9: Parts and structure of stomach

Above: Diaphragm

Below: Small intestine and transverse colon

Left: Spleen

Right: Liver

The stomach wall is composed of same four basic layers as rest of the alimentary tract but the smooth muscle layer consists of three layers—outer layer of longitudinal fibres, middle layer of circular fibres and inner layer of oblique fibres. This type of muscle arrangement has churning and peristaltic movements. In empty stomach, mucosa is thrown into large longitudinal folds called **rugae,** which disappear when stomach is distended. Below the surface of mucous membrane **gastric glands** are present that have specialised cells for secreting gastric juice. There are mucus neck cells which secrete mucus. Chief cells secrete pepsinogen and oxyntic cells secrete HCl.

Blood supply: Stomach gets its arterial supply from the three branches of **coeliac trunk,** a branch of abdominal aorta. Veins drain into the **portal vein.**

Lymph drains into the coeliac group of lymph nodes.

Sympathetic nerves supply the blood vessels and also carries pain impulses.

Vagus is secretory to the glands and causes peristalsis and inhibits the pyloric sphincter as well.

Intestines

Intestines follow the stomach. There are two parts of intestines—small intestine and large intestine. Their differences shown in Table 10.1.

Small Intestine

It is the intestine between pylorus of stomach and ileocaecal valve. It is 5 metres long. The mucosal folds run circularly across the wall and are permanent. It is subdivided into 3 parts—proximal 25 cm is **duodenum,** middle 2/5th is **jejunum** and distal 3/5th is **ileum.**

Duodenum

Duodenum is C-shaped with **head of pancreas** lying in its concavity. The **bile duct** and the **pancreatic duct** open by a **common opening** into the **duodenum,** 10 cm from the pylorus at **major duodenal papilla.**

Jejunum and Ileum

These two parts form most of the small intestine. These are suspended from the posterior abdominal wall by a fold of peritoneum called **the mesentery.**

The digestive process that begins in stomach is continued in the small intestine. This is also the main site of absorption of the products of digestion.

Small intestine wall is composed of same four basic layers as rest of alimentary tract. Mucosa of small intestine is thrown into permanent ridges called **circular or Kerckring's folds.** These folds enhance the absorption of nutrients by increasing the surface area and also promote mixing of chyme (digested liquid food).

The mucosa has 0.5–1 mm finger like projections, **villi.** These vastly increase the surface area for absorption and digestion. The villi are lined by various types of cells. Absorptive cells are of simple columnar epithelium with tiny **microvilli** (1 μm long)

Table 10.1: Differences between small and large intestines

Small intestine	Large intestine
1. 5 metres long	1.5 metres long
2. Lies in the central part of abdomen	Lies along the periphery of abdomen
3. Has less capacity of distending	Has more capacity of distending
4. Mucosa shows villi	No villi present
5. Taenia or sacculations are absent	Taenia and sacculations both are present
6. Appendices epiploicae absent	Appendices epiploicae as tags of fat present

on their free border, forming a fuzzy line called **brush border** along intestinal lumen. Each villus encloses a network of blood and lymph capillaries. The lymph capillaries are called **lacteals.** Nutrients absorbed by epithelial cells covering the villus pass through wall of a capillary or lacteal to enter blood or lymph, respectively.

Arterial blood supply is from the superior mesenteric artery which gives 12–15 branches for small intestine and 3 branches for large intestine as well. **Veins** drain into superior mesenteric vein which with splenic vein forms the portal vein.

The **lymph vessels** drain into para-aortic lymph nodes and from there into the upper part of cisterna chyli, at the beginning of the thoracic duct.

Nerve supply is from vagus and sympathetic nerves. These nerves form plexuses within the wall of intestine. These are submucosal or **Meissner's plexus** and myenteric or **Auerbach's plexus** in between two coats of muscularis externa. These plexuses cause peristaltic movement for propelling the contents of small intestine towards large intestine.

Large Intestine

It is the last part of the digestive tube and follows the small intestine. It starts at ileocaecal junction. Its parts are caecum, vermiform appendix, colon, rectum and anal canal (Fig. 10.1).

Caecum

Lies in the right iliac fossa. The ileocaecal valve guards the opening of ileum into the caecum, and 2 cm below this opening is the opening of the vermiform appendix. It is continuous with the ascending colon.

Vermiform Appendix

It is the narrowest part of the digestive tube. It is usually 8 cm long and 0.5 cm wide. It has a base and a tip. The tip may occupy different positions.

Arterial supply is from appendicular artery, one of the caecal branches of superior mesenteric artery.

Colon

It forms the greatest length of large intestine, and is subdivided into **ascending colon** on right side of abdominal cavity, **transverse colon** across the abdomen, **descending colon** on the left side and **pelvic colon** in the pelvis (Fig. 10.1).

The large intestine shows the same basic layers of tissue. In colon the longitudinal muscle fibres are thickened in three thick bands called **taeniae coli,** situated at regular intervals around it. They stop at the junction of the sigmoid colon and rectum. These bands of muscle are slightly shorter than the total length of colon, they give a sacculated or puckered appearance forming a series of pouches called **haustra.** Small pouches of visceral peritoneum filled with fat are attached to taeniae coli and are called **appendices epiploicae.**

Arterial supply of ascending and most of the transverse colon is by superior mesenteric artery. Rest of the colon is supplied by inferior mesenteric artery. **Veins** drain into the portal vein. **Lymph vessels** drain into the para-aortic lymph nodes.

Parasympathetic nerve supply to ascending and most of transverse colon is from vagus, while to small left part of transverse colon, descending and pelvic colon is from **pelvic splanchnic nerve** (sacral 2, 3, 4 segments). **Sympathetic nerves** relax the smooth muscle and constrict ileocaecal and internal anal sphincters.

Rectum and Anal Canal

Rectum starts at the middle of sacrum and is 15 cm long. It follows forward curvature of sacrum and coccyx and ends 2.5 cm below and in front of coccyx where it continues as anal canal.

Anal canal is the last 4 cm of digestive tube. From the anorectal junction it passes downwards and backwards to the anus. In the wall of anal canal, the inner circular layer of smooth muscle becomes thickened to form **internal anal sphincter** while outside this is **external anal sphincter** of skeletal muscle. Internal sphincter is supplied by autonomic nerves while external anal sphincter by inferior rectal nerve.

Rectum and anal canal has the same basic 4 layered structure like other parts of digestive tract.

The lining membrane of anus consists of stratified squamous epithelium continuous with skin beyond external anal sphincter.

The **mucous membrane** of anal canal shows in upper part three folds which keep it mostly closed. These are due to plexus of veins. If enlarged these form **haemorrhoids or piles** which may cause pain or bleeding or both.

Rectum and anal canal are supplied by **superior rectal artery** (continuation of inferior mesenteric artery), **middle and inferior rectal arteries,** branches of internal pudendal artery.

Veins draining along superior rectal artery end in portal vein, while those running along middle and inferior rectal arteries end in pudendal and systemic veins. Thus anal canal is a site of **porto-systemic anastomosis.**

LIVER

The liver is the largest gland in the body weighing about 1500 g and receives 1500 cc of blood per minute.

Liver lies under the diaphragm, in right hypochondriac/epigastric and partly into left hypochondriac regions. It extends into the thoracic cavity up to 5th rib and receives protection from the costal cartilages. It may be felt below the right costal margin on deep inspiration (Fig. 10.1).

The liver is kept in position by 2–3 hepatic veins which enter the inferior vena cava, by intra-abdominal pressure and by peritoneal folds forming supporting ligaments that attach the liver to inferior surface of diaphragm. The liver has anterior, superior, posterior, right lateral surfaces which are continuous with each other.

Relations of Liver

Anterior: Anterior abdominal wall and diaphragm

Posterior: Oesophagus, gall bladder, aorta, inferior vena cava

Above: Diaphragm

Below: Stomach, duodenum, right kidney and suprarenal gland

Laterally: lower ribs.

Liver biopsy is done through **right 8th intercostal space** in full expiration to avoid injury to lung.

Liver also has an inferior or visceral surface which is related to various abdominal viscera. In addition, this surface shows a horizontal 5 cm fissure called the **porta hepatis.** Porta hepatis is the gateway of liver. Portal vein and hepatic artery enter the liver while hepatic ducts leave the liver. Attached to the margins of porta hepatis is a fold of peritoneum the **lesser omentum** which extends from the liver to the lesser curvature of stomach.

Liver is divided into four lobes—right lobe (largest), left lobe, caudate lobe, quadrate lobe (Fig. 10.10). The caudate and quadrate lobes are seen on posterior surface.

Arterial supply of the liver is from common hepatic artery of coeliac trunk of the aorta (20%) while venous drainage via hepatic veins is into inferior vena cava. It receives 80% of blood from digestive tract via the portal vein.

Portal vein is formed behind the neck of pancreas by union of superior mesenteric and splenic veins. Like any artery it divides into right and left branches before entering the liver.

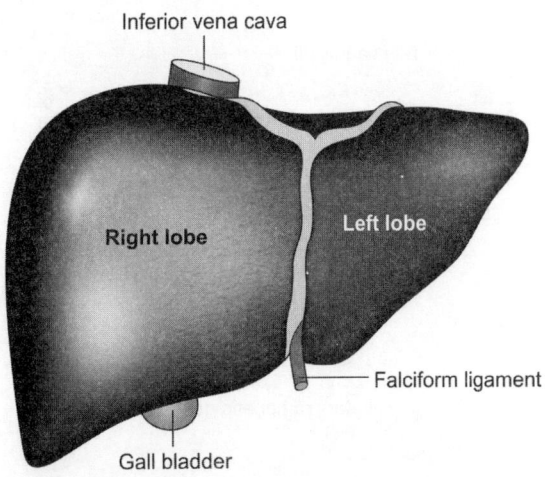

Inferior vena cava

Right lobe

Left lobe

Falciform ligament

Gall bladder

Fig. 10.10: The liver: anterior view

The liver is made up of hexagonal hepatic lobules about 1 micron in diameter. Lobules are made up of cubical cells, **hepatocytes** arranged in pairs of columns radiating form a **central vein.** Between two pairs of columns of cells there are **sinusoids** (blood vessels with incomplete walls). Sinusoids contain a mixture of blood from branches of hepatic artery and portal vein (Fig. 10.11). Blood drains from sinusoids into **central vein.** These join with veins from other lobules, forming larger veins and eventually become **hepatic veins** which leave the liver and empty into inferior vena cava.

Bile canaliculi run between liver cells. Thus each column of hepatocytes has a blood sinusoid on one side and a bile canaliculus on the other. The canaliculi join to from larger bile canals and eventually they form right and left **hepatic ducts** which drain bile from liver.

The combination of bile ductule, branch of hepatic artery and portal vein is known as **portal triad.** At the angles of lobule lie six portal triads. Blood flows from portal triad into hepatic sinusoid and towards the central vein. Bile flows **centrifugally** (from centre to periphery) from bile canaliculi to bile ductule.

Lymph flow from liver is large and is about 0.75 mL/minute. It drains in to nodes in porta hepatis and finally reaches the thoracic duct.

Sympathetic nerves enter the liver with the hepatic artery to control the lumen of the vessels. Pain fibres are carried along the phrenic nerve (C3, 4) which supplies peritoneum over the gall bladder. Pain of gall bladder is referred to tip of right shoulder as the supraclavicular nerves also have same root value (C3, 4).

EXTRAHEPATIC BILIARY APPARATUS

Components of this apparatus are gall bladder, right and left hepatic ducts which leave porta hepatis and soon join to form **common hepatic duct,** which is 4 cm long.

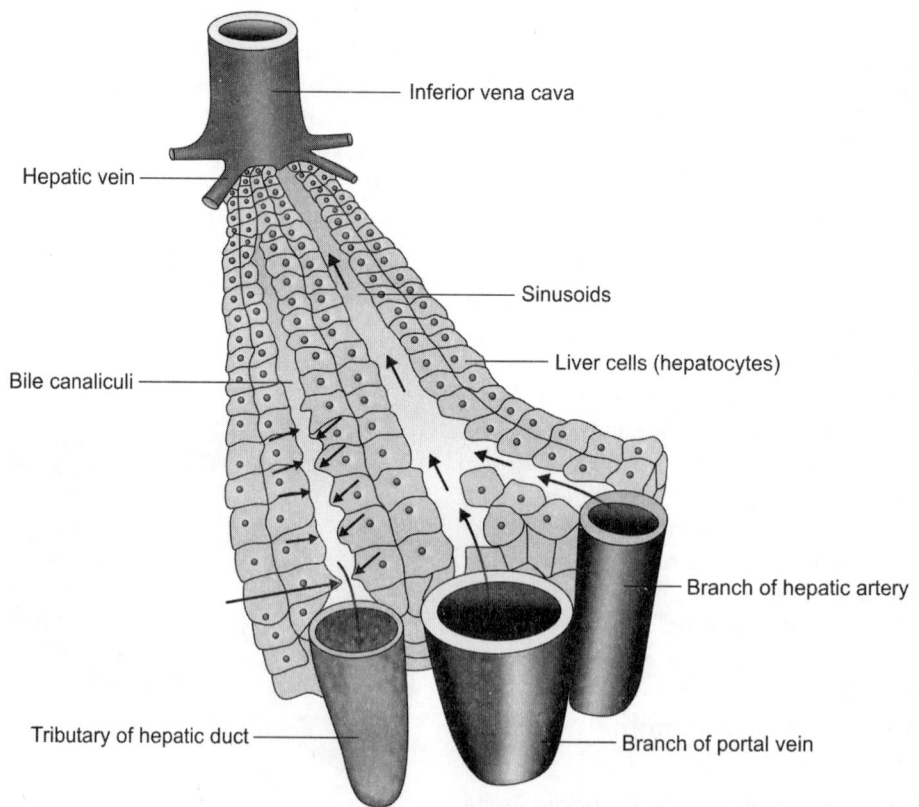

Fig. 10.11: Blood supply of liver

The gall bladder is 7 cm long and lies on the under surface of liver.

Cystic duct about 3 cm long from the neck of gall bladder joins the common hepatic duct to form the bile duct.

The bile duct is 8 cm long. The bile duct and the main pancreatic duct open together at the major duodenal papilla into the second part of the duodenum.

All these components carry the bile produced in the liver. Bile runs in distinct channels and does not mix with the blood (Fig. 10.12). It helps in the digestion of fats.

Gall Bladder

Gall bladder is pyriform organ 7 cm long with a capacity of 50 mL. It is present in a depression on the inferior surface of the liver. It acts as a storage and concentrating organ for bile. Its parts are the fundus, body, which narrows to form the neck, which continues as the cystic duct. Cystic duct allows two way traffic to bile (Fig. 10.12).

Arterial supply of gall bladder is through the cystic artery arising from the right hepatic artery. **Cystic vein** drains into right branch of portal vein. **Lymph** from extrahepatic biliary apparatus drains into lymph nodes in the porta hepatis. **Pain fibres** from gall bladder

and the ducts run with sympathetic nerves. It is referred to tip of right shoulder as the supraclavicular nerves also have same root value (C3, 4). Pain of biliary colic enters the spinal cord via 7th to 9th thoracic nerves.

Mucosa of gall bladder consists of simple columnar epithelium. Submucosa is absent. Muscular layer is of smooth muscle fibres with an additional layer of oblique fibres. Outer most layer is of peritoneum.

PANCREAS

Pancreas is a gland present across the upper part of posterior abdominal wall from right to the left side. It contains both exocrine secretion for digestion of carbohydrates, fats and proteins as well as endocrine secretion, from islets of Langerhans, which act on the carbohydrate metabolism (Fig. 10.12).

Pancreas is 15 cm long, and consists of a **head, neck, body** and **tail.** It lies behind the peritoneum. Head of pancreas lies in the 'C' of the duodenum. Bile duct runs behind head of pancreas. An **uncinate process** from the lowest part of head passes to left behind superior mesenteric vessels. **Neck** is small segment behind which superior mesenteric vein and splenic vein join to form the portal vein.

Body is triangular in shape and is related to the splenic artery along the upper border, transverse mesocolon along the anterior border. The **tail** is the part lying anterior to left kidney reaching up to the hilum of spleen.

Exocrine secretions of pancreas are secreted by secretory cells present in the lobules (acini). Each lobule is drained by a tiny duct and these eventually unite to form pancreatic duct. Secretions are delivered to duodenum by the **main** and **accessory pancreatic ducts.**

Main pancreatic duct and common bile duct open in the **hepatopancreatic ampulla,** which enters the duodenum at major duodenal papilla situated at a distance of 10 cm from the pylorus. Duodenal opening of ampulla is controlled by **sphincter of Oddi.**

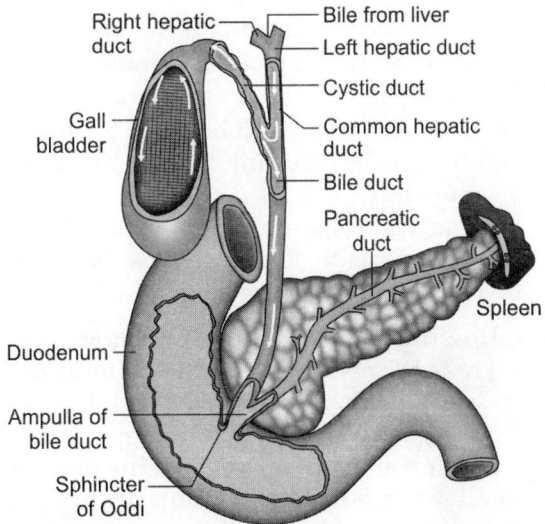

Fig. 10.12: Extrahepatic biliary apparatus and pancreas

Blood supply to pancreas is by splenic and mesenteric vessels.

SPLEEN

The spleen is the largest lymphoid organ of the body. It is purplish red, highly vascular organ lying at the back of left hypochondriac region (*see* Fig. 4.11).

It is situated well under cover of the costal margin, between the diaphragm on one side and kidney, stomach, colon and tail of pancreas on the other side. These four viscera make impressions on the visceral surface of spleen. This surface also has a deep fissure, the **hilum,** for the passage of splenic vessels. Spleen is 2.5 cm thick, 7.5 cm broad, 12.5 cm long, weighs 200 g and lies between 9th and the 11th ribs. The spleen is supported by peritoneal ligaments, i.e. gastrosplenic and lienorenal ligaments.

Spleen is supplied by the tortuous **splenic artery** from coeliac trunk, which runs along the upper border of pancreas to the hilum.

Splenic vein runs behind the pancreas to join superior mesenteric vein and so forms the portal vein.

Lymph vessels leave the hilum and drain into coeliac nodes.

Spleen is covered by a dense connective tissue **capsule. Trabeculae** extend inwards from capsule. Cellular material of spleen is divided into **white pulp** and **red pulp.** Red pulp consists of blood filled venous sinuses and white pulp is of lymphatic tissue, comprise lymphocytes and macrophages.

Spleen is part of the lymphatic system and its functions are:

1. *Phagocytosis:* Leukocytes platelets are phagocytosed in spleen. Old and abnormal RBCs are destroyed in spleen and break-down products (bilirubin and iron) are passed to the liver.
2. *Storage of blood:* Spleen contains up to 350 mL blood. In shock, sympathetic stimulation can return a large part of this volume to circulation.
3. *Immunity:* Spleen contains B- and T-lymphocytes which are important in immune response to infections.
4. *Erythropoiesis:* RBC production occurs in spleen and liver in fetal life and in adults also in times of great need.
5. *Storage of platelets.*

DIGESTION AND ABSORPTION

The food consists of nutrients like carbohydrates, proteins, fats and small quantities of vitamins and minerals. Most of these have to be broken down into simpler substances so that these can be absorbed and transported to the tissues.

Mouth

About 1.5 litres/day saliva is secreted by the 3 sets of salivary glands in the mouth. It lubricates and moistens the food and chewing (mastication) converts it into a soft mass of **bolus.**

The secretory function of salivary glands are under the stimulatory and inhibitory control of parasympathetic and sympathetic nervous system respectively.

Sight, smell and thought of delicious food produces saliva. 99.5% saliva is water and rest is made up of mucin, salts, proteins and amylase (ptyalin).

Functions of Saliva

1. Salivary amylase digests the cooked starch into maltose.
2. It acts as cleansing agent for the mouth.
3. It keeps the mouth moist and lubricated.
4. It helps in getting the taste of food.
5. Food in the mouth is lubricated by saliva before it can be made into a bolus ready for swallowing.
6. Enzyme lysozyme and immunoglobulin A in saliva provide defence against bacterial invasion.

Swallowing and its three stages: Mouth, pharynx and oesophagus participate in the process of swallowing.

Once the food is masticated and made into bolus by mixing with saliva, then the process of swallowing is initiated voluntarily.

The bolus is pushed into the pharynx with the help of tongue and cheeks. Once the bolus reaches the pharynx the palatoglossal arches close the way back to the mouth. This is the first stage of swallowing.

Almost at the same time, soft palate closes off the nasopharynx to prevent the bolus entering the nose. Epiglottis moves backwards to close the opening of larynx like a lid. This is second stage of swallowing. This stage is controlled by swallowing centre in medulla oblongata and lower pons of brain. The muscles of pharynx push the bolus down through the upper oesophageal sphincter.

Bolus itself stimulates peristalsis of oesophageal wall which pushes the bolus into stomach through oesophagus. Bolus takes 4–8 seconds to travel the entire length of oesophagus and reaches the stomach by relaxation of cardiac sphincter. This is the third stage of swallowing.

Stomach

Its size is determined by the amount of food ingested. The stomach has several functions:

1. It serves as a temporary store for food and delivers its contents slowly into the intestines.
2. It initiates the digestion of proteins.
3. Gastric secretions are highly acidic and kill harmful micro-organisms carried with the food.
4. It secretes gastric juice which contains intrinsic factor for the absorption of vitamin B_{12}.
5. Mechanical breakdown of food contents by the peristaltic movements of stomach. The addition of gastric juice liquefy the contents to **chyme.**

The gastric juice is thin, colourless liquid with acidic pH of 2.0. Daily secretion of gastric juice is about 2 litres. Some amount of gastric juice is always present in the stomach. However, the quantity of juice depends on the amount and type of food ingested.

The acidity is due to the presence of hydrochloric acid (HCl). It also contains mucus, water, minerals, gastric lipase and inactive enzyme like pepsinogen. Water and minerals are secreted by gastric glands. Mucus is secreted by **goblet cell,** hydrochloric acid and intrinsic factor by **parietal cells** and pepsinogen by **chief cells** in gastric glands.

Hydrochloric acid kills the bacteria present in the food and provides acidic medium to activate pepsinogen into pepsin. Pepsin begins the digestion of proteins and breaks proteins to polypeptides. Gastric lipase breaks down triglycerides in fat molecules.

The gastric juice is secreted from the mucous membrane of the stomach and it takes place in 3 phases:

1. *Cephalic phase:* Sight, smell, thought of food stimulates secretion of gastric juice. It occurs before the food reaches the stomach.
2. *Gastric phase:* Secretion of gastric juice due to processing of food in the stomach. Even after completion of the meal, the secretion of gastric juice continues under the stimulation of hormone **gastrin.**

   Gastrin is released into the blood from the antrum of stomach, and reaches the fundic cells of stomach. The hormone stimulates the parietal cells of mucosa which synthesises hydrochloric acid from the chlorides of blood. Excessive acidity inhibits the release of gastrin.
3. *Intestinal phase:* As and when the partially digested food reaches the small intestine, another hormone **enterogastrone** is released from intestinal mucosa which acts on stomach and suppresses the gastric motility and gastric secretion.

Mucus lubricates the lining of stomach wall and protects against protein digesting enzymes and hydrochloric acid.

Diet rich in carbohydrate leaves the stomach in 2–3 hours, high protein diet and fatty meals take longer time to leave stomach.

The partially digested food which is ready to enter duodenum is referred as **chyme.**

Pancreas

Daily 1.2–1.5 litres pancreatic juice is secreted by the pancreas. The stimulus for the secretion comes from the entry of chyme into the duodenum.

Pancreatic juice has alkaline pH, and is made up of water, minerals and digestive enzymes, such as **amylase, trypsin, chymotrypsin, carboxypeptidase, elastase** and **lipase. Amylase** hydrolyses starch into sugars. **Lipase** breaks lipids into fatty acids, glycerol and monoglycerides. However, this step requires emulsification of fats in the presence of bile salts. Emulsification increases the surface area of fat droplet so that lipase can hydrolyse it. 80% of fat digestion is due to the pancreatic lipase.

Proteases digest proteins to polypeptides and amino acids. Proteases like trypsin, chymotrypsin are secreted as inactive enzymes so that the gland itself is not digested. Once released from the gland trypsinogen is activated to trypsin by the **enterokinase** to enable the protein digestion. **Trypsin** acts on inactive precursors called chymotrypsinogen, procarboxypeptidase and proelastase to produce chymotrypsin, carboxypeptidase and elastase respectively Presence of acidic chyme from stomach in duodenum stimulates the production of **secretin** and **cholecystokinin** (CCK) hormones from endocrine cells in wall of duodenum. These hormones in turn stimulate the production of pancreatic juice. CCK secretin form the hormone complex, **enterogastrone.** Secretin secretion of pancreatic juice is rich in bicarbonate ions. CCK stimulates secretion of pancreatic juice rich in digestive enzymes.

Liver

It performs the following functions:

1. It converts glucose into glycogen for storage in presence of insulin. The bulky appearance of liver is due to glycogen. Glucagon converts liver glycogen to glucose.
2. It catabolises various nutrients and produces heat.
3. Amino acids and nucleic acids are broken down to urea and uric acid in the liver.
4. The liver cells secrete bile which contains bile pigment (bilirubin), bile salts and cholesterol. Gall bladder acts as a storehouse for bile.

5. It also stores iron and vitamins like B_{12}, A, D, E, K.
6. It is the major site for the synthesis of plasma proteins like albumin and blood clotting factors.
7. Toxic substances like drugs, chemicals, food additives are converted to less harmful and water soluble substance by liver. Thus, the toxins are easily eliminated in the urine. Metabolism of alcohol takes place in the liver.
8. Thyroid hormones and steroids are metabolised in liver.

Secretion of Bile

About 800–1000 mL bile is secreted daily. The secretion of bile is a continuous process. Increased blood flow to the liver increases bile secretion and vice versa.

Bile is a yellowish green liquid and has alkaline pH and has no digestive enzymes. It has bile acids like taurocholic acid, glycocholic acid, and their salts like sodium taurocholate and sodium glycocholate. Cholesterol and lecithin are also components of bile.

Bile enters duodenum during digestion, otherwise it is kept stored in the gall bladder (Fig. 10.12).

Presence of chyme in the duodenum causes contraction of gall bladder and release of bile through bile duct into the duodenum. The quantity of bile released depends on the fat content of diet. More the dietary fat, more is the release of bile. CCK hormone causes contraction of gall bladder and relaxation of sphincter of hepatopancreatic ampulla, allowing the bile to flow into duodenum.

Functions of Bile

1. Bile salts are required for the emulsification of fats, i.e. reduce the size of globules, increasing their surface area and their absorption.
2. It is used as a carrier for the elimination of bile pigment, bilirubin which is formed from the breakdown of haemoglobin. Bilirubin is broken down to stercobilin in intestine and excreted in faeces.

3. Bile acts as a medium for excretion of toxins and cholesterol.
4. Bile salts make fatty acids soluble, enabling both these and fat soluble vitamins (e.g. vitamins A, D, E and K) to be readily absorbed.

Small Intestine

Daily secretion of intestinal juice is 1–2 litres. It secretes digestive enzymes, such as sucrase, maltase, lactase, lipase, peptidases along with water and mucus.

The duodenal contents are carried forward with the help of peristaltic and segmentation movements of intestinal wall. Segmentation movement consists of a series of local constrictions of the intestinal wall which occur rhythmically at points where food material is present. This movement mixes the chyme with digestive juices and brings the food in close contact with the intestinal mucosa for absorption.

The last phase of digestion and absorption of carbohydrates, proteins and fats take place in the villi of small intestine.

The acidic chyme which comes to the small intestine combines with bile, pancreatic juice and intestinal juice.

Any microbes escaping from the killing action of gastric juice will be eradicated by the lymph follicles.

The alkaline pancreatic juice combines with acidic chyme and makes it alkaline. Alkaline pH is most suitable for the action of digestive enzymes from pancreas and intestine. Once the pancreatic juice reaches the intestine, protein digesting enzymes are activated, which then hydrolyse proteins.

In final phase of digestion:
- Proteins are digested by proteases to amino acids.
- Carbohydrates are digested by amylase (salivary and pancreatic) to sugars.
- Fats are hydrolysed by **lipase** to fatty acid and glycerol.
- Lactose is broken down by **lactase** to glucose and galactose.
- Sucrose digested by **sucrase** to glucose and fructose.
- Maltose is broken by **maltase** to glucose.

Absorption in Small Intestine

All the mechanical and chemical phases of digestion from mouth through the small intestine change the food into a form that can pass through epithelial cells lining mucosa and into underlying blood and lymphatic vessels **(absorption)**.

These forms are monosaccharides (glucose, galactose and fructose) from carbohydrates; single amino acids, dipeptides and tripeptides from proteins; and fatty acids, glycerol and monoglycerides from triglycerides.

Absorption of about 90% of nutrients occurs in small intestine and the other 10% occurs in stomach and large intestine. Undigested food particles in small intestine pass to the large intestine, e.g. cellulose (Table 10.2).

Absorption occurs by two processes:

1. *Diffusion:* Monosaccharides, amino acids, fatty acids and glycerol diffuse along their

Table 10.2: Digestion of carbohydrates, proteins and fats

Mouth	Stomach	Small intestine
Carbohydrates are partially digested to disaccharides by salivary amylase	Pepsin hydrolyses proteins to proteases and peptides	Pancreatic amylase completely digests carbohydrates to disaccharides
Fats and proteins are not digested	Gastric lipase digests very little of dietary fat	Trypsin, chymotrypsin act on peptides, proteins and produce free amino acids and smaller peptides Maltase, lactase, sucrase act on disaccharides and liberate glucose, fructose and galactose Peptidases release free amino acids Bile and lipase digest fat to glycerol and free fatty acids

concentration gradient into intestinal epithelial cells from intestinal lumen.

2. *Active transport:* Monosaccharides, amino acids, fatty acids and glycerol are also actively transported into villi.

Normally, all the digested carbohydrates and 95–98% proteins are absorbed in small intestine. About 95% of lipids present in small intestine are absorbed. Mono-saccharides and amino acid pass into capil-laries in villi and fatty acids and glycerol into lacteals.

Large Intestine

The secretion of large intestine does not contain any enzymes but has mucin, water, salts and alkaline pH.

Water, minerals, drugs are absorbed by the large intestine. Contents of ileum are fluid but due to absorption of water, semisolid consis-tency of faeces is achieved.

Large intestine accommodates useful bacteria like *E. coli, Enterobacter aerogenes, Streptococcus faecalis*. Bacteria in large intestine decompose bilirubin to **stercobilin,** which give faeces their brown colour. The friendly bacteria synthesise useful substances such as B group vitamins and vitamin K, which are absorbed by the large intestine.

Defaecation

The anal canal is guarded by internal and external sphincter muscles. Normally rectum is empty. Various stimuli start the peristaltic action and faeces enter the rectum. This irritates the sensory nerve endings of rectum giving desire to defaecate. Defaecation is associated with voluntary contraction of abdominal muscles, descent of diaphragm and peristalsis of colon and relaxation of internal and external anal sphincters. The entry of chyme into caecum from ileum is regulated by ileocaecal sphincter. As food passes, it fills the caecum and accumulates in ascending colon. Peristalsis occurs in large intestine at a slower rate. Large intestine also shows charac-teristic **haustral churning.** In this process, haustra remain relaxed and become distended when they fillup. When distension reaches a certain point, walls contract and squeeze the contents into next haustrum. **Mass peristalsis** also occurs in large intestine in which a strong peristalsis in middle of transverse colon forcing its contents into rectum. Food in stomach initiates this **gastrocolic reflex** in colon and it takes place 3–4 times a day, during or immediately after a meal.

Absorption of Other Nutrients

Water is absorbed through pores of cell membrane by diffusion and it is maximum in the small intestine. In fact, osmotic effect of a solute being absorbed causes the passive absorption of water. Small amounts of water is also absorbed in large intestine. The entire length of small intestine as well as large intes-tine participates in the process of water absorption. About 9.3 litres of fluid enters small intestine (ingestion of liquids 2.3 litres and gastrointestinal secretions 7.0 litres), small intestine absorbs about 8.3 litres of fluid and large intestine absorbs 0.9 litre. Only 0.1 litre (100 mL) of water is excreted in faeces each day.

Electrolytes: Small intestine is the site for the absorption of electrolytes. They combine with water molecule in solution and absorbed by diffusion, through the pores of cell membrane. The diffusion continues as long as electrolyte concentration is higher in the intestinal lumen than the cells. Sodium is passively absorbed by diffusion. Bicarbonate, chloride either passively follow sodium or is actively transported.

The absorption of calcium, iron, potassium and phosphate takes place from small intestine by active transport. It is a carrier mediated transport, located in the villus and requires energy, e.g. calcium is transported by calcium binding protein.

Absorption of vitamins: Water soluble vita-mins (B and C) do not need bile salts for absorption. Fat soluble vitamins (A, D, E, K) need bile salts for absorption. These are absor-bed by simple diffusion. Vitamin B_{12} combines with intrinsic factor produced by stomach and combination is actively transported in ileum by active transport (Table 10.3).

Table 10.3: Absorption of vitamins in GIT

Organ	Water soluble vitamins absorbed	Fat soluble vitamins absorbed
Duodenum	Dietary B group vitamins such as folic acid, pyridoxine, niacin, thiamine and vitamin C	Dietary vitamin D
Small intestine colon	Dietary riboflavin Friendly bacteria synthesize vitamin B_{12} which is absorbed at the same site	Dietary vitamins A, E and K. Bacteria synthesise vitamin K and is absorbed

FOOD AND DRUG INTERACTION

Definition

Food and drug interaction is a change in drug effect on the body when a drug is taken with certain food or beverage. Food can cause reaction that changes the effect of medicine. This can increase, decrease or delay the absorption of drug or can cause adverse effect.

Taking a medicine with food can cause your body not to absorb the medicine. For example, while taking ACE inhibitors, avoid food rich in potassium such as banana, coconut water, etc. On the other hand some medicine are better absorbed when taken with food. If not taken with food it may cause nausea or vomit.

Food and drug interaction happens when a drug is taken orally, it travels to the liver. In the liver specific enzymes breakdown and metabolise the drug and process the chemical.

Introducing new substance at the same time, which is not beneficial can potentially interfere with these enzymes. When this happens medicine becomes ineffective or its effect gets diluted

How does drug interaction occur?
There are several mechanisms by which drug interacts with food or other substances. An interaction can result when there is increase or decrease in:
- Absorption of a drug in the body
- Distribution of the drug in the body
- Metabolism made by the body for the drug
- Elimination of the drug from the body.

Why food and drug interaction is important?
1. It affects how medication works by changing levels of drug in the body
2. It puts you at risk for side effects and toxicity
3. It worsen a medical condition one may already have
4. It can increase the cost or delay healthcare.

Drug can alter food intake and nutritional status
1. Appetite increased or decreased, unusual food cravings
2. Metaboilic rate increased or decreased
3. Taste or smell altered
4. Oral side effects like dry mouth, mouth pain
5. Difficulty in swallowing
6. Nausea, vomiting and diarrhoea.

Factors that affect drug interaction:
It is important to have information for food and drug interaction. Personal traits also play an important role in it:
1. *Genetic:* Individual genetic make up can make the same drug work differently on different bodies. Some people can process certain medicine more quickly than others.
2. *Weight:* Some drugs are dosed according to weight while others are not. Weight can affect the dose and could also increase or decrease the risk of drug interaction.
3. *Age:* As body ages interaction also changes, some of which may affect how our body responds to medication. Kidney, liver and circulatory system may also slow down with age. This can slow the breakdown and removal of drugs from the body and may also affect how long drug stays in the body.
4. *Sex:* Difference between sexes such as anatomy and hormones can play a part in drug interaction. For example, the recommended dose of Zolpede (Ambien) for female is nearly half the dose of man.

5. *Life style diet and exercise:* Certain diets can be problematic when combined with certain medication. For example, researches have shown that high fat intake can reduce the response of brochodilators, which people suffering from asthma use for treatment. On the other hand exercise can also change how medicine works. For example, people who use insulin to treat diabetes can experience hypoglycaemia during exercise. They may need to adjust the time to eat and take insulin.

6. *How long drug stays in the body:* The right dose of medication depends how body absorb and processes the drug. That is why it is important that treating physician is aware of all the medication patient is taking before prescribing a new medicine.

How to minimise food and drug interaction?

1. Correct dose of the medicine
2. Follow the prescribed route of medication
3. Follow time interval between doses
4. Whether the medicine is to be taken with food, before food or after food

Persons at highest risk for food and drug interaction:

1. Person who require long-term drug therapy
2. Taking many drugs including alcohol
3. Those persons who have poor or marginal nutrition
4. Elderly who have several risk factors
5. Person who has immature or impaired metabolic system.

Tips to remember when taking medication:

1. Read the prescription label and understand it
2. Read all directions, warnings and precautions
3. Take medicine with full glass of water unless told otherwise
4. Do not break, crush or stir the medicine in food unless instructed
5. Do not mix the medicine in hot drinks as heat may keep the drug from working
6. Never take medicine with alcohol.

Drugs with side effects and nutritional implications are shown in Table 10.4.

Table 10.4: Drugs with side effects and nutritional implications

Medication	Side effects	Nutritional implications
Monoamine oxidase inhibitors (MAOI) (antidepressants) Isocarboxazid Phenelzine Tranylcypromine	Sudden high blood pressure may occur alcohol and may increase depressants effect Caffeine may increase blood pressure and cardiac arrhythmia	Avoid foods rich in **tyramine** for example, cheese, yeast, meat stock, smoked or pickeled meat, fermented sausages and salami, beer, wine, avocado, banana, raisins, excess of caffeine like tea, coffee and chocolates
Theophylline (asthma, pulmonary disease)	Avoid caffeine	Caffeine foods like tea, coffee and chocolates can increase heartbeat, nervousness, nausea, vomiting, headache
Alendronate sodium/ Ibandronate sodium (osteoporosis)	Follow instructions	Take medicine first thing in the morning with full glass of water. Do not lie down take food after one hour
Warfarin coumarin (blood thinner/anti-coagulant)	Anorexia, nausea, diarrhoea, abdominal cramps	Eat small frequent meals fluid and electrolyte replacement in case of diarrhoea. Avoid vit. K rich foods, cranberry juice, cauliflower, cabbage, broccoli, raw tomatoes, tomato soup, spinach, green tea, spring onions, brussels, sprouts, soybean oil, wheat grass, liver, bacon, swisschard fish, alcohol, avocado kale, turnip greens

Contd...

Table 10.4: Drugs with side effects and nutritional implications (Contd...)

Medication	Side effects	Nutritional implicationa
Atorvastatin, provastatin, simvastatin Socorro (lipid altering agents inhibitors of HMG-CoA reductase)	Constipation/diarrhoea, gas, pain in upper abdomen	Avoid grapefruit (chakotra) Eating low fat food and avoid alcohol
Lisinopril, captopril, ramipril (angiotensin converting enzymes ACE inhibitors) BP medicine	May increase serum potassium level May decrease serum **sodium** Nausea, metallic taste in mouth	Maintain adequate hydration Avoid salt substitute with potassium Avoid potassium supplements Avoid foods rich in potassium coconut water, banana, green leafy vegetables, orange, tomato juice
Aspirin, diclofenac, ibuprofen, ketoprofen (nonsteroidal anti-inflammatory drug NSAID)	Can cause stomach bleeding	To be taken with food or milk
Acetaminophen	Can cause liver damage	To be taken with food. Avoid alcohol
Cetirizine, clemastine, faxofenadine Triprolidine	Drowsiness	Avoid alcohol
Erythromycin		Avoid fruit juices, wine. As it decreases its effectivity
Tetracycline		Avoid dairy products. To be taken 1 hour before food or 2 hours after food, take medicine with full glass of water
Livothyroxin (hypothyroidism)		To be taken first thing in the morning with full glass of water avoid walnut, soybean flour.

CLINICAL ASPECTS

Mouth

Angular stomatitis: The angles of mouth show painful cracks due to vitamin B deficiency or infection by herpes simplex virus. It usually occurs after an attack of common cold or influenza.

Aphthous stomatitis: Recurrent painful oral ulcers develop inside the mouth. They are often associated with vitamin B complex deficiency.

Fungal infection of mouth: It occurs in bottle fed babies and in elderly people with low immunity. It is usually caused by *Candida albicans.*

Cancer of mouth: This mostly occurs in people who keep betel nut in their mouth for long periods. Chronic irritation of delicate mucous membrane of mouth and tongue results in squamous cell carcinoma.

Glossitis: Inflammation of the tongue causes areas of redness on the tongue, which are quite painful. The tongue becomes smooth in deficiency of vitamin B. In anaemia, the undersurface of tongue looks pale. Chronic irritation due to sharp edge of the tooth or betel nut may cause cancer which spreads fast and is usually fatal.

Tumours of salivary glands: Pleomorphic adenoma is benign tumour consisting of epithelial and connective tissue cells and it usually occurs in parotid gland. Malignant tumour may also develop in any salivary gland.

During embryonic development, roof of mouth (hard palate) develops as two separate halves (right and left) and before birth these two fuse along the midline. The upper lip/hard palate may show a developmental defect due to incomplete fusion in the form of **cleft lip or cleft palate** (partial or complete or both).

In the newborn baby with cleft palate, there is communication between mouth and nasal cavity. These children when fed with milk, get choked as the milk enters the nasal cavity, pharynx, larynx and there is defective speech.

Teeth: Teeth are the hardest tissues of our body. They are used in medicolegal practice for identification and age determination.

In **caries,** the enamel gets removed and the nerves get exposed, causing severe pain.

The gums may get inflamed. The condition is called **'gingivitis'.** Teeth provide proper shape to the face and must be maintained well.

1. *Mumps:* Viral infection of the parotid (especially), submandibular and sublingual glands is called mumps. The virus may also spread to the testis, ovary, brain and pancreas.
2. *Tonsillitis and adenoids* occur at the oropharyngeal junction.

Oesophagus

1. **Oesophagus** may get partly fibrosed if caustic materials are taken accidently leading to narrowing **(stricture)** and difficulty in swallowing.
2. The lower end of oesophagus may develop dilatation of veins in liver fibrosis **(cirrhosis).** These veins may rupture to cause haemetemesis (vomiting of blood).

Reflux Oesophagitis

Persistent regurgitation (back-flow) of acidic gastric juice into oesophagus causes irritation and painful ulceration. It may lead to haemorrhage and fibrosis leading to narrowing **(stricture).**

Achalasia

There is constriction of cardiac sphincter of oesophagus due to malfunction of myenteric plexus because of which there is blockage of passage of ingested material into stomach. The oesophagus becomes dilated. It may lead to dysphagia (difficulty in swallowing), regurgitation of gastric contents.

Tumours of Oesophagus

Malignant tumours are more common. They usually occur at the distal end of oesophagus and at the level of larynx and bifurcation of the trachea. It leads to the obstruction of the oesophagus. The tumour may spread to the adjacent structures.

Stomach

Gastritis

It occurs when there is imbalance between corrosive action of gastric juice and protective effect of mucus on gastric mucosa. The insufficient amount of mucus in stomach leads to damage of surface epithelium from hydrochloric acid.

Acute gastritis develops due to regular, prolonged use of aspirin and other non-steroidal anti-inflammatory drugs (NSAIDs); excessive intake of alcohol, heavy cigarette smoking, food poisoning, ingestion of corrosive acids and alkalis.

Chronic gastritis is a milder form. It may follow acute attacks or autoimmune disease.

Vomiting

Vomiting/emesis is the forcible expulsion of contents of upper gastrointestinal (GI) tract (stomach and sometimes duodenum) through the mouth. It usually occurs due to irritation of stomach. Nurses have to observe, record and report about the vomiting of the patient for treatment.

An ulcer is crater like lesion in membrane. Ulcers that develop in areas of the GI tract exposed to acidic gastric juice are called peptic ulcers.

Helicobacter pylori is the most frequently seen increases of peptic ulcer. This bacteria produces ammonia which damages the protective layer of the stomach.

The stomach bears the brunt of all wrong types of food including too hot/too cold food or fluids. The ulcers in the stomach occur along its lesser curvature and in first few centimetres of duodenum in alcoholics and heavy smokers. People with erratic eating habits with erratic timings are also subjects of peptic ulcers. The ulcers may cause bleeding or perforation. If untreated, the chronic ulcers may become cancerous.

Small Intestine

1. *Typhoid fever* is caused by *Salmonella typhi*. It occurs due to intake of contaminated water. It causes ulcers in the small intestine. It may affect the liver, spleen and gall bladder.
2. *Tuberculosis* also affects the intestine. The most common site is ileocaecal junction. TB intestine causes intestinal obstruction.
3. *Food poisoning* by *E. coli* causes vomiting and diarrhoea.
4. *Cholera* is caused by *Vibrio cholerae* and causes severe vomiting, diarrhoea and dehydration. It needs urgent attention and transfusion of intravenous fluids to correct dehydration.
5. *Hernia* is the protrusion of a part of small intestine through a weakness in the wall of abdominal cavity. It is mostly inguinal or femoral and occurs more commonly in male or female respectively. It is reducible to begin with, but may become irreducible or obstructed to give rise to complications.

Large Intestine

1. *Caecum* is the beginning of large intestine. It is a common site of **intestinal tuberculosis.**
2. *Appendicitis:* Inflammation of vermiform appendix results in appendicitis. In its early stages, there is pain around umbilicus while in later stage, it gets localised in the right iliac fossa. Its complications may lead to abscess formation at various sites in abdomen, peritonitis, fibrous adhesions between bowel loops leading to obstruction. The removal of appendix is called **'appendicectomy'.**
3. *Dysentery* is either bacterial or amoebic according to the nature of causative agent. **Bacterial dysentery** is caused by **Shigella**

while the **amoebic dysentery** is caused by *Entamoeba histolytica* with mucus.
4. *Cancer of the colon* is a common entity in people who eat less of fibre in their diet. It is less common in India as Indians eat vegetables, which contain good amount of fibres.
5. *Malabsorption:* Due to various defects in the intestinal mucous membrane or glands related to it there is decreased absorption of glucose, fatty acids, amino acids and water from the intestine. This results in severe weakness and nutritional deficiencies.
6. *Haemorrhoids* (piles) results from enlargement and inflammation of rectal veins. These develop when veins are put under pressure and become engorged with blood. Such a distended vessel oozes blood.

Glands

Pancreas

Inflammation of pancreas is called **'pancreatitis'.** It may be acute or chronic leading to damage to pancreas. Most commonly it is caused by gallstones and alcoholism. Severity of disease is related to amount of pancreatic tissue destroyed. Malabsorption syndrome develops due to defective digestion. Lack of insulin causes diabetes.

Liver

Liver is like the 'reserve bank' of our body. Most of the nutrients are deposited here to be used if and when necessary.

1. *Cirrhosis* results from long term inflammation caused by a variety of agents in which liver tissue is destroyed and replaced by fibrous tissue. Various causes of cirrhosis are alcoholism, hepatitis B and C virus infection, parasitic infections of liver, chemicals that destroy hepatocytes. Symptoms include jaundice, oedema in legs and uncontrolled bleeding due to oesophageal varices, ascites (collection fluid in peritoneal cavity).
2. *Hepatitis* is inflammation of liver that can be caused by viruses, drugs and chemicals

including alcohol. Viral infections are the most common cause and include type A, B, C and E. The viruses enter the liver cells and cause degenerative changes and inflammation ensues. As groups of cells die, areas of necrosis develop and lobules become distorted. Fibrosis develops in damaged area and adjacent hepatocytes proliferate. Type A and E virus spread by hands, food, water contaminated by infected faeces. Type B and C virus spread by blood and blood products. Most patients suffering from hepatitis A and E virus recover. Infection by hepatitis B and C leads to chronic liver disease, cirrhosis and may lead to liver cancer.

3. *Jaundice* results from abnormal bilirubin metabolism and excretion. Bilirubin which is produced in liver due to breakdown of haemoglobin is excreted in bile after conjugation in liver. Jaundice results from abnormalities in the metabolism of bilirubin, e.g. excess breakdown of RBCs, impaired conjugation or defective excretion of bilirubin and obstruction to flow of bile from liver to duodenum. Jaundice can be due to infection of liver. The bilirubin level in the blood rises and it gets deposited in various tissues, e.g. skin, conjunctiva and brain.

Gall Bladder

Since it stores bile, it is subjected to inflammation, called **'cholecystitis'**. The pain may radiate to the tip of right shoulder.

The bile gets concentrated in gall bladder. At times the salts may precipitate to cause multiple gallstones. This condition is called **'cholelithiasis'**. Surgical removal of gall bladder is called **'cholecystectomy'**.

Obesity

When the weight is more than 20–25% of normal weight, the person is said to be obese. Obesity itself is a disease as it leads to diabetes, hypertension, arthritis and heart disease. Weight reduction should be slow and sustained. It must not be too fast, as the weight lost tends to come back.

Kwashiorkor

It is a disorder in which diet is deficient in protein intake despite normal caloric intake. Clinical features are ascites, enlarged liver, lower than normal body temperature, oedema in lower limbs and sometimes mental retardation.

Marasmus

It results from inadequate intake of both protein and calories. Clinical features are growth retardation, low body weight, muscle wasting and thin, and dry skin.

Anorexia Nervosa

It is psychiatric disorder characterised by self-induced weight loss leading to amenorrhoea (absence of menstruation), osteoporosis. It is seen in young, single females.

Peritoneal Dialysis

Peritoneum acts as a selective permeable membrane. In kidney failure, special fluid is injected into the peritoneal cavity. This special fluid removes the urea, etc. from blood. Then, the fluid is removed.

Points to Remember

1. In human teeth erupt two times only. These are called milk teeth and permanent teeth.
2. There are nine regions in the anterior abdominal wall.
3. Most dilated part of digestive system is the stomach.
4. Liver is the largest gland of the body.
5. Pancreas secretes insulin. Lack of insulin results in diabetes.

MCQs

1. **Parts of pharynx from above downwards are:**
   (a) Nasopharynx, laryngopharynx, oropharynx
   (b) Oropharynx, laryngopharynx, nasopharynx
   (c) Nasopharynx, oropharynx, laryngopharynx

2. **Subdivisions of abdominal cavity are:**
   (a) Eight
   (b) Seven
   (c) Nine
   (d) Ten

3. **Synthesis of bile occurs in:**
   (a) Liver
   (b) Gall bladder
   (c) Pancreas
   (d) Duodenum

4. **Part of large intestine that is joined to rectum is called:**
   (a) Ascending colon
   (b) Transverse colon
   (c) Descending colon
   (d) Sigmoid colon

Ans.   1 c   2 c   3 a   4 d

Endocrine System

Most of the functions in the human body are regulated by two main systems—autonomic nervous system, and endocrine system.

These two systems mostly work independently to maintain the homeostasis of the internal environment. The autonomic nervous system is concerned with rapid changes while the endocrine system is involved in slower and more precise adjustments.

Endocrine system consists of widely separated endocrine glands. Each endocrine gland is composed of specialised secretory cells, which secrete a chemical substance called hormone and release it into the blood stream directly. These glands do not have a duct system, so are also known as ductless glands. The hormone released is carried by the bloodstream to another (target) organ or tissue where it exerts its effects by affecting cellular growth and metabolism. Endocrine glands though work independently, their balanced action is necessary to maintain body homeostasis (Fig. 11.1).

Most hormones released are either derived from amino acids or steroids (Fig. 11.2).

All endocrine glands have different embryologic origin, differ histologically and are located in different parts of the body. The various endocrine glands are:

1. Hypothalamus pituitary gland
2. Thyroid gland
3. Parathyroid glands
4. Adrenal/suprarenal glands
5. Islets of Langerhans in pancreas
6. Pineal gland
7. Ovaries (in female)
8. Testes (in males)
9. Placenta
10. Juxtaglomerular apparatus in kidney.

HYPOTHALAMUS AND PITUITARY GLAND

Hypothalamus is present in the floor of the third ventricle of brain. It is the **master gland** of the endocrine system. It secretes two true hormones, i.e. **oxytocin** and **antidiuretic**

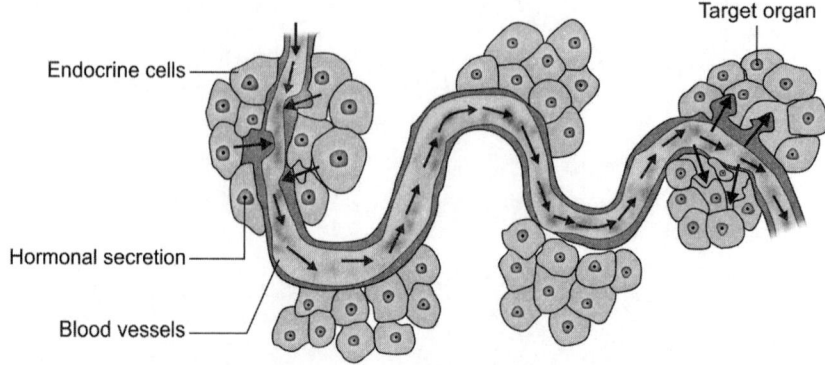

Fig. 11.1: Endocrine gland

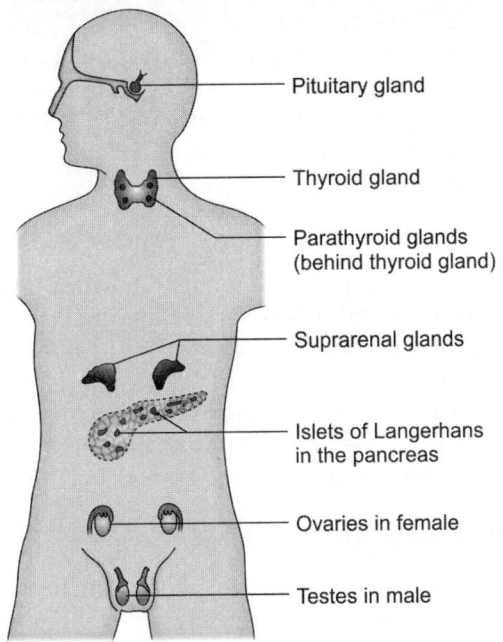

Fig. 11.2: Components of endocrine system

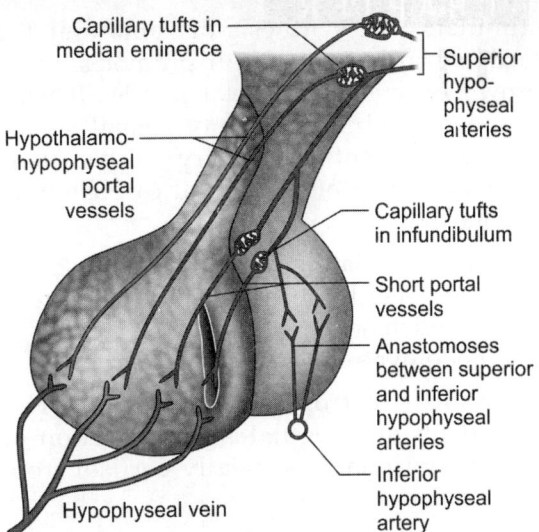

Fig. 11.3: The lobes of the pituitary gland and their relationship with the hypothalamus

hormone **(ADH)**. It also secretes the releasing and inhibiting factors to control the trophic hormones released from the anterior pituitary and thereby control the activity of most of the endocrine glands.

   Pituitary gland (hypophysis cerebri) is a small ovoid structure attached to the base of the brain. It lies in the hypophyseal fossa located on the superior surface of the body of sphenoid bone. It lies below the hypothalamus to which it is attached by a stalk. It weighs about 500 mg and has three distinct parts (Fig. 11.3).

1. *Anterior pituitary* (adenohypophysis): Constitutes 80% of pituitary gland. It contains five different types of glandular cells. It is richly supplied by blood vessels and is linked with hypothalamus through the blood vessels. This link is called **hypothalamohypophyseal portal vessels** through which products of hypothalamus are brought to the anterior pituitary.

2. *Posterior pituitary* (neurohypophysis): Constitutes 20% of pituitary gland. It consists of nervous tissue and blood vessels. There are **no glandular cells.** It does not synthesise any hormone. It is linked with

hypothalamus by a **neural hypothalamo-hypophyseal tract.** The hormones ADH and oxytocin are synthesised in hypothalamus and transported by neural tracts to posterior pituitary and are released from there.

3. *Intermediate lobe:* It is a thin strip of tissue between anterior and posterior lobes. Its function in humans is not known.

Anterior Pituitary

Some of the hormones secreted by the anterior pituitary stimulate or inhibit secretion by other endocrine glands while others have a direct affect on target tissues. The various releasing/inhibiting hormones released by the hypothalamus release/inhibit specific hormones from anterior pituitary. The trophic hormone released from the anterior pituitary in turn stimulates the target gland to produce and release its hormone. Rise in blood level of that hormone inhibits the secretion of releasing factor by hypothalamus **(negative feedback mechanism).** Low level of hormone in blood stimulates the release of appropriate releasing hormone from hypothalamus.

Growth hormone (GH) is the most abundant hormone synthesised by the anterior pituitary. It is important for the growth and development in the body. GH does not act itself but it stimulates the synthesis of **somatomedin** (active principle of GH). It promotes linear growth of bones and skeletal muscles. It helps in growth and maturation of genital organs and development of secondary sex characters. It also affects protein, fat and carbohydrate metabolism.

Thyroid stimulating hormone (TSH) stimulates and regulates the activity of thyroid gland which secretes hormones T_4 and T_3 (tetraiodothyronine and triiodothyronine).

Adrenocorticotrophic hormone (ACTH) stimulates and regulates the secretion of steroid hormones especially cortisol from adrenal cortex.

Prolactin stimulates milk production **(lactation)** and has a direct effect on breasts immediately after childbirth.

Gonadotrophins are released from anterior pituitary after puberty. **Follicle stimulating hormone** (FSH), in both sexes, stimulates production of gametes (ova or spermatozoa). **Luteinising hormone** (LH) and FSH in females stimulate the secretion of oestrogen and progesterone during menstrual cycle. In males, LH also called **interstitial cell stimulating hormone** (ICSH) stimulates interstitial cells of testes to produce the hormone testosterone.

Posterior Pituitary

It releases oxytocin and ADH hormone. These hormones act directly on target tissues.

1. *Oxytocin* acts on uterine smooth muscle and muscle cells of the lactating breast. During childbirth it stimulates the uterine contractions and causes expulsion of fetus. It stimulates contraction of myoepithelial cells surrounding the mammary ducts to facilitate ejection of milk.

2. *Antidiuretic hormone* (ADH) reduces the urine output. It causes an increase in the permeability to water of the distal convoluted and collecting tubules of nephrons of the kidney. It is responsible for 20% reabsorption of total volume reabsorbed in kidneys. Thus, it is responsible for

maintaining water and acid–base balance of the body. In high concentration, it causes contraction of smooth cells of blood vessels of skin and abdominal organs, thus raising the blood pressure. So, it is also called **vasopressin.**

Intermediate Lobe

It probably produces **melanocyte stimulating hormone** (MSH). MSH stimulates melanocyte cells in deeper layers of epidermis to synthesise **melanin.** This hormone is more important in lower animals for increasing/ decreasing the amount of melanin in the skin for safety reasons.

THYROID GLAND

Thyroid is an endocrine gland, which pours its secretion directly into the blood. There is no duct in this gland (Fig. 11.1). The gland lies in front of the trachea and larynx in neck, and is enclosed in deep cervical fascia. So, the gland moves during swallowing (Fig. 11.4).

It weighs about 25 g. It comprises two lobes and median isthmus. The two lobes are joined by a narrow isthmus, lying in front of trachea. The lobes are roughly cone shaped, about 5 cm long and 3 cm wide. It is related to two

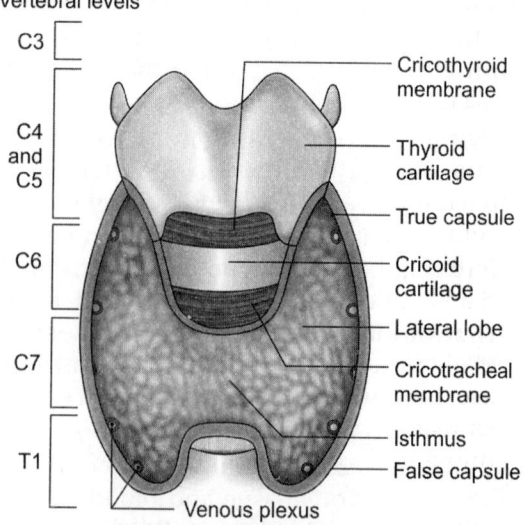

Vertebral levels

C3

C4 and C5

C6

C7

T1

Cricothyroid membrane

Thyroid cartilage

True capsule

Cricoid cartilage

Lateral lobe

Cricotracheal membrane

Isthmus

False capsule

Venous plexus

Fig. 11.4: Thyroid gland from front

tubes—trachea, oesophagus; two nerves—external laryngeal and recurrent laryngeal and their accompanying arteries. Superior thyroid artery runs with external laryngeal nerve and inferior thyroid artery runs with recurrent laryngeal nerve.

Arterial blood supply is through superior and inferior thyroid arte ries. The **venous drainage** is by thyroid veins, which drain into internal jugular veins.

Thyroid gland is made of numerous **follicles** lined by cuboidal to columnar epithelial cells. The cells selectively take up iodine from blood. Iodin e plus tyrosine amino acid synthesise triiodothyronine (T3) and tetraiodothyronine/thyroxine (T4). These two hormones are kept in combination with globulin to form **thyroglobulin** in the lumen of the follicle to be released, if and when required. Thyroglobulin is broken to active hormones according to the need of the body.

Between the follicles are cells called **parafollicular cells (C cells),** which secrete the hormone calcitonin.

Functions

Thyroid gland maintains and regulates basal metabolic rate of the body. It increases cellular metabolic activities in all body tissues except brain, spleen, lungs and retina, thus increasing heat production.

It stimulates haemopoiesis, vitamin B_{12} absorption from intestine. It also stimulates oogenesis and spermatogenesis. T3 and T4 also regulate metabolism of carbohydrates, proteins and fats. These hormones are essential for normal growth and development of skeleton and nervous system.

Calcitonin has effect on calcium metabolism and its effects are opposite to that of parathyroid hormone secreted from parathyroid glands. It acts on bone and kidneys to decrease the raised blood calcium level. It reduces reabsorption of calcium from bones and inhibits reabsorption of calcium by renal tubules.

Functions of thyroid gland secretion, i.e. T3 and T4 are controlled by thyroid stimulating hormone (TSH) of anterior pituitary gland. Increased levels of T3 and T4 decrease TSH secretion and vice versa. Secretion of TSH is also stimulated by thyroid releasing hormone (TRH) from hypothalamus.

PARATHYROID GLANDS

These are four pea-shaped glands situated two each on the posterior surface of the each lobe of thyroid gland. These are supplied by branches of inferior thyroid artery (Figs 11.5A and B).

The gland secretes a hormone, **parathormone/parathyroid hormone (PTH),** which maintains blood calcium level.

Secretion of this hormone increases the level of serum calcium. It acts by increasing the amount of calcium absorbed from small intestine and reabsorbed from renal tubules. It also stimulates resorption of calcium from bones by stimulating osteoclasts (bone destroying cells). Thus, it regulates blood calcium level which is important for muscle contraction and blood clotting.

SUPRARENAL/ADRENAL GLANDS

This pair of endocrine gland lies above the kidneys (Fig. 11.2). Each gland is made up of peripheral cortex and a central medulla. They are about 4 cm long and 3 cm thick.

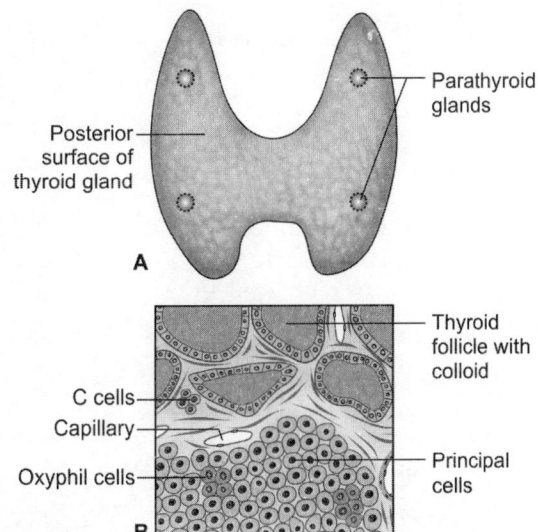

Figs 11.5A and B: Thyroid and parathyroid glands

The cortex and medulla are structurally and functionally different from each other. Both of these function to combat stress.

Cortex has three zones each with different secretions:

1. *Outermost zone* is **zona glomerulosa** which secretes mineralocorticoids. **Aldosterone** is the main mineralocorticoid. It is concerned with regulation of water and electrolyte balance in the body. It stimulates the reabsorption of sodium (Na^+) by renal tubules and excretion of potassium (K^+) in the urine. With Na^+ reabsorption there is retention of water also, so it regulates blood volume and blood pressure also. Secretion of aldosterone is stimulated by high blood potassium and angiotensin.

2. *Middle zone* is **zona fasciculata** which secretes glucocorticoids. These are essential for life. They regulate metabolism and responses to stress. Main glucocorticoids are cortisol, corticosterone and cortisone. Metabolic side effects of glucocorticoids are **gluconeogenesis** (formation of glucose from proteins), **hyperglycaemia** (raised blood glucose level), **catabolism** (breakdown) of proteins, **lipolysis** (breakdown of triglyceride fats into fatty acids and glycerol for energy production). It also promotes reabsorption of sodium and water from renal tubules. Glucocorticoids also delay wound healing, suppress immune response and prevent deposition of calcium in bones.

3. *Innermost zone* is **zona reticularis.** It secretes sex hormones [androgens, dehydroepiandrostenedione (DHEA)] are synthesized in adrenal cortex. These are converted into testosterone in peripheral tissues and exert their effect.

Medulla secretes epinephrine/adrenaline and norepinephrine/noradrenaline (Fig. 11.6).

Both epinephrine and norepinephrine are synthesised from amino acid tyrosine. **Epinephrine** is a hormone of emergency though it is not absolutely essential for life. **Norepinephrine** is released from postganglionic neurotransmitter at sympathetic division of autonomic nervous system. Epinephrine and some norepinephrine are released in blood from adrenal medulla during stimulation of the sympathetic nervous system. They are hormones of emergency, together they help the body during the conditions of **fight or flight** after initial sympathetic stimulation by increasing the heart rate and blood pressure, increasing

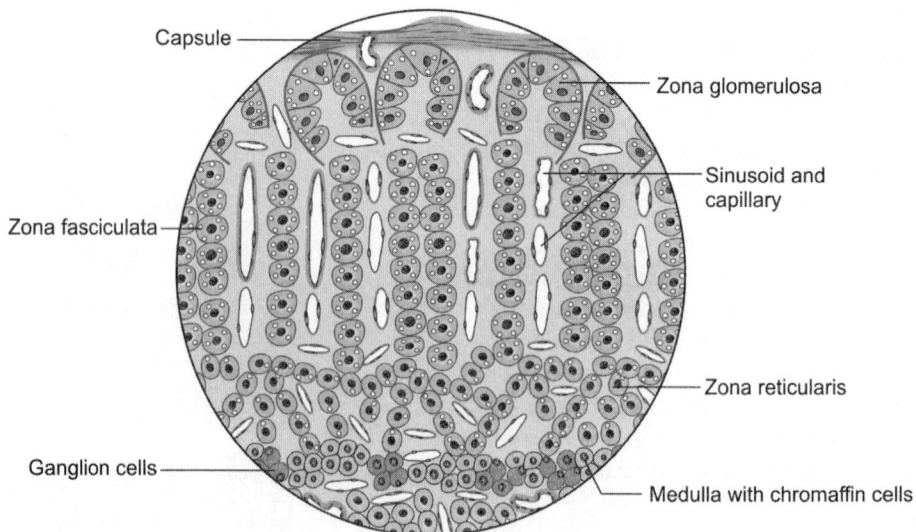

Fig. 11.6: Structure of suprarenal gland

Labels: Capsule, Zona glomerulosa, Sinusoid and capillary, Zona fasciculata, Zona reticularis, Ganglion cells, Medulla with chromaffin cells

metabolic rate, dilating the pupils and diverting the blood to essential organs, e.g. heart, brain and skeletal muscles.

Summary of effects of noradrenaline and adrenaline are:

1. Constriction of blood vessels of skin, digestive system
2. Dilating coronary arteries
3. Increasing heart rate
4. Dilating the bronchioles
5. Dilating the pupils
6. Decrease rate of digestion
7. Converting glycogen to glucose.

PANCREAS—ISLETS OF LANGERHANS

Pancreas is unique as it is both an exocrine and endocrine gland. The **pancreatic acini** secreting **pancreatic juice** form the exocrine part as it is carried by the pancreatic duct to the duodenum. The endocrine part is islets of Langerhans, whose cells secrete glucagon (by α cells), insulin (by β cells) and somatostatin (by δ cells) (Fig. 11.7). Normal blood glucose level is 80–120 mg%. Blood glucose level is maintained by the opposing actions of insulin and glucagon—insulin decreases blood glucose levels while glucagon increases it.

Insulin increases the cell membranes permeability for glucose in muscles and adipose tissue. It increases glucose utilization in them. It also increases conversion of glucose to glycogen (glycogenesis) in liver and skeletal muscle, increases protein and lipid synthesis, decreases **glycogenolysis** (breakdown of glycogen) and gluconeogenesis.

Glucagon increases blood glucose level by glycogenolysis in liver and skeletal muscles and gluconeogenesis. It also increases lipolysis in adipose tissues.

Somatostatin inhibits the secretion of both insulin and glucagon.

PINEAL GLAND

It is about 1 cm long and found attached to the roof of third ventricle of brain.

Melatonin hormone is secreted by the pineal gland. It probably causes:

1. Inhibition of growth and development of sex organs before puberty.
2. Because of its neural connection with hypothalamus it coordinates **circadian** (events that occur at approximately 24 hours interval) and **diurnal** (events that occur during daytime) rhythm of many tissues.

OVARIES, TESTES AND PLACENTA

Described in Chapter 12, 'Reproductive System'.

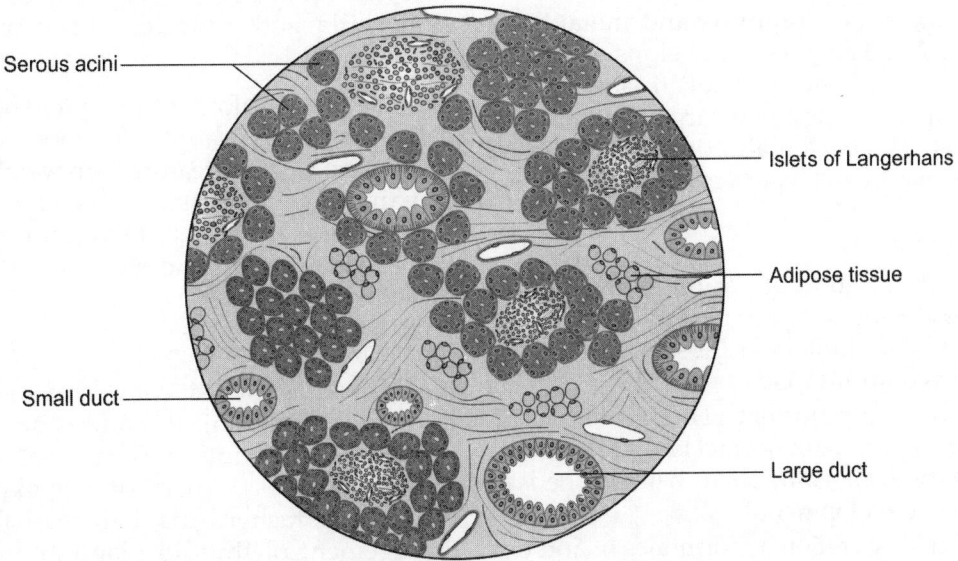

Fig. 11.7: Pancreatic acini and islets of Langerhans

JG APPARATUS IN KIDNEYS

Described in Chapter 6, 'Urinary System'.

Local Hormones

Histamine: It is synthesised by the mast cells. It increases capillary permeability

Serotonin: Present in brain and platelets. It causes contraction of smooth muscles.

Prostaglandins: These cause vasoconstriction, bronchospasm, etc.

CLINICAL ASPECTS

Endocrine diseases result from either overproduction (hypersecretion) or under-production (hyposecretion) of hormones.

Diseases of Pituitary Gland

Gigantism and Acromegaly

It is a result of prolonged hypersecretion of GH from anterior pituitary. Usually, it results from a tumour of GH secreting cells.

Excess of GH during childhood before fusion of metaphysis and epiphysis results in **gigantism.** The individual has abnormal increase in stature due to skeletal overgrowth but body proportions are normal.

Acromegaly results when there is hypersecretion of GH after puberty and ossification is complete, i.e. epiphysis and metaphysis have fused. The person develops abnormal thickening of bones and soft tissues leading to prominent mandible, enlargement of hands and feet. The person also develops enlarged tongue and liver. Hypertension may develop.

Hypopituitarism

Deficient secretion of various hormones of pituitary leads to hypopituitarism. If all the hormones of pituitary are absent, it is known as **panhypopituitarism.**

Deficient secretion of GH in childhood lead to short stature with normal body proportion **(pituitary dwarfism).** There will also be lack of sexual development.

Deficient secretion of hormones of anterior pituitary in adults Sheehan's syndrome results

from infarction due to shock. If it develops after severe haemorrahge during or after childbirth, there will be lactation failure also besides the clinical features of hypothyroidism and adrenal insufficiency.

Diabetes insipidus results from hyposecretion of ADH. There is excretion of excessive amounts of dilute urine causing dehydration, extreme thirst.

Diseases of Thyroid Gland

Goitre

There is enlargement of the thyroid gland without signs of hyperthyroidism. Secretion of T4 and T3 is reduced and their low levels stimulate TSH secretion resulting in enlargement of thyroid gland. Enlarged gland may cause pressure on adjacent tissues leading to difficulty in swallowing and breathing, hoarseness of voice. It is usually due to iodine deficiency.

Hypothyroidism

It results from insufficient secretion of T4 and T3.

Cretinism develops when deficiency of thyroxine (T4) occurs in fetal life or early childhood. It leads to decreased (retarded) physical and mental development, coarse dry skin, enlarged tongue and prominent abdomen.

Myxoedema develops when thyroid hormone deficiency occurs in adults. It is more common in females. Clinical features are weight gain, constipation, depression, dry skin, broad bloated face, tiredness, intolerance to cold. Body hair is sparse and short. Heart rate is slow (bradycardia).

Hyperthyroidism

It results from excessive levels of T4 and T3 hormones. The clinical features are due to increased metabolic rate. The patient presents with weight loss, warm sweaty skin, heat intolerance, tachycardia, hair loss. There is enlargement of thyroid gland and **exophthalmos** (eyeballs appear protruded out).

Diseases of Parathyroid Glands

Hyperparathyroidism

Excessive secretion of PTH causes resorption of calcium from bones, raising the blood calcium level (hypercalcaemia). There is formation of renal stones, calcification in soft tissues, muscle fatigue, polyuria and extreme thirst. The condition is called osteitis fibrosa cystica.

Hypoparathyroidism

Deficiency of PTH causes abnormally low levels of blood calcium (hypocalcaemia). There is tetany, seizures, premature cataract and mental disturbances. "Tetany" results in painful spasms of skeletal muscle.

Diseases of Adrenal Gland

Diseases of Adrenal Cortex

Deficiency of glucocorticoids occur leading to low blood glucose, muscle weakness and decreased gluconeogenesis. Hyposecretion of both glucocorticoids and mineralocorticoids lead to **Addison's disease**. Clinical features of Addison's disease are muscle weakness and wasting, loss of appetite, increased pigmentation of skin, tiredness, mental confusion, hypotension, menstrual disturbances and electrolyte imbalance.

Hyposecretion of mineralocorticoids result in low blood sodium and raised blood potassium with hypotension, dehydration.

Hypersecretion of glucocorticoids lead to **Cushing's syndrome**. Clinical features include painful adiposity of face **(moon face)**, neck and abdomen, excessive protein catabolism leading to muscle wasting, osteoporosis, hyperglycaemia, susceptibility to infection due to depressed immune response, mental disturbances.

Hypersecretion of mineralocorticoids due to excessive aldosterone leads to excessive reabsorption of sodium chloride and water from kidneys causing hypertension and increased blood volume, increased potassium excretion leading to hypokalaemia which causes muscle weakness, cardiac arrhythmia. Hyposecretion of mineralocorticoids result in low blood sodium and raised blood potassium with hypotension, dehydration.

Diseases of Adrenal Medulla

The disorders affecting the adrenal medulla (pheochromocytoma) usually result in excessive secretion of epinephrine and norepinephrine. Clinical features are hypertension, hyperglycaemia, excessive sweating and increased metabolic rate.

Diseases of Islets of Langerhans

Diabetes Mellitus

It is usually due to deficiency or absence of insulin or to insulin resistance, i.e. impaired insulin activity. Deficiency of insulin leads to disruption of carbohydrate and fat metabolism. Diabetes be classified into:

1. *Type I, insulin dependent diabetes mellitus (IDDM):* Seen in children and young adults. It is of sudden onset. Deficiency of insulin is due to destruction of β islet cells.
2. *Type II, non-insulin dependent diabetes mellitus (NIDDM):* This type involves 80% of cases and tends to develop in persons over 45 years. In this type, the insulin secretion may be below or above normal. It is due to insulin resistance, i.e. there is change in cell membrane which blocks the insulin assisted movement of glucose into cells.
3. *Secondary diabetes:* It develops secondary to drug intake, pregnancy or other endocrinal disturbances.

Metabolic Effects of Diabetes Mellitus

1. *Hyperglycaemia:* Blood glucose level remains high after meal due to defective glucose uptake and use by cells, decreased conversion of glucose to glycogen and increased gluconeogenesis because of deficiency of intracellular glucose.
2. *Glycosuria and polyuria:* Excessive glucose filtered out by kidneys is not reabsorbed because it exceeds the renal threshold leading to glycosuria. Excessive glucose in filtrate raises the osmotic pressure which decreases tubular water reabsorption and urine volume is increased (polyuria). Polyuria leads to hypovolaemia and excessive thirst.

3. Ketoacidosis occurs due to excessive formation of ketone bodies due to breakdown of body fats.

4. Weight loss occurs due to increased protein and fat breakdown.

Complications of Diabetes Mellitus

1. *Diabetic ketoacidosis:* Seen in IDDM. It occurs due to increased insulin requirement or insulin resistance.

2. *Hypoglycaemia:* Seen in IDDM. It is due to excess insulin administration than needed to balance the food intake.

3. *Cardiovascular disturbances:* Atherosclerosis occurs in peripheral vessels and capillaries leading to myocardial infarction, gangrene, loss of sight due to retinopathy, neuropathy and renal failure.

4. Diabetics are highly susceptible to **infections.**

Points to Remember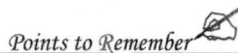

1. Endocrine glands pour their secretion directly into blood.
2. Pancreas is both an exocrine and an endocrine gland.
3. 2 pairs of arteries supply the thyroid gland while 3 pairs of veins drain the gland.
4. Suprarenal gland comprises an outer cortex and an inner medulla.
5. Medulla of suprarenal secretes adrenaline/noradrenaline.

MCQs

1. Anterior pituitary is also called:
(a) Adenohypophysis
(b) Neurohypophysis
(c) Corpus callosum
(d) Arachnoid villi

2. Pineal gland is located at:
(a) Epithalamus
(b) Thalamus
(c) Hypothalamus
(d) Subthalamus

3. All the following hormones are secreted by anterior pituitary *except*:
(a) Growth hormone
(b) FSH
(c) Prolactin
(d) Insulin

4. Milk ejecting hormone is:
(a) Progesterone
(b) Oestrogen
(c) Melatonin
(d) Oxytocin

Ans. 1 a   2 a   3 a   4 d

Reproductive System

The living beings have the property of reproduction by which they give rise to offsprings. In human beings, both males and females produce specialised germ cells called **gametes.** The male gametes are called **spermatozoa** (produced by testes) and the female gametes are called ova (produced by ovaries). These contain the genetic material/genes, on chromosomes, which pass inherited characteristics to the next generation.

FEMALE REPRODUCTIVE SYSTEM

Reproductive system in female comprises internal pelvic genital organs and external genital or perineal genital organs.

Internal genital organs are a pair of ovaries, pair of fallopian or uterine tubes, a single uterus and vagina (Figs 12.1A and B).

External genital organs include the:
- Mons pubis
- Labia minora
- Labia majora
- Clitoris
- Bulb of the vestibule, greater vestibular glands and the vestibule of the vagina (Fig. 12.6A and B).

Internal Genital Organs

Ovary

Each ovary is an almond-shaped structure, 3 cm long, 2 cm wide and 1 cm thick, lying

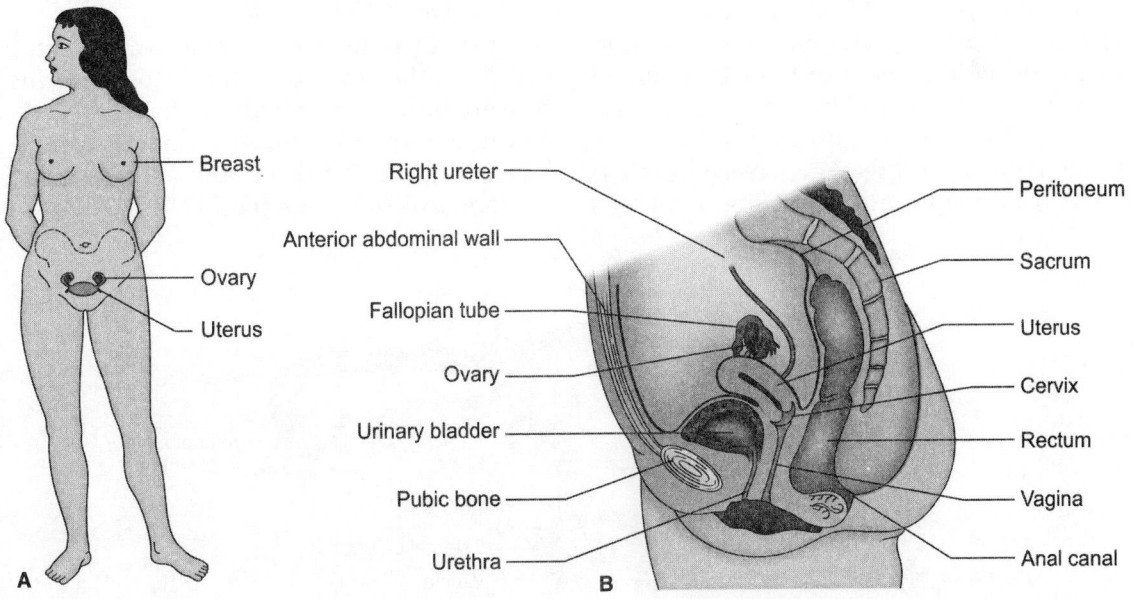

Figs 12.1A and B: (A) Organs of female reproductive system and (B) sagittal section of female pelvis

near the side wall of pelvis. It is suspended by a fold of peritoneum from the back of broad ligament. Fallopian tube almost embraces the ovary all over except the lateral surface. The ovary has a **hilum** for the entry and exit of vessels, nerves and lymphatics (Fig. 12.2).

Ovary receives **arterial supply** from ovarian artery which arises from aorta at the level of 2nd lumbar vertebra. It also supplies lateral part of the fallopian tube. Left ovarian vein drains into left renal vein while right one drains into inferior vena cava. Lymph drains into lateral aortic and preaortic lymph nodes.

Ovary consists of two layers of tissue. Outer **cortex** contains **ovarian follicles,** in various stages of maturity, each of which contains an ovum. During child bearing years, every 28 days, one ovarian follicle matures, ruptures and releases its ovum into peritoneal cavity. This is called ovulation. **Medulla** lies in centre and consists of fibrous tissue, blood vessels and nerves. Ovary also produces hormones like oestrogen and progesterone.

The oestrogen and progesterone along with prolactin, follicle-stimulating hormone (FSH) and Luteinising hormone (LH) from the anterior pituitary regulate the menstrual cycle, maintain pregnancy and prepare the mammary glands for lactation. They also promote development and maintenance of feminine secondary sex characters (development and enlargement of breasts, feminine pattern of growth of pubic and axillary hair, increased fat deposition in subcutaneous tissue at hips and breasts, increase in rate of growth in height and widening of pelvis).

Ovaries also produce **relaxin** (relaxes uterine smooth muscle during pregnancy, increases flexibility of pubic symphysis during pregnancy and helps dilate uterine cervix during labour and delivery) and **inhibin** (inhibits secretion of FSH from anterior pituitary).

Menopause: This stage occurs between 45 years and 55 years and is the end of child bearing period. Oestrogen and progesterone become less and less and menstruation stops. Ovaries do not respond to LH and FSH of the hypophysis cerebri.

Uterus

The uterus (womb) is a muscular organ composed of smooth muscle fibres. It is flattened pear-shaped organ 7.5 cm long, 5.0 wide and 2.5 cm thick (3" × 2" × 1"). It is present between urinary bladder and rectum. It is divided into three parts: (1) fundus, (2) body and (3) cervix (Fig. 12.2).

1. *Fundus* is the part which projects above the opening of fallopian tubes.

2. *Body* is the main part and projects above the urinary bladder. It is narrowest inferiorly at internal os. The cavity is triangular.

3. *Cervix* is the narrow lower end and opens into the upper part of the vagina at the external os (Fig. 12.3).

The body of uterus is bent forwards on the cervix at the level of internal os and this forward inclination of body of uterus on cervix constitutes **anteflexion. Anteversion** is angle between the long axis of body of uterus and the long axis of vagina (Fig. 12.4).

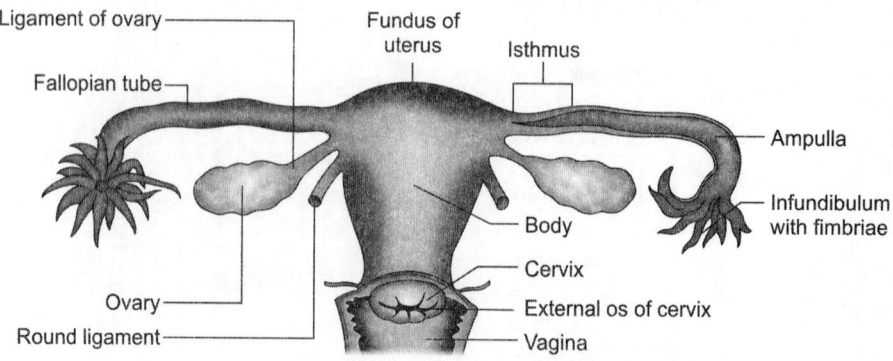

Fig. 12.2: Female internal genital organs

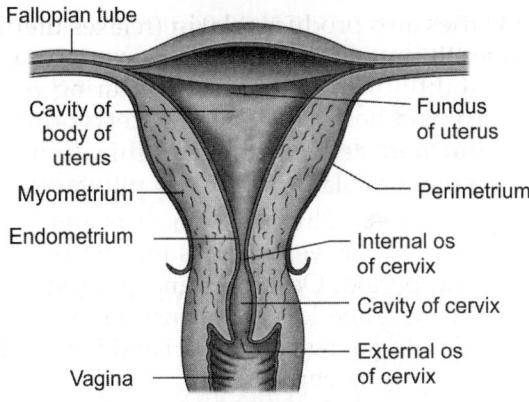

Fig. 12.3: Parts and structure of uterus

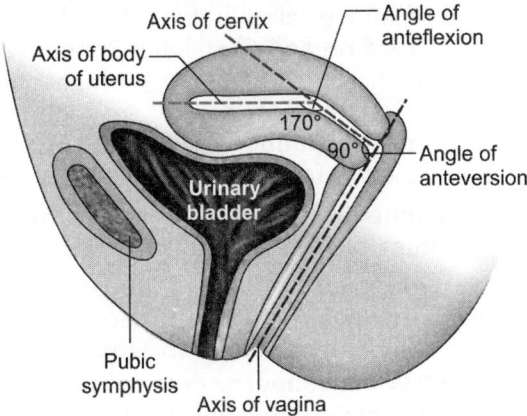

Fig. 12.4: Angulation of uterus and vagina

Peritoneal relations: Uterus is suspended from each side of the pelvis by a double-fold of peritoneum, the **broad ligament.** In its upper free margin lies the **fallopian tube** which is 10 cm long. The lateral end of **fallopian tube** has a number of **fimbriae.** These fimbriae lie near the side wall of pelvis below the ovary so that the ovum at ovulation can easily be picked up (taken) by the tube.

The anterior layer of broad ligament provides a fold in which runs the round ligament of uterus, which passes through the inguinal canal to fuse with the labia majora.

The posterior layer of broad ligament provides another fold for the ligament of ovary and ovary itself.

Supports of the uterus:

1. *Muscular supports:* **Levator ani, urogenital diaphragm** and **perineal body** with number of perineal and pelvic floor muscles attached to it.

2. *Ligaments:*
   a. *Lateral ligaments or cervical ligaments* pass from cervix of uterus and vagina laterally to the lateral pelvic wall.
   b. *Uterosacral ligaments* pass from the cervix and vagina backwards to the sacrum (Fig. 12.5).
   c. *Pubocervical ligaments* pass from the pubic bone to the cervix.
   These ligaments support the uterus.

3. Angulation of uterus, angle of anteversion (Fig. 12.4).

4. Peritoneal folds like broad ligaments.

5. Round ligaments.

Structure:

1. Walls of uterus are composed of three layers of tissue: (1) perimetrium, (2) myometrium and (3) endometrium. **Perimetrium** consists of peritoneal covering. Bulk of uterine wall consists of smooth muscle called the **myometrium** (Fig. 12.3). The mucous membrane lining myometrium internally is called **endometrium.** It is composed of columnar epithelium, tubular glands and stroma.

2. *Arterial supply* to uterus is by uterine arteries (branches of internal iliac arteries). Uterine artery crosses the ureter and runs on the side of the uterus in a tortuous manner. It supplies cervix, body, fundus of uterus and medial part of fallopian tube. **Venous drainage** occurs into internal iliac veins. **Lymphatic drainage** occurs to aortic lymph

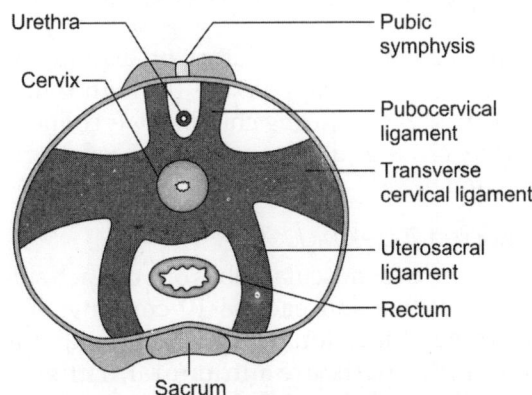

Fig. 12.5: Ligamentous supports of uterus

nodes and lymph nodes associated with iliac blood vessels. Some lymphatics pass to the superficial inguinal nodes.

Function: Uterus prepares itself for implantation of fertilised ovum **(zygote),** so that zygote fully develops into a foetus and is delivered as a newborn baby.

Vagina

It is female organ of copulation. It is a muscular tube 10 cm long-lying obliquely behind pubic symphysis and in front of rectum and anal canal (Figs 12.1B and 12.2).

The menstrual products are discharged from it. It is lined by stratified squamous epithelium and an underlying connective tissue stroma with no glands. In reproductive age group (15–49 years), pH of vagina is maintained between 3.5 and 4.9 by *Lactobacillus acidophilus* (Doderlein's bacilli) bacteria.

Hymen: It is a thin layer of mucous membrane which covers the opening of vagina. It gets perforated at menarche due to menstrual flow. It gets torn at the time of intercourse or by strenuous exercises. The condition of the hymen is not a reliable sign of virginity.

Around the upper end of vagina, into which the cervix of the uterus projects, are the **fornices.** They are the right, left, anterior and posterior fornix. The posterior fornix is the deepest. Lower end of vagina opens into the perineum.

It is supplied by uterine and vaginal branches of internal iliac vessels. Lymphatic drainage is through deep and superficial iliac glands.

It functions as a copulatory organ and also provides an elastic passage through which baby passes out during childbirth. It connects the external and internal organs of reproduction.

Fallopian Tube/Oviduct

These are two muscular tubes one on each side of the uterus and each is 10 cm long. It is subdivided into four parts. From medial to lateral the **parts** are intramural, isthmus, ampulla and infundibulum. The end of each tube has the finger like projections called **fimbriae.** The fertilisation occurs normally in the ampulla of the tube. If implantation occurs in the tube itself, it is known as **ectopic pregnancy.** Such tube mostly ruptures, leading to severe bleeding.

Function: It carries the secondary oocyte from ovary to uterus. If fertilisation is to occur, it occurs in the ampullary part of the tube.

Nerve supply of female internal genital organs: Uterus is supplied by autonomic nerves. Sympathetic from lumbar 1, 2 segments and parasympathetic from sacral 2, 3, 4 segments. Most of vagina is also supplied by autonomic nerves. Lower end of vagina is supplied by branches of pudendal nerve posteriorly and by ilioinguinal nerve anteriorly.

External Genital Organs

Mons pubis is a mound of hairy skin and subcutaneous fat in front of pubic symphysis.

Labia majora are two fatty cutaneous folds which pass backwards from mons pubis (Fig. 12.6A).

Labia minora are two cutaneous folds, without fat lying internal to labia majora. These form the boundary of vestibule of the vagina. Vagina, urethra and ducts of greater vestibular glands open into the vestibule. Just inside the vaginal orifice, a fold of mucous membrane, the hymen obstructs the opening.

Clitoris lies at the anterior end of labia minora. It is formed by two small **corpora cavernosa**

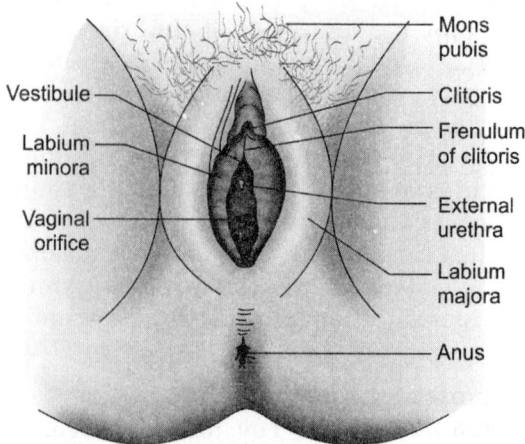

Fig. 12.6A: Female external genital organs

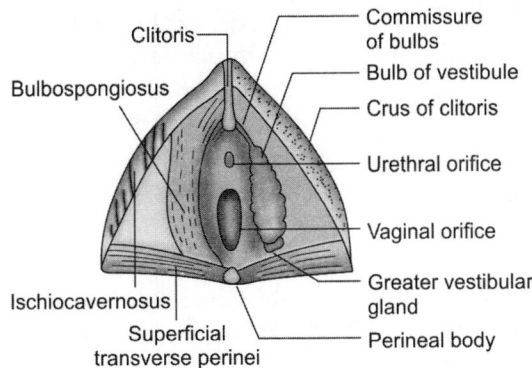

Clitoris

Bulbospongiosus

Commissure of bulbs

Bulb of vestibule

Crus of clitoris

Urethral orifice

Vaginal orifice

Greater vestibular gland

Ischiocavernosus

Superficial transverse perinei

Perineal body

Fig. 12.6B: Structure of clitoris

and two **bulbs of the vestibule** (Fig. 12.6B). It corresponds to penis in the male but clitoris has no corpus spongiosum and is not traversed by the urethra. It has no reproductive significance.

Greater vestibular glands lie under cover of the back part of bulb of vestibule. Their duct, 2 cm long-opens into the vagina.

FEMALE REPRODUCTIVE CYCLE

There are cyclical changes in the ovary and uterus every 26–30 days in females during the child bearing period. As a result of these changes, there is release of secondary oocyte from ovary, in addition to secretion of oestrogen and progesterone hormones from ovaries **(ovarian cycle).** Simultaneously, under the influence of hormones from ovary there are changes in the endometrium of uterus **[uterine (menstrual) cycle]** to prepare it for the arrival of a fertilised ovum that will develop there until birth.

Immediately after the menses, under the influence of FSH of anterior pituitary, the ovarian follicles start to develop into primary follicles. These change to secondary follicles and only one of these develops into **Graafian follicle.** Some cells of the follicles secrete oestrogen. Oestrogen causes **proliferative changes** in the uterine endometrium and it becomes thicker. Short, straight endometrial glands develop.

Approximately on the 14th day of the cycle, the Graafian follicle ruptures releasing the secondary oocyte. This occurs under the influence of LH of anterior pituitary. Then onwards the follicle is called **corpus luteum** and secretes the hormone progesterone. Progesterone is responsible for the **secretory changes** in the endometrium. The endometrium becomes oedematous and endometrial glands enlarge and secrete increased amounts of watery mucus (Fig. 12.7).

If pregnancy ensues, the corpus luteum continues to function for 3 months. The corpus luteum is supported by human chorionic gonadotrophin (hCG) secreted by developing embryo. If there is no pregnancy, corpus luteum degenerates on 28th day of the cycle. At the site of degenerated corpus luteum, an inactive mass of fibrous *tissue* forms, called the **corpus albicans.** Lack of hormones induces menstruation. During **menstrual phase,** the functional layer of endometrium is shed. This lasts for 4–5 days (first day of menstruation is day 1 of a new cycle). Menstrual flow consists of 50–150 mL of blood, tissue fluid, mucus and epithelial cells shed from the endometrium. Menstrual flow passes out from the uterine cavity through the cervix and vagina to the exterior.

Ovulation

It takes place between 12 days and 14 days prior to the next menstrual cycle. Graafian follicle ruptures to release secondary oocyte in a process called ovulation.

During ovulation, the body temperature rises by 0.5–1.0°C.

BREAST/MAMMARY GLAND

The breast is present both in males and females, but is rudimentary in males and children. It is well-developed in the female after puberty.

The breast is modified sweat gland. It is an important accessory organ of female reproductive system and provides nutrition to the newborn in the form of milk.

The breast lies in the superficial fascia of the pectoral region. A small extension of the breast called the **axillary tail of Spence,** pierces the deep fascia and lies in the axilla.

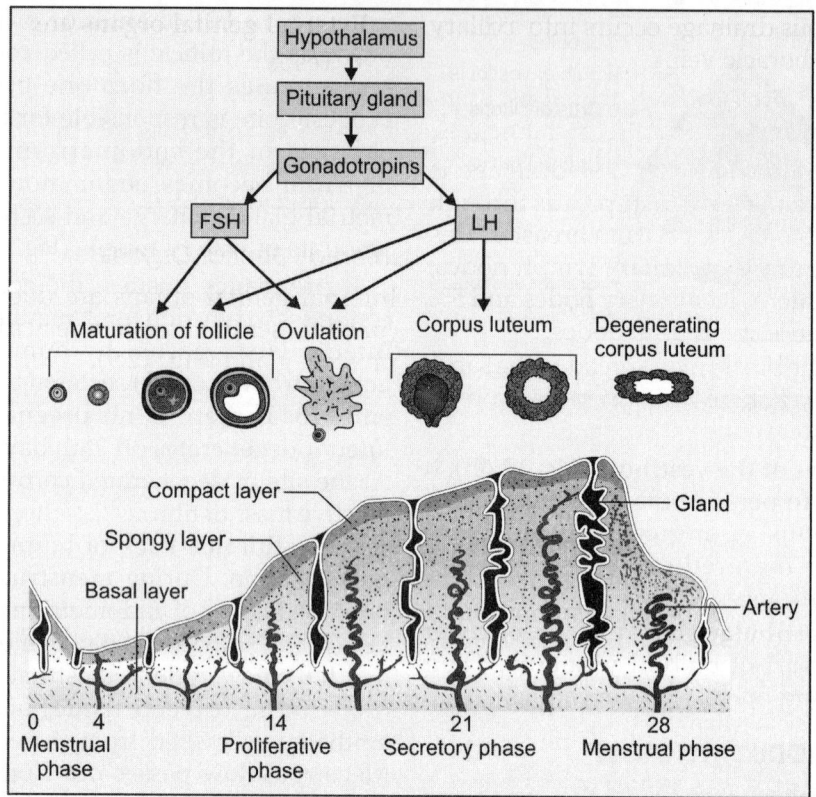

Fig. 12.7: Effects of hormones leading to ovarian cycle including phases of endometrium in menstrual cycle

It extends vertically from the second to the sixth ribs. Horizontally, it extends from lateral border of sternum till the mid-axillary line.

The deep surface of the breast is related to pectoralis major and serratus anterior muscles.

Structure of the Breast

The structure of breast is divided into skin, parenchyma and stroma. The skin covers the gland and presents a conical projection called the **nipple,** situated at the level of 4th inter-costal space. Nipple is pierced by 15–20 lacti-ferous ducts.

The skin around the base of the nipple is pigmented, circular and is known as the **areola.**

The parenchyma is made up of glandular tissue. The gland comprises 15–20 **lobes.** Each lobe is made up of lobules which are formed by various acini. The glands drain into **lacti-ferous sinuses** which open onto the nipple (Fig. 12.8).

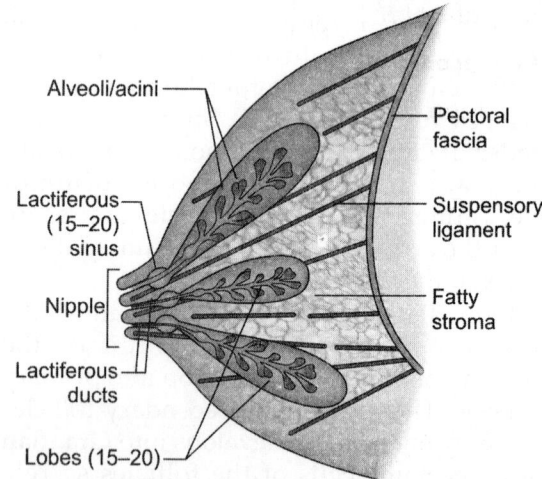

Fig. 12.8: Structure of the breast

The stroma is the supporting framework of the gland. It is made up of fibrous as well as fatty tissue.

Blood supply: The breast is supplied by branches of axillary and internal thoracic arteries. Venous drainage occurs into axillary and internal thoracic veins.

Nerve supply: Breasts are supplied by branches from 4th, 5th and 6th intercostal nerves.

Lymphatic drainage: Lymphatic drainage is important as cancer of breast spreads through lymphatics. 75% of lymph from breast drains into various groups of axillary lymph nodes, 20% into the internal mammary nodes and 5% into the posterior intercostal nodes.

Cancer of the breast may spread to the same side axillary lymph nodes. It may also spread to opposite breast and opposite side axillary lymph nodes.

For early diagnosis every female must palpate her both breasts every month to note any growth.

The essential function of breast is the synthesis, secretion and ejection of milk. These functions called **lactation** are associated with pregnancy and childbirth. **Milk secretion** is stimulated by hormone **prolactin** from anterior pituitary with contributions from progesterone and oestrogen. The **ejection** of milk is stimulated by **oxytocin** released from posterior pituitary in response to the sucking of an infant on the mother's nipple (suckling).

MALE REPRODUCTIVE SYSTEM

Male reproductive system consists of following internal and external genital organs.

External genital organs are:
- Testis
- Epididymis
- Ductus deferens (partly)
- Spermatic cord
- Penis (Fig. 12.9).

Internal Genital Organs

Internal genital organs are ductus deferens (partly), seminal vesicle, ejaculatory duct, prostate gland (Fig. 12.9).

External Genital Organs

Scrotum: It is a pouch in the perineum and is divided into two compartments by a raphe. Each compartment contains one testis, one epididymis and part of ductus deferens. Scrotum lies below symphysis pubis and behind the penis.

Testis

The testis is an oval egg-shaped structure 4 cm long, 2.5 cm wide and 3 cm thick, suspended by the **spermatic cord** into the **scrotum.**

Each testis is covered by three layers of tissue. Outermost is a sac of peritoneum called the **tunica vaginalis.** Testis during foetal life descends from the upper part of posterior abdominal wall through lower part of anterior abdominal wall into the scrotum taking peritoneal covering and blood vessels with it.

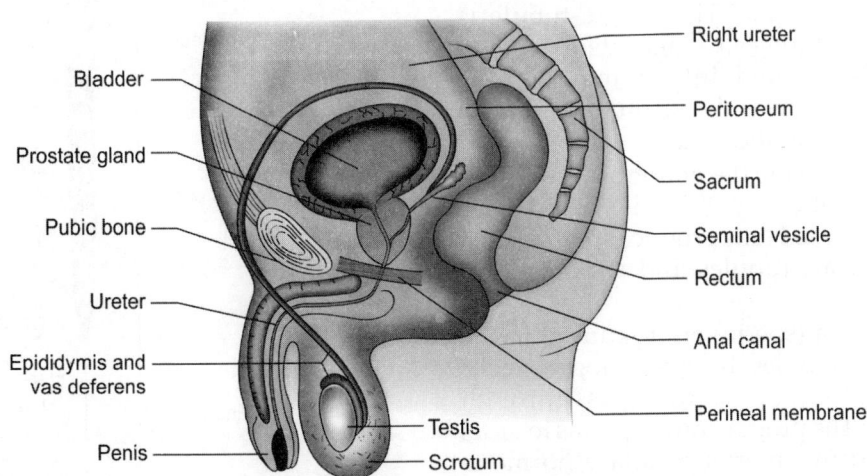

Fig. 11.9: Sagittal section of male pelvis

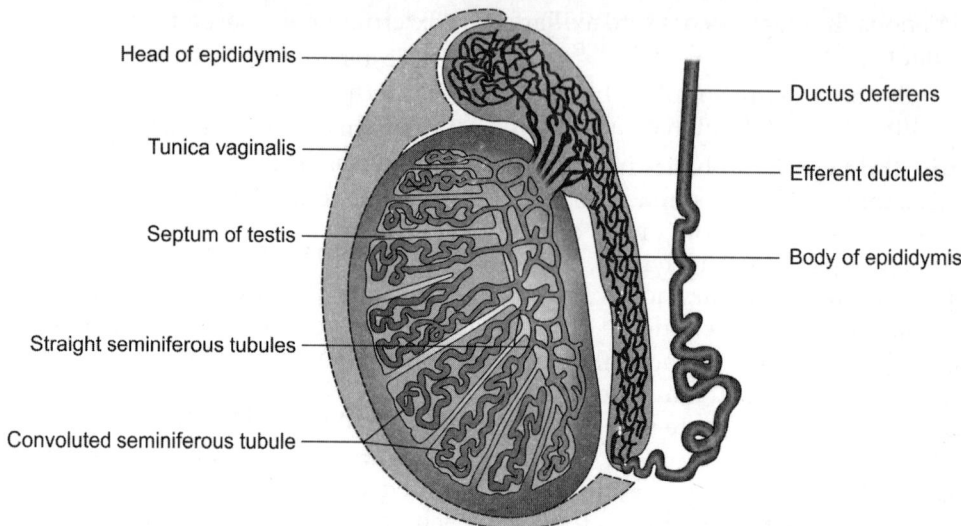

Fig. 12.10: Longitudinal section of a testis and ductus deferens

Tunica albuginea lies beneath the tunica vaginalis and fibrous septa from it divide the testis into lobules.

Innermost is **tunica vasculosa** consisting of a network of capillaries supported by delicate connective tissue (Fig. 12.10).

Each testis is made up of 200–300 lobules. Each **lobule** has 1–4 convoluted loops called **seminiferous tubules.** Each tubule is composed of **germinal epithelial cells** (spermatogenic cells) and **Sertoli cells.** Between tubules are **interstitial cells of Leydig** that secrete hormone testosterone after puberty.

At upper pole of testis tubules combine to form a single tubule. This single tubule is about 6 metres long. It is repeatedly folded and tightly packed into a mass called **epididymis.** It leaves the scrotum as **ductus deferens** in spermatic cord.

Testis lies outside the abdominal cavity as lower temperature by 2–4°C is required for spermatogenesis. Testis produce spermatozoa in seminiferous tubules and are stored in epididymis.

Spermatozoa (sperm) are produced in the seminiferous tubules by spermatogenic cells of testis and mature as they pass through epididymis. The production of sperms in testis is controlled by anterior pituitary hormone FSH. Sertoli cells support and protect developing sperms.

Spermatozoa: Each spermatozoon is made up of a head, middle piece and a tail (Fig. 12.11). The head contains a nucleus. Anterior to nucleus is the acrosome with enzymes, which help in penetration of sperm into secondary oocyte. Middle piece contains mitochondria. The tail pushes the sperm along its way.

The main hormone produced by testis is **testosterone,** a male sex hormone/androgen. Testosterone regulates the production of sperms, stimulates the development and

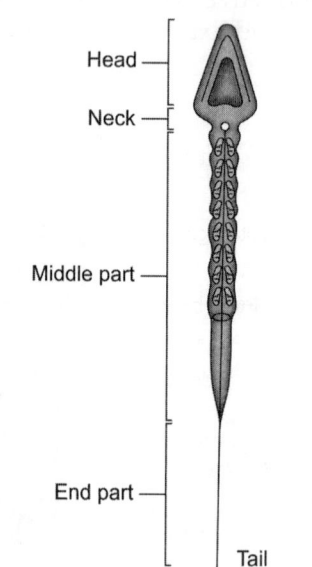

Fig. 12.11: Parts of a spermatozoa

maintenance of masculine secondary sex characteristics (deepening of voice, beard growth, growth of pubic, axillary and chest hair, muscular and skeletal growth resulting in wide shoulders and narrow hips, thickening of skin, enlargement of penis, scrotum and prostate gland. It also contributes to sexual drive in both males and females (adrenal cortex is the source of androgens in females) and also stimulate protein synthesis.

Epididymis

Each epididymis is attached to the back of its own testis, and comprises head, body and tail which continues as the ductus deferens.

Epididymis is a single highly coiled tube. It stores the sperms. In addition, sperms mature here.

Ductus Deferens

It is also known as **vas deferens.** It is thick muscular tube and is the continuation of tail of epididymis. It partly lies with external genitalia and partly with the internal genital organs.

Vas deferens in its external part forms important component of spermatic cord, runs through the inguinal canal, and the side wall of the pelvis and crosses the pelvic floor to reach back of urinary bladder. There it is joined by duct of seminal vesicle to form the **ejaculatory duct,** which opens into the prostatic urethra. It carries the maturing spermatozoa from epididymis till the prostatic urethra.

Spermatic cord suspends the testis in the scrotum. Besides vas deferens it contains testicular artery and vein, lymphatics and autonomic nerves.

Blood supply: Testis and epididymis are supplied by the testicular artery, a branch of abdominal aorta at level of 2nd lumbar vertebra. The artery is long and enters the spermatic cord to reach the testis and epididymis. Testicular vein on left side drains into left renal vein and on right side drains into inferior vena cava.

Lymphatic drainage: Lymphatics of testis drains into para-aortic nodes, while that of skin of scrotum drains into inguinal nodes.

Prostate

It is a glandular organ situated in the lowest part of pelvis, below the bladder, surrounding first 3 cm of urethra. It is 4 cm wide, 3 cm long and 2 cm deep. It lies in front of rectum and rests on the levator ani muscles (Figs 12.9 to 12.12).

Prostate contains glands present within the mixture of fibrous and smooth muscles. The secretion of glands forms 30% of the seminal fluid.

Prostate is small till puberty. Testosterone secreted by the testis enlarges the size of prostate. The secretion of prostatic gland is discharged into the prostatic urethra through its 10–12 ducts. It helps in maturation of spermatozoa.

Its arterial supply is from branches of inferior vesical and from middle rectal artery. Veins drain finally into the internal iliac veins.

Seminal Vesicle and Ejaculatory Duct

The **seminal vesicles** are a pair of pouch like structures with smooth muscle. It is 4–5 cm long. Each vesicle lies against the back of bladder. The duct of seminal vesicle joins with vas deferens to form **ejaculatory duct.** This duct is 2 cm long and runs through the prostate to open into prostatic urethra. The genital ducts of both sides drain into the urinary tract, so the urethra serves as a common channel for semen and urine.

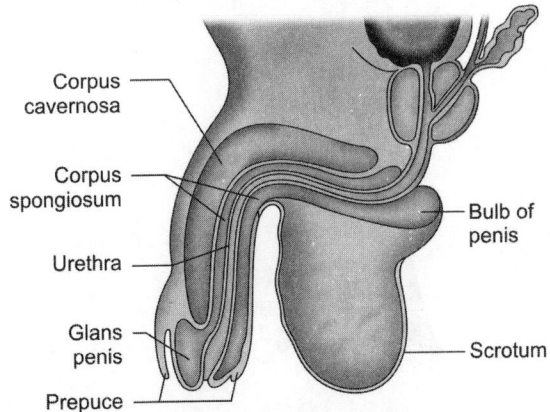

Corpus cavernosa

Corpus spongiosum

Urethra

Glans penis

Prepuce

Bulb of penis

Scrotum

Fig. 12.12: Section of the prostate gland and associated reproductive structures

Secretions of the seminal vesicles add to the volume of semen and help in maturation of spermatozoa.

Urethra and Penis

Male urethra provides a common passage for the flow of urine and semen. It is about 19–20 cm long.

Penis is the male organ of copulation and contains the longest, spongy part of the urethra. Penis is made of three spongy erectile tissue: (1) one central, (2) the **corpus spongiosum** with urethra and (3) on each side the **corpus cavernosum** (Fig. 12.13). Urethra opens on the **glans penis,** the expanded end of corpus spongiosum. Just above the glans, the skin is folded upon itself and forms a movable double layer, the **prepuce.**

Blood supply of penis is by internal pudendal vessels.

Nerve supply is by autonomic and somatic nerves.

Penis functions as a tube for the passage of urine most of the time, and for passage of semen whenever required.

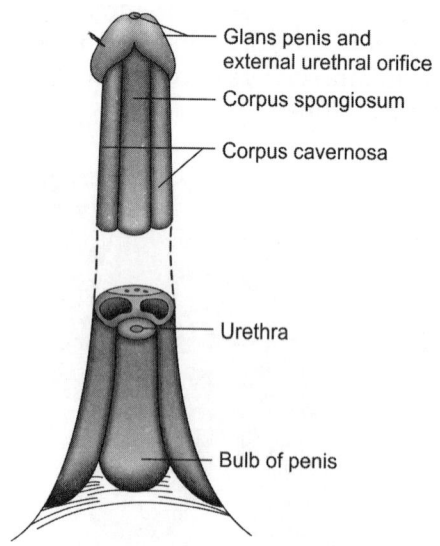

- Glans penis and external urethral orifice
- Corpus spongiosum
- Corpus cavernosa
- Urethra
- Bulb of penis

Fig. 12.13: Structure of the penis

HUMAN SEXUAL RESPONSE

During sexual intercourse (coitus) between male and female, sperm are ejaculated from the male urethra into the vagina. During this act, the physiological and emotional changes are experienced by both males and females and these are termed human sexual response.

FERTILIZATION, IMPLANTATION AND DEVELOPMENT

The spermatozoa are viable in the female reproductive tract for a period of 48 hours and secondary oocyte is fertilisable for only 24 hours. Seminal fluid contains millions of spermatozoa. However, very few of them reach the site of fertilisation. Spermatozoa undergo changes in female reproductive system in a process called **capacitation.**

CLINICAL ASPECTS

Sexually Transmitted Diseases (STDs)

STDs are a group of communicable diseases that are transmitted predominantly by sexual contact. These are caused by a wide range of bacterial, viral, protozoal and fungal agents. They have a higher incidence in 20–30 years age group. Syphilis, gonorrhoea, chlamydia and human immunodeficiency virus (HIV) constitute major STDs in India.

Syphilis

Syphilis is caused by spirochaete *Treponema pallidum*. The organism after penetrating the genital mucosa produces local as well as distant lesions.

Primary syphilis occurs approximately 3 weeks after sexual contact with an infected individual. A single, firm, non-tender, raised lesion (chancre) forms at the site of organism invasion on penis, cervix, anus or vaginal wall. It ulcerates and heals spontaneously in 2–8 weeks.

Secondary syphilis occurs 2–10 weeks after primary stage. It consists of skin rash, lesions on mucous membrane, fever, lymph node enlargement. These lesions resolve spontaneously.

Tertiary syphilis occurs years after primary stage and lesions are seen in aorta, heart, central nervous system, bones and liver.

Gonorrhoea

It is caused by pyogenic bacteria *Neisseria gonorrhoeae*. In males, it leads to suppurative urethral infection, which spreads to epididymis, prostate and seminal vesicles if untreated. In females, there is infection of cervix, fallopian tubes, ovaries and peritoneum.

Chlamydia

It is caused by *Chlamydia trachomatis*. In females, it infects the cervix and ascends to cause pelvic inflammation. In males, it causes urethritis and epididymitis.

AIDS

Acquired immune deficiency syndrome (AIDS) is caused by a retrovirus HIV. In AIDS, there is breakdown of body's immune system, leaving the victim vulnerable to a number of life-threatening opportunistic infections. Neurological disorders develop due to infection of neurons in brain.

Sexual transmission is most common method of transmission and is responsible for 75% of all cases. It can also be transmitted via blood transfusion, sharing of needles by intravenous drug abusers and from mother to child by breast milk or across the placenta before birth.

HIV virus infects the CD4+ T lymphocytes in blood and the number of helper T cells is decreased. This leads to profound suppression of immunity.

Initially, there is fever, weight loss, diarrhoea, skin rash, myalgia, sore throat 3–6 weeks after infection followed by generalised lymph node enlargement. In final phase, there is breakdown of host defences and development of clinical disease. The patient presents with long-lasting fever (>1 month), fatigue, weight loss and diarrhoea. Gradually, the CD4+ T lymphocyte count falls below 500 cells/microlitre and opportunistic infections develop. Opportunistic infections are the cause of death in 80% AIDS patients.

Female Reproductive System

Pelvic Inflammatory Disease

It is inflammatory condition of female pelvic organs, usually caused by bacterial infection. It usually begins as vulvovaginitis (inflammation of vulva and vagina) and spreads to cervix, uterus, uterine tubes and ovaries. Clinical features are fever, foul smelling vaginal discharge, pain in lower abdomen, abnormal uterine bleeding. Complications include infertility intestinal obstruction due to adhesions.

Imperforate hymen: Hymen is a membrane close to lower end of vagina. It allows the menstrual flow to come out. If hymen is so complete and does not even allow the menstrual flow to come out, the condition is called 'imperforate hymen'.

Rape

Sexual intercourse with a female without consent, i.e. forced penetration of penis into vagina is called rape.

Ovary

Ovary is subjected to tumours, which may be benign or malignant. Benign tumours are more common and dermoid cysts are the most common type.

Malignant ones are epithelial cell tumours or luteal cell tumours. Ovary is also a common site of metastases from the tumour of stomach, pancreas or breast.

Uterus

1. *Fibroid* is a very common clinical entity. These are benign tumours of myometrium (smooth muscle). They are of variable size and are usually multiple. They are common in reproductive period (15–49 years). Clinical features are discomfort, frequency of micturition, irregular periods, painful periods (dysmenorrhoea) and reduced fertility.

2. *Endometrial cancer:* Uterus may also be the site of **endometrial cancer.** It is seen in women 50–60 years of age, who are obese,

hypertensive or diabetic. It may spread to liver, lungs and bones via blood or lymph.

3. *Cancer of the cervix* is extremely common. It starts from the cervical epithelium, involving its whole thickness. It may spread locally to body of uterus, vagina, bladder or rectum. It occurs most commonly between 35 years and 50 years of age. It is more frequent in women who have started sexual activity at an early age, who have many partners or who have many pregnancies. Human papilomavirus infection is also associated with this cancer. There may be metastases in the bones, liver or lungs.

Uterus is supported by muscles of pelvic diaphragm and also by urogenital diaphragm. Many strong ligaments also provide support. If these muscles get injured (during delivery) or ligaments get overstretched, the uterus descends downwards. This condition is known as **prolapse of the uterus.**

4. *Endometritis:* It is inflammatory condition of endometrium usually caused by bacterial infection. It occurs most frequently after childbirth or abortion. Clinical features are fever, abdominal pain, foul smelling vaginal discharge and enlargement of uterus. It may lead to sterility. Infection may spread to myometrium, perimetrium, uterine tubes and surrounding pelvic tissues.

5. *Endometriosis:* There is growth of endometrial tissue outside uterus. It occurs most commonly in ovaries, uterine tubes and other pelvic structures. This tissue like the endometrial tissue in uterus, is responsive to fluctuations in sex hormone levels of menstrual cycle. Clinical features are pain, swelling, haemorrhage. It may lead to fibrosis and pelvic adhesions.

Fallopian Tubes

1. *Salpingitis:* Inflammation of fallopian tube is called **'salpingitis'.** It is usually due to spread of infection from uterus. If not completely treated, the tube may get blocked, leading to infertility.

2. *For female sterilisation,* 1.5–2 cm of lateral part of fallopian tube is removed bilaterally and their ends are ligated separately. This prevents the oocyte being fertilized by the spermatozoa.

3. *Ectopic pregnancy:* The fertilisation of oocyte takes place in the lateral part of the fallopian tube. Then, it migrates to the uterine cavity. In some cases, the zygote stays in the fallopian tube and cells multiply. Such a pregnancy is called 'ectopic pregnancy'. Such pregnancy ends within 2–3 months by rupture of tube and it can cause severe haemorrhage.

Mammary Gland (Breast)

Gynaecomastia

There is a proliferation of breast tissue in men. It is usually benign and affects one breast only. It is common in a young adult and older men. Common causes are drug intake, e.g. digoxin; cirrhosis of liver and endocrine disorders leading to high oestrogen levels.

Mastitis

Inflammation of the breast can be non-suppurative (during lactation due to congestion of breast) or suppurative (due to pyogenic bacteria). Suppurative mastitis is due to infection by *Staphylococcus aureus* and *Streptococcus pyogenes.* The infection enters through the nipple abrasion and spreads along the mammary ducts of lobe causing pus formation in one or more lobes of the gland. Clinical features are localised swelling and redness. If it does not resolve, an abscess may form. While draining the abscess, the incision should be radial so as not to damage more than one lactiferous duct.

Tumours

Most breast tumours (90%) are benign. **Fibroadenoma** is the most common type. They usually occur after puberty. Malignant tumours are usually found in upper outer quadrant of the breast. It is commonly seen after 35 years of age. These are painless nodules in one of the breasts only. Early spread via lymphatic vessels is common to axillary and internal mammary nodes. It can spread even to opposite breast and opposite axillary lymph nodes. Local spread may occur to skin, muscle and pleura. Factors predisposing to it are genetic component, disorders leading to high oestrogen levels, early menarche, late menopause and no pregnancies. Early diagnosis and treatment can prevent its spread. Every adult woman must palpate both her breasts with the palm of her hands, to detect any nodule at an early stage.

Male Reproductive System

1. *Phimosis:* When the skin of prepuce cannot be retracted, leading to narrowing of urethral orifice, the condition is called phimosis.

2. *Urethritis:* Urethra may get infected by infection descending from urinary bladder. Urethra may also get infected during catheterization, and infection may ascend up to other organs like seminal vesicles, prostate, testis and epididymis. Gonococcal infection due to sexually transmitted infection may also cause urethritis. Chronic infection may lead to urethral constriction due to fibrosis.

Testis

1. *Orchitis:* Inflammation of testis is called orchitis. It may be an ascending infection from the urethra or occur secondary to mumps.

2. *Undescended testis:* Testis develops in the lumbar region and then descends down via the inguinal canal. If it does not descend and remain in lumbar or inguinal region, the condition is called undescended testis. There is increased risk of infertility and testicular cancer in undescended testis.

3. *Hydrocele:* There is collection of fluid in the tunica vaginalis (extension of peritoneal cavity) surrounding the testis.

4. *Testicular tumour:* The testicular tumours are mostly malignant. These are common in undescended or ectopic testis.

Prostate

Prostatitis: Acute or chronic inflammation of prostate is called prostatitis.

Benign enlargement of prostate: Median lobe of prostate gland enlarges to cause obstruction to the internal urethral orifice. This causes back pressure to cause hydronephrosis of kidney. It is common in men over 50 years of age. In benign enlargement, the prostate gland needs to be removed partially.

Malignant tumours of prostate: The peripheral glands of prostate are affected by cancer. The cancer spreads by venous plexus into bones especially the vertebral column. It also spreads to neighbouring organs. It is common in men over 50 years of age.

Points to Remember

1. Male gonad (testis) lies outside the abdominal cavity as spermatogenesis needs lower temperature by 2–3°C.

2. Male urethra carries urine and seminal fluid at different time.

3. Clitoris does not contain urethra.

4. Vasectomy and tubectomy are important family welfare methods.

MCQs

1. **Angle of anteversion between uterus and vagina is:**
   - (a) 80°
   - (b) 120°
   - (c) 90°
   - (d) 60°

2. **Most important ligamentous support of uterus is:**
   - (a) Pubocervical ligament
   - (b) Uterosacral ligament
   - (c) Transverse cervical ligament
   - (d) Rectouterine fold of peritoneum

3. **Hormones required for ovulation are:**
   - (a) Oestrogen
   - (b) LH
   - (c) FSH
   - (d) FSH and LH

4. **Narrowest part of male urethra is:**
   - (a) Prostatic part
   - (b) Membranous part
   - (c) Internal urethral orifice
   - (d) External urethral meatus

5. **Structure of penis is:**
   - (a) Two corpora cavernosa, one corpus spongiosum
   - (b) Two corpora cavernosa, two corpus spongiosum
   - (c) One corpus spongiosum, two corpora cavernosa
   - (d) Only two corpus cavernosa

Ans ! 1 c   2 c   3 b   4 d   5 a

PRACTICAL PART

The Skeleton

Label the Bones in the Diagram

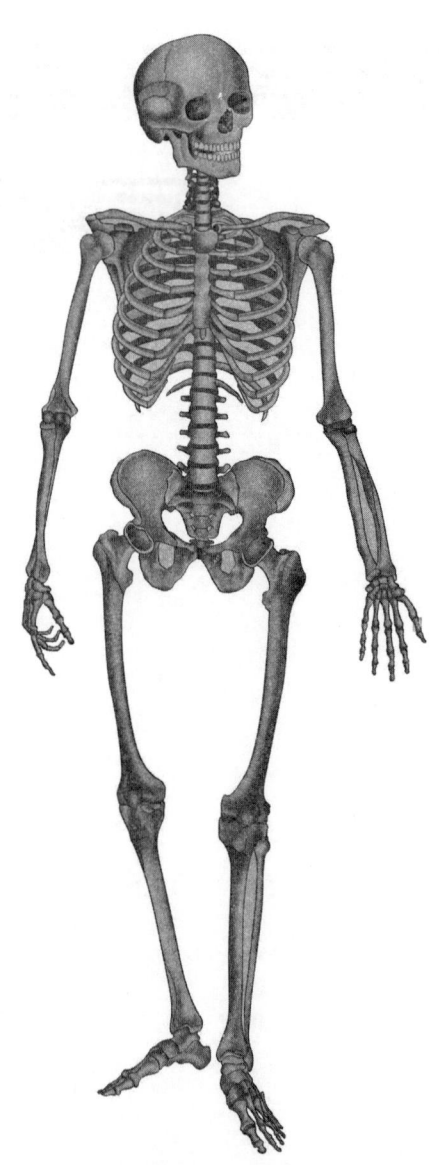

Enumerate Four Functions of Skeleton

Fig. 13.1: Skeleton

UPPER LIMB

Label the Joints of Upper Limb in Fig. 13.2

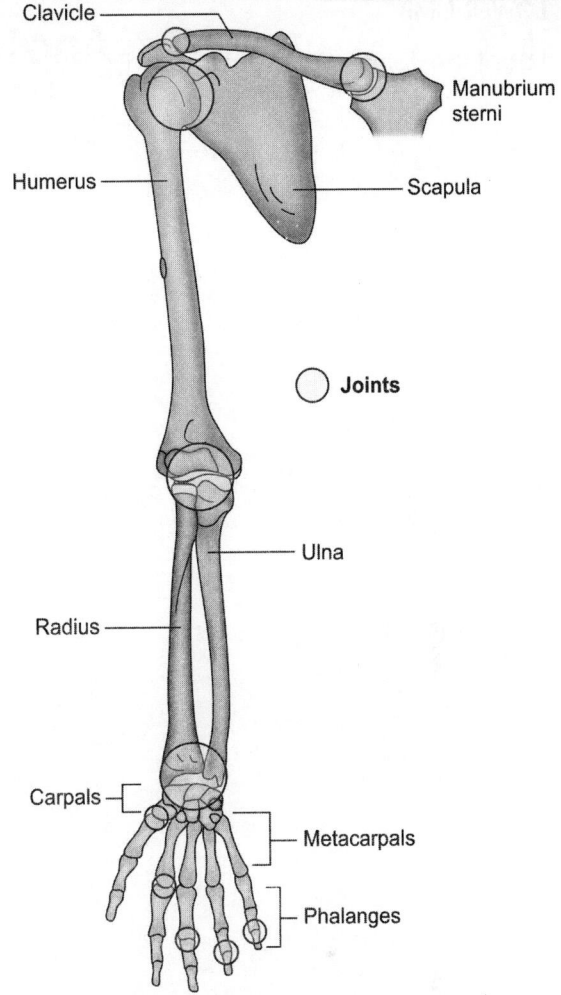

Fig. 13.2: Bones of upper limb

Bones of the upper limb are:
- Clavicle   – 1
- Scapula   – 1
- Humerus   – 1
- Radius   – 1
- Ulna   – 1
- Carpal bones   – 8
- Metacarpals   – 5
- Phalanges   – 14

LOWER LIMB

Label the Joints of Lower Limb in Fig. 13.3

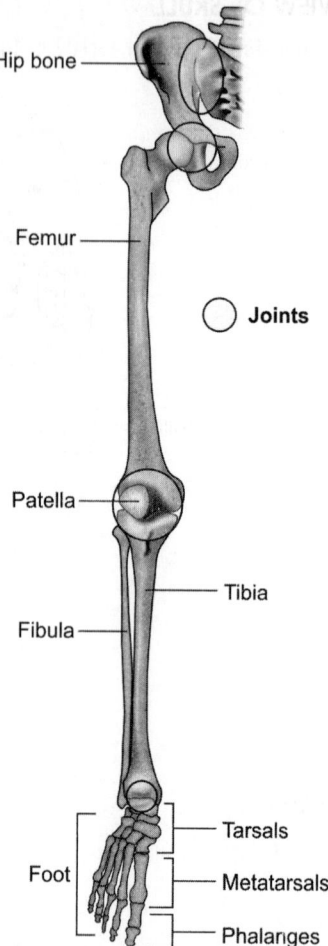

Fig. 13.3: Bone of lower limb

Bones of the lower limb are:
- Hip bone — 1
- Femur — 1
- Patella — 1
- Tibia — 1
- Fibula — 1
- Tarsals bones — 7
- Metatarsal — 5
- Phalanges — 14

LATERAL VIEW OF SKULL

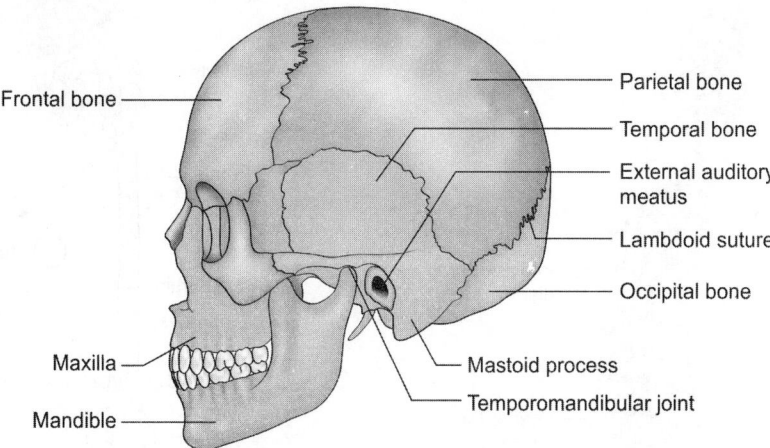

Fig. 13.4: Study the lateral view of skull

CRANIAL FOSSAE

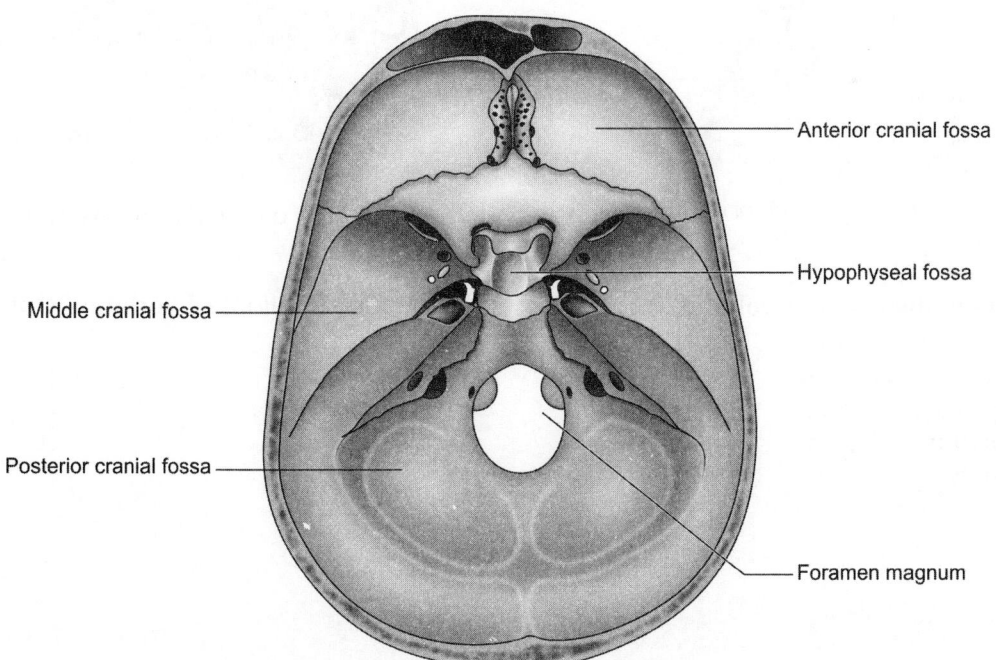

Fig. 13.5: Study the cranial fossae

VERTEBRAL COLUMN

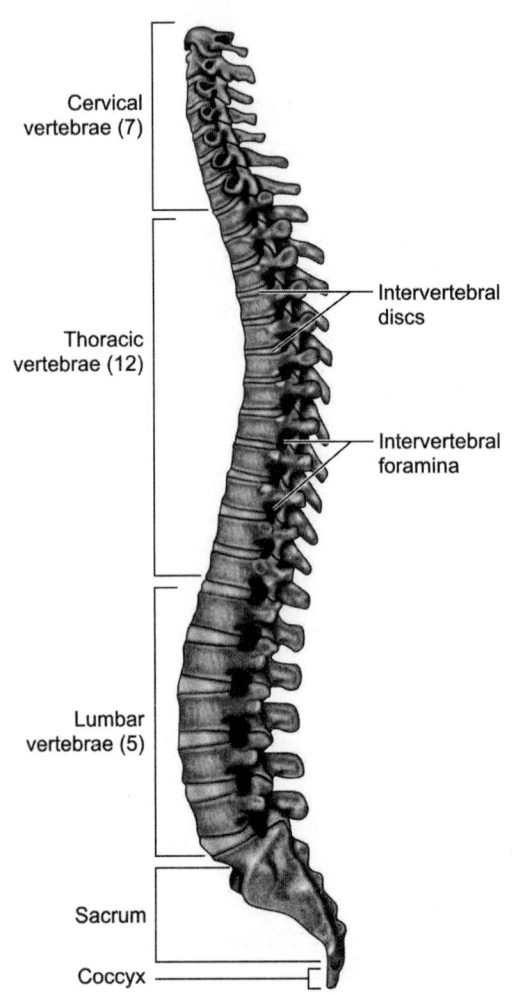

Fig. 13.6: Vertebral column

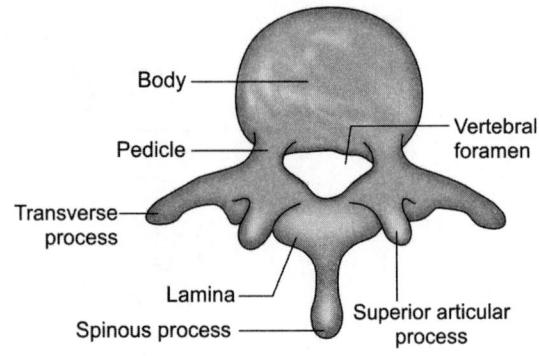

Fig. 13.7: Typical vertebra

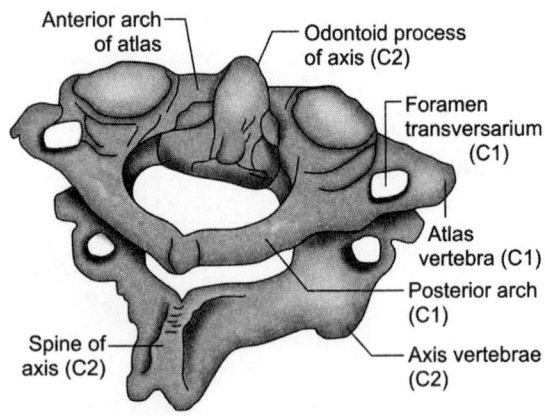

Fig. 13.8: 1st and 2nd cervical vertebrae

Bones of the vertebral column are:
- Cervical vertebrae   – 7
- Thoracic vertebrae   – 12
- Lumbar vertebrae   – 5
- Sacrum   – 1
- Coccyx   – 1

Write Three Functions of Vertebral Column

THORACIC CAGE

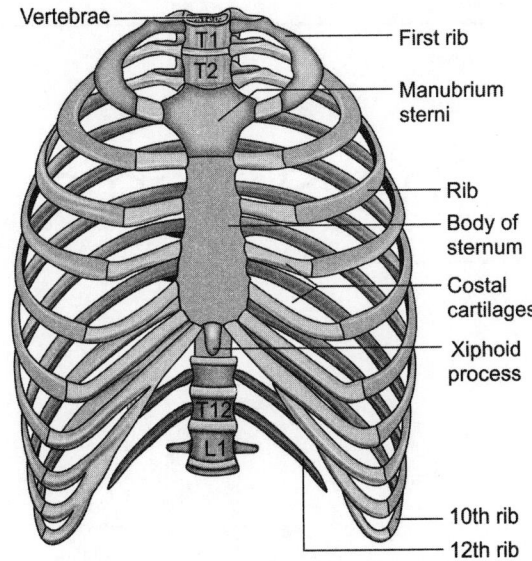

Fig. 13.9: Bones of the thoracic cage

Bones of the thoracic cage are:
- Sternum   – 1
- Ribs   – 12 pairs
  - Vertebrosternal (true)   7 pairs
  - Vertebrochondral (false)   3 pairs
  - Vertebral (floating)   2 pairs

Write Functions of Thoracic Cage

The Systems

DIGESTIVE SYSTEM

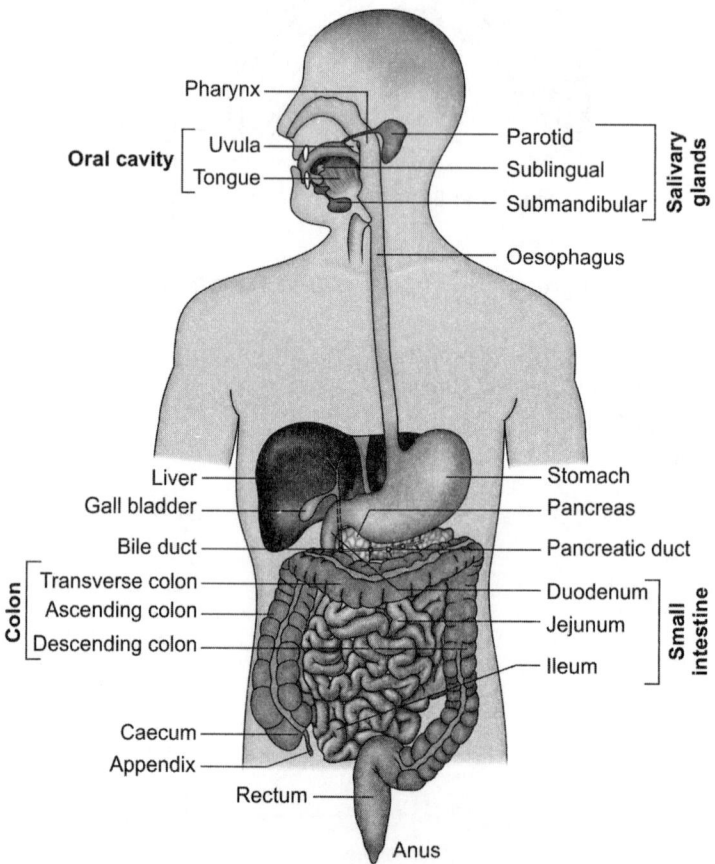

Pharynx

Oral cavity — Uvula
Tongue

Parotid
Sublingual
Submandibular

Salivary glands

Oesophagus

Liver
Gall bladder
Bile duct

Colon — Transverse colon
Ascending colon
Descending colon

Stomach
Pancreas
Pancreatic duct

Duodenum
Jejunum
Ileum

Small intestine

Caecum
Appendix

Rectum

Anus

Fig. 14.1: Digestive system

Exercise

1. Identify the parts of digestive system from the Fig. 14.1.
2. Write the functions of:
   a. Stomach
   b. Small intestine
   c. Large intestine
   d. Liver and gall bladder
   e. Pancareas

CIRCULATORY SYSTEM

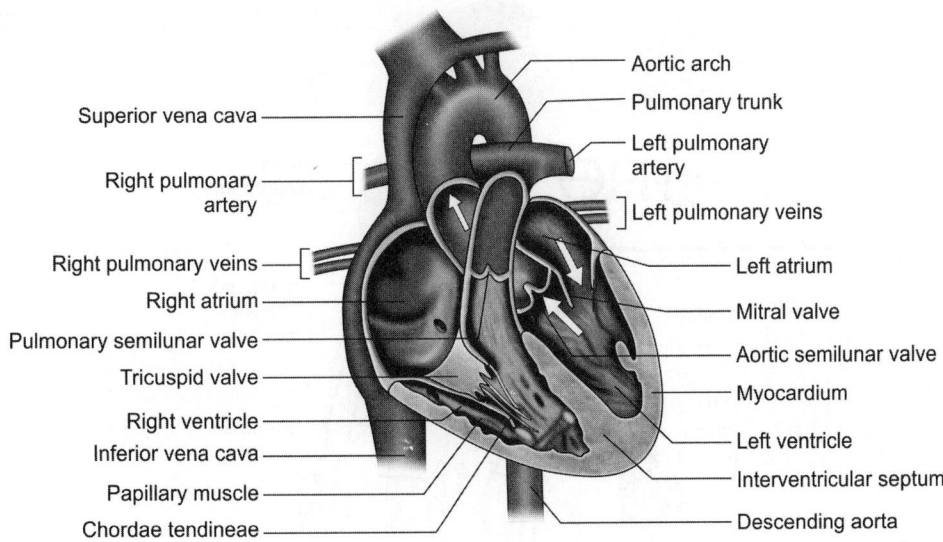

Fig. 14.2A: Heart

Exercise

1. Name the chambers of the heart.
2. Which chamber receives venous blood of the whole body except the lungs?
3. Name the chamber and artery which send venous blood to the lungs.
4. Which veins bring oxygenated blood from lungs to heart?
5. Which is the thickest chamber of heart?
6. Which is the thickest artery of the body?

ARTERIAL SYSTEM

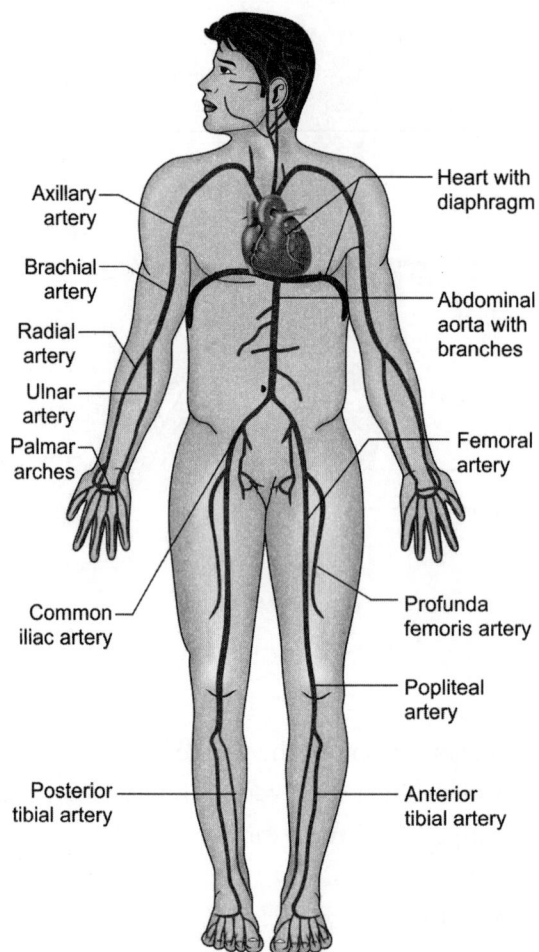

Fig. 14.2B: Arterial system *(For colour Fig. see Plate 3)*

Exercise

1. Circulatory system comprises:
   a. Heart
   b. Arteries
   c. Capillaries
   d. Veins
2. Identify the arteries and learn their names.
3. Learn the circulation of blood from Chapter 4.

VENOUS SYSTEM

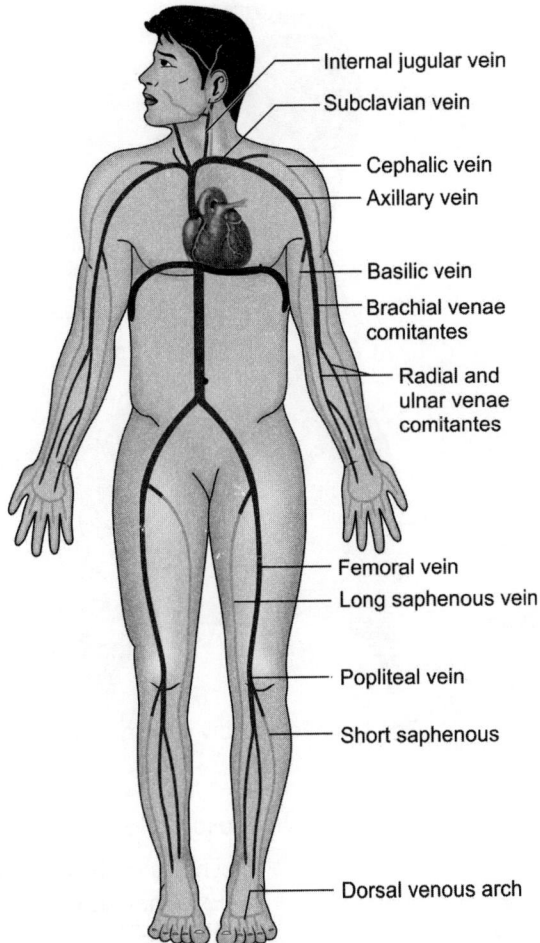

Internal jugular vein

Subclavian vein

Cephalic vein

Axillary vein

Basilic vein

Brachial venae
comitantes

Radial and
ulnar venae
comitantes

Femoral vein

Long saphenous vein

Popliteal vein

Short saphenous

Dorsal venous arch

Fig. 14.2C: Venous system *(For colour Fig. see Plate 3)*

Exercise

1. Learn the names of veins of the whole body.

RESPIRATORY SYSTEM

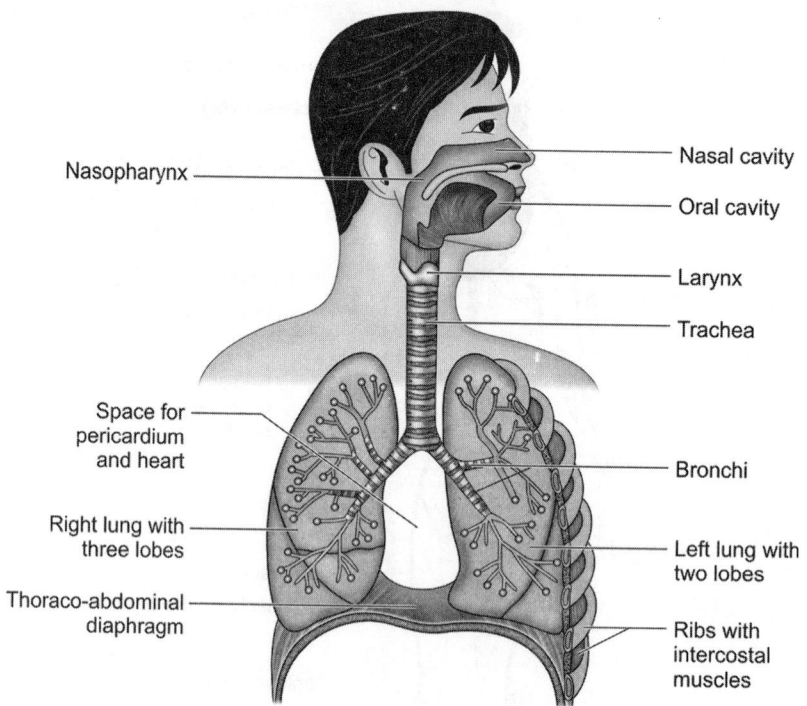

Nasopharynx —————————————— Nasal cavity

———————————————— Oral cavity

———————————————— Larynx

———————————————— Trachea

Space for
pericardium
and heart ————————

———————————————— Bronchi

Right lung with ————————
three lobes

———————————————— Left lung with
two lobes

Thoraco-abdominal ————————
diaphragm

———————————————— Ribs with
intercostal
muscles

Fig. 14.3: Respiratory system

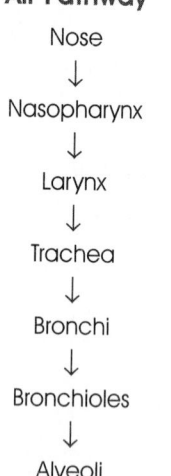

Air Pathway

Nose
↓
Nasopharynx
↓
Larynx
↓
Trachea
↓
Bronchi
↓
Bronchioles
↓
Alveoli

Muscles for Respiration

1. Thoraco-abdominal diaphragm.
2. External, internal and innermost intercostal muscles.

Exercise

1. Identify the parts of respiratory system.

URINARY SYSTEM

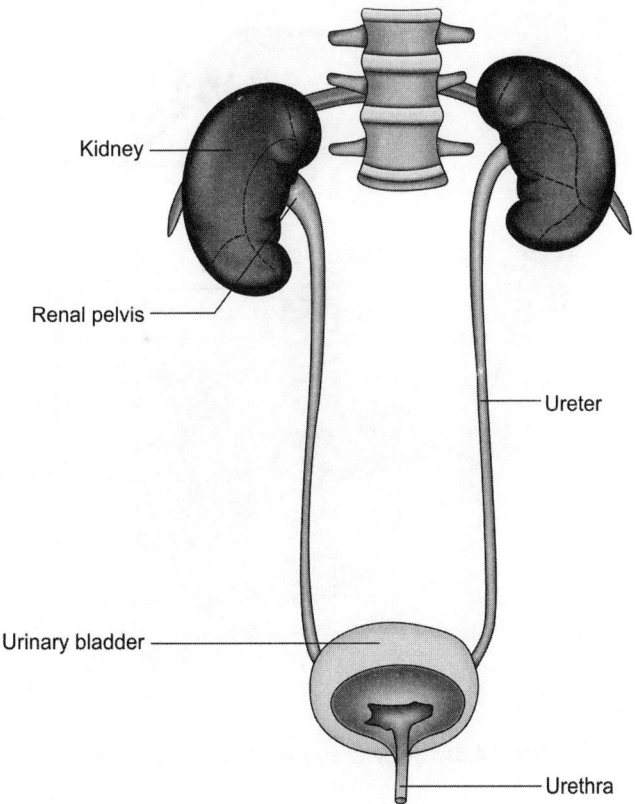

Fig. 14.4: Parts of urinary system

Exercise

1. Identify:
   a. Kidneys (two)
   b. Ureters (two)
   c. Urinary bladder (one)
   d. Urethra (one)
2. Name the borders and surfaces of kidney.
3. Name the structures present at the hilum of kidney.

FEMALE REPRODUCTIVE SYSTEM

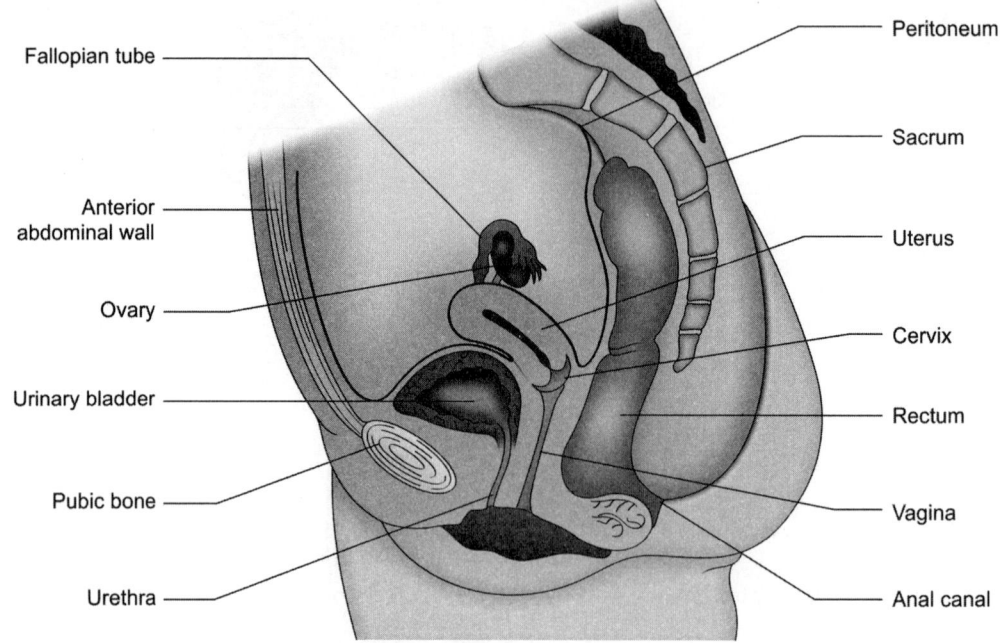

Fig. 14.5A: Sagittal section of female pelvis

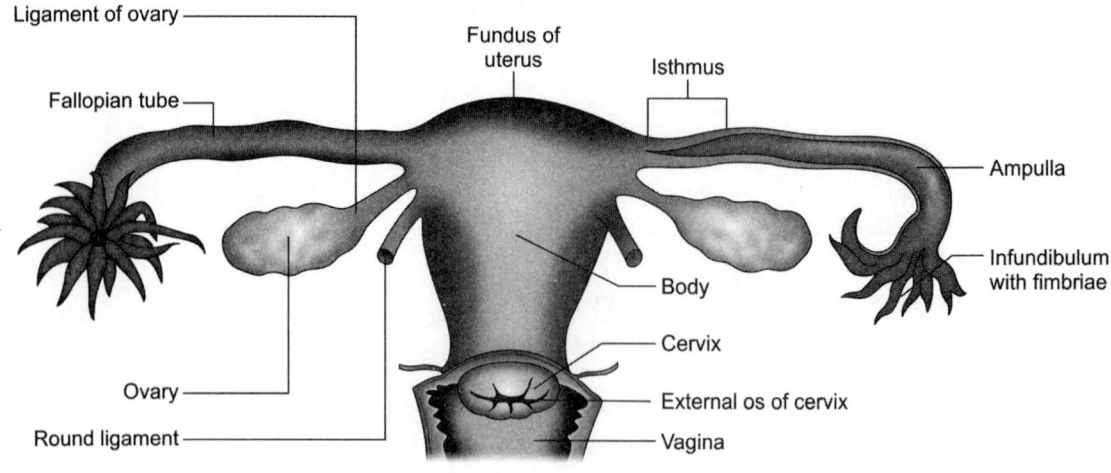

Fig. 14.5B: Parts of internal genital organs

Exercise

1. Identify the parts of female reproductive system in Figs 2.5A and B.

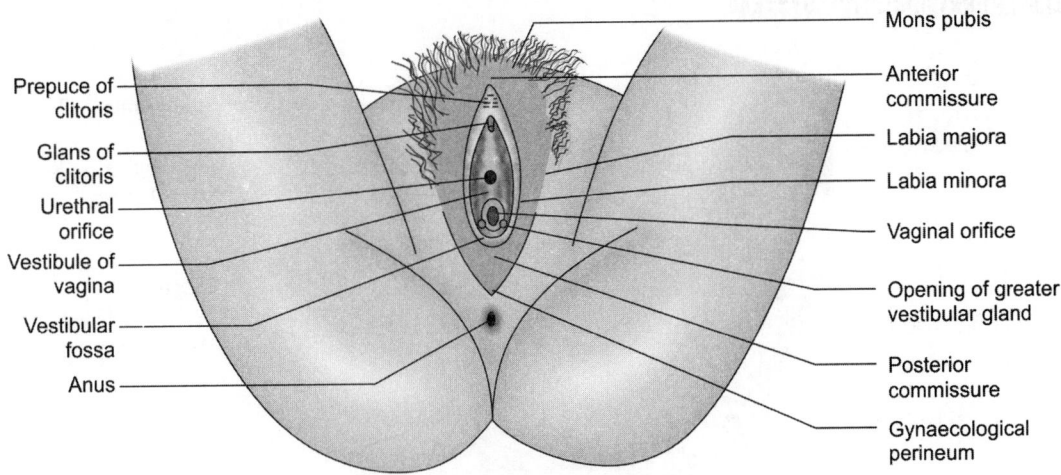

Fig. 14.5C: Female external genital organs

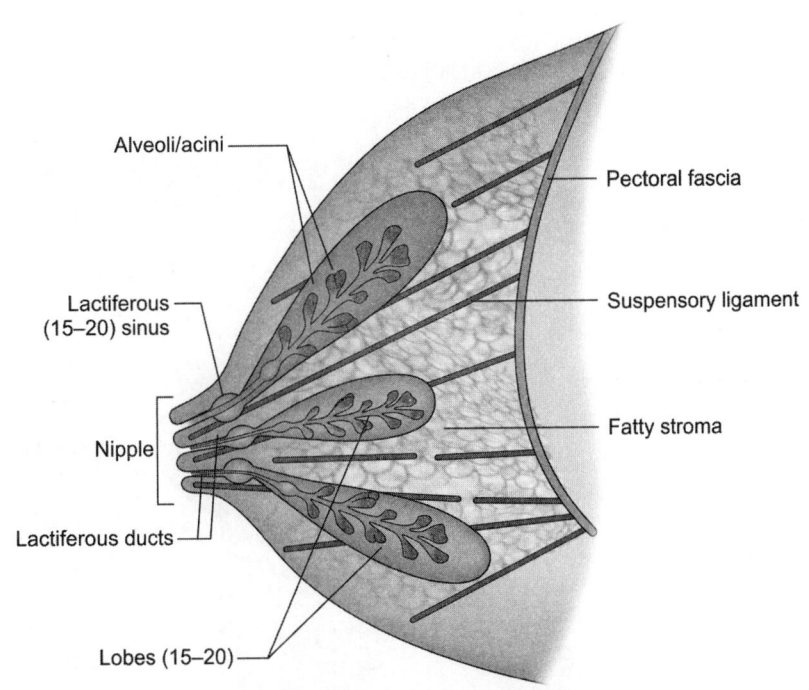

Fig. 14.5D: Structure of mammary gland

Exercise

1. Enumerate the functions of:
   a. Ovary   c. Fallopian tube
   b. Uterus, vagina   d. Mammary gland
2. What is tubectomy?

MALE REPRODUCTIVE SYSTEM

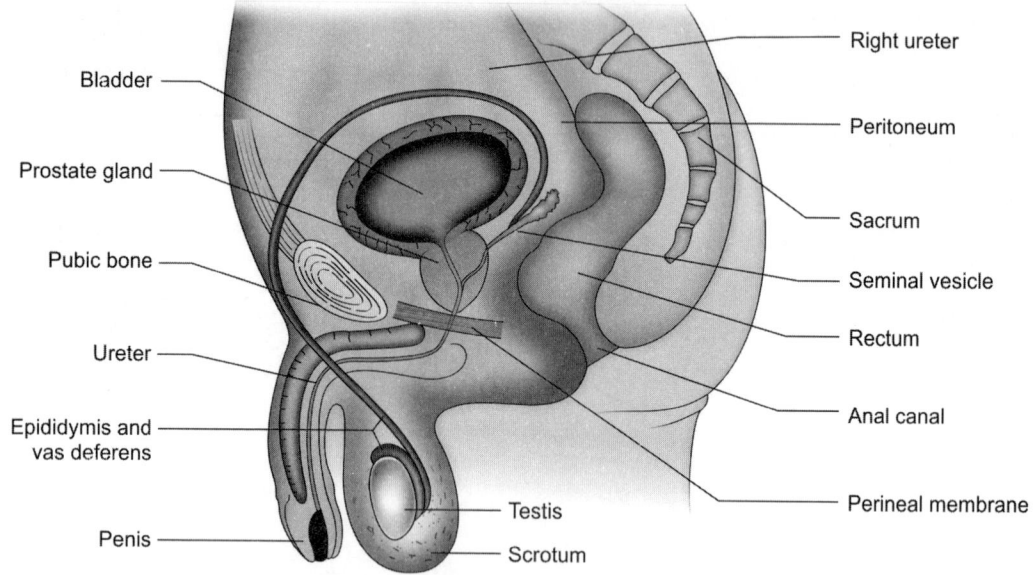

Fig. 14.6A: Sagittal section of male pelvis

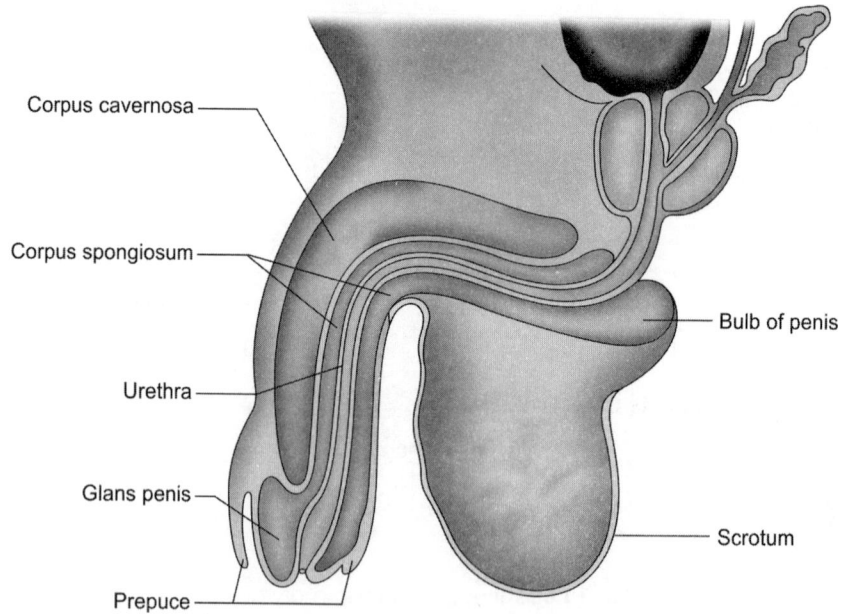

Fig. 14.6B: Parts of male genital system

Exercise

1. Identify the parts of male reproductive (genital) system in Figs 2.6A and B.

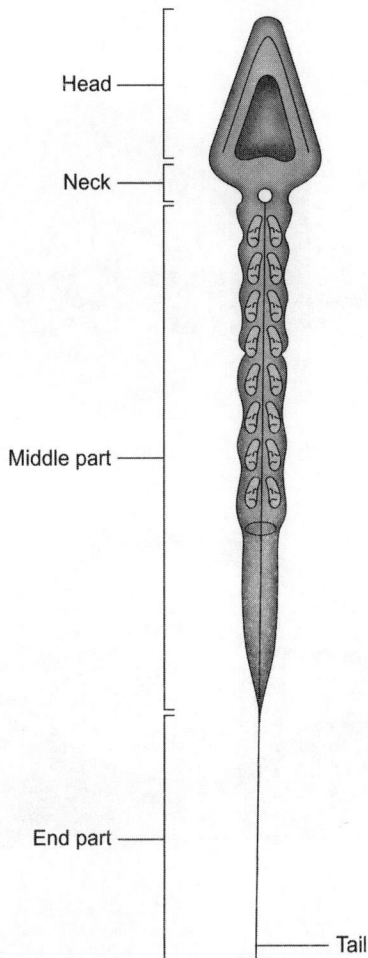

Fig. 14.6C: Parts of spermatozoa

Exercise

1. Identify and learn the parts of spermatozoa.
2. What are the functions of:
   a. Testis   d. Prostate
   b. Epididymis   e. Penis
   c. Vas deferens
3. What is vasectomy?

SPECIAL SENSES

THE EYE

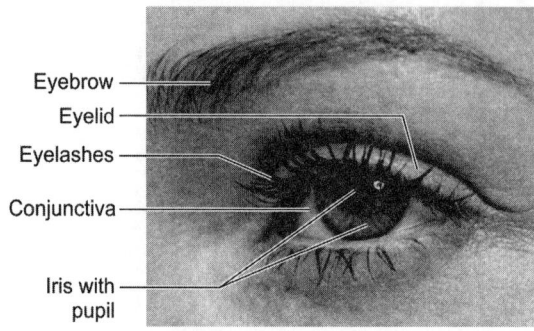

Eyebrow
Eyelid
Eyelashes
Conjunctiva
Iris with pupil

Fig. 14.7A: Parts of eye as seen from outside *(For colour Fig. see Plate 3)*

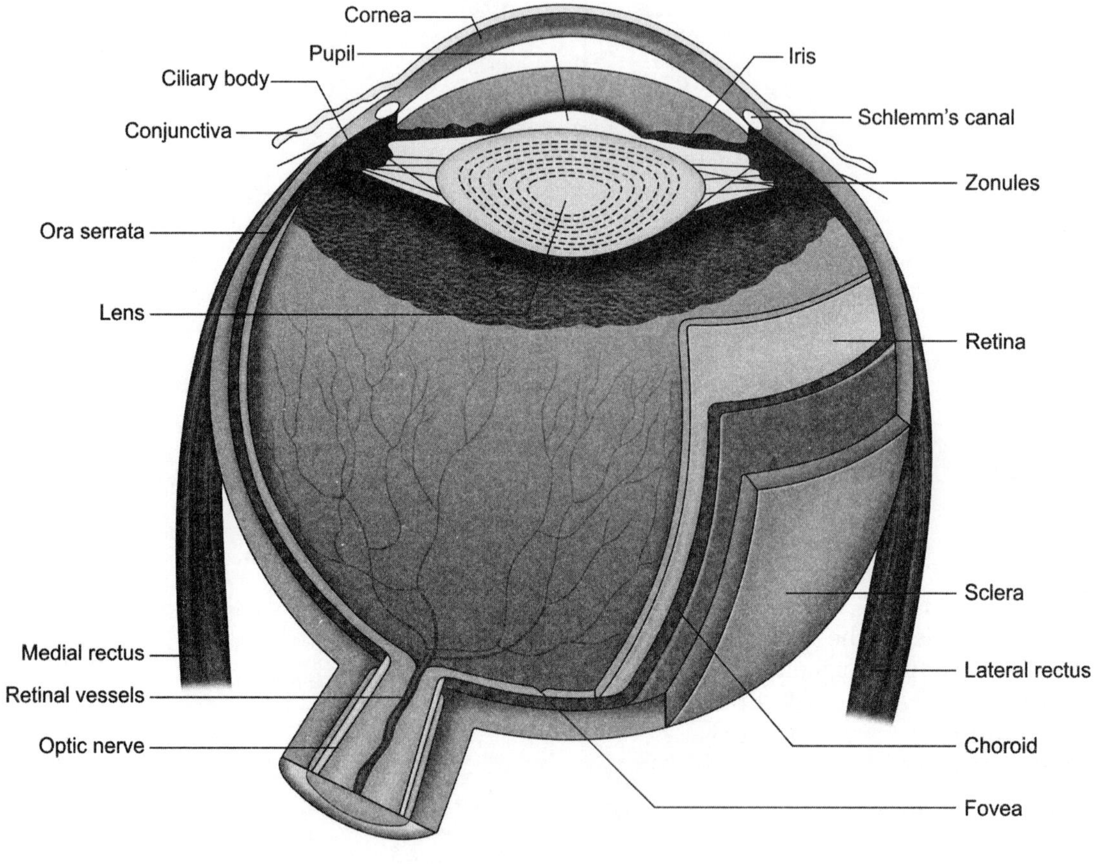

Cornea
Pupil
Ciliary body
Conjunctiva
Ora serrata
Lens
Medial rectus
Retinal vessels
Optic nerve

Iris
Schlemm's canal
Zonules
Retina
Sclera
Lateral rectus
Choroid
Fovea

Fig. 14.7B: Layers of the eyeball

Exercise

1. Identify parts of the eye and learn them in Fig. 14.7A.
2. Identify the layers of the eyeball in Fig. 14.7B.

THE EAR

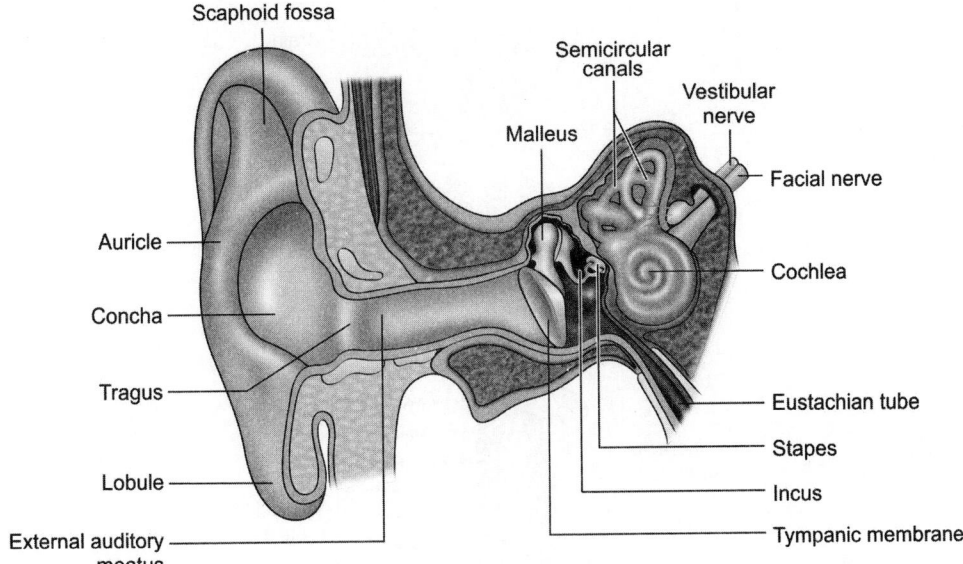

Fig. 14.8A: Parts of the ear

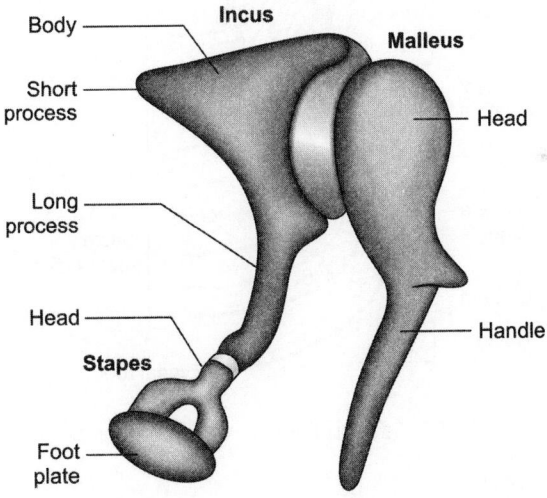

Fig. 14.8B: Ossicles *(For colour Fig. see Plate 3)*

Exercise

1. Trace the path of sound waves from external ear till the vestibulocochlear nerve.

CENTRAL NERVOUS SYSTEM (CNS)

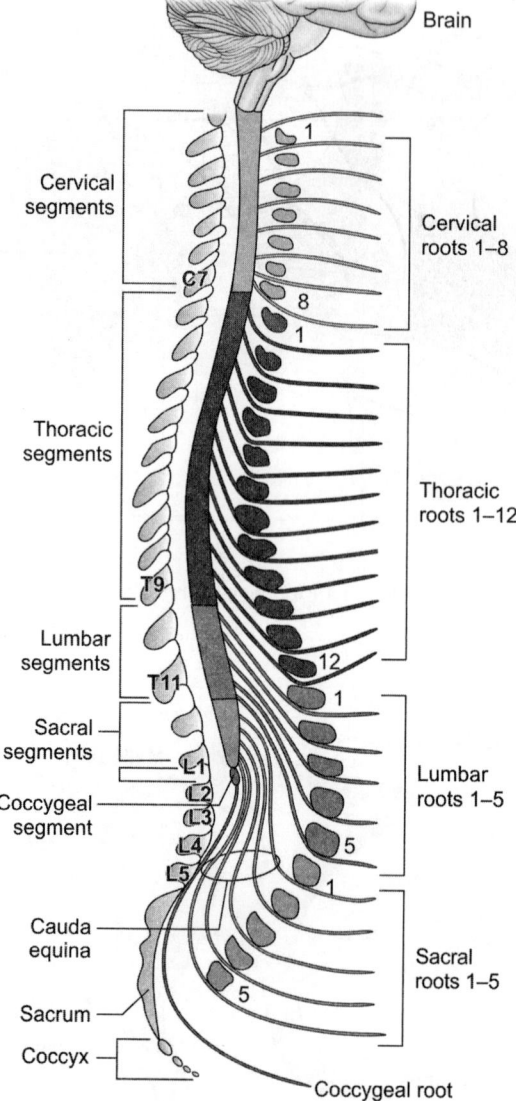

Fig. 14.9A: Section through vertebral canal

Exercise

1. How many spinal nerves are present.

2. Name the types of spinal nerves.

CEREBRAL HEMISPHERE

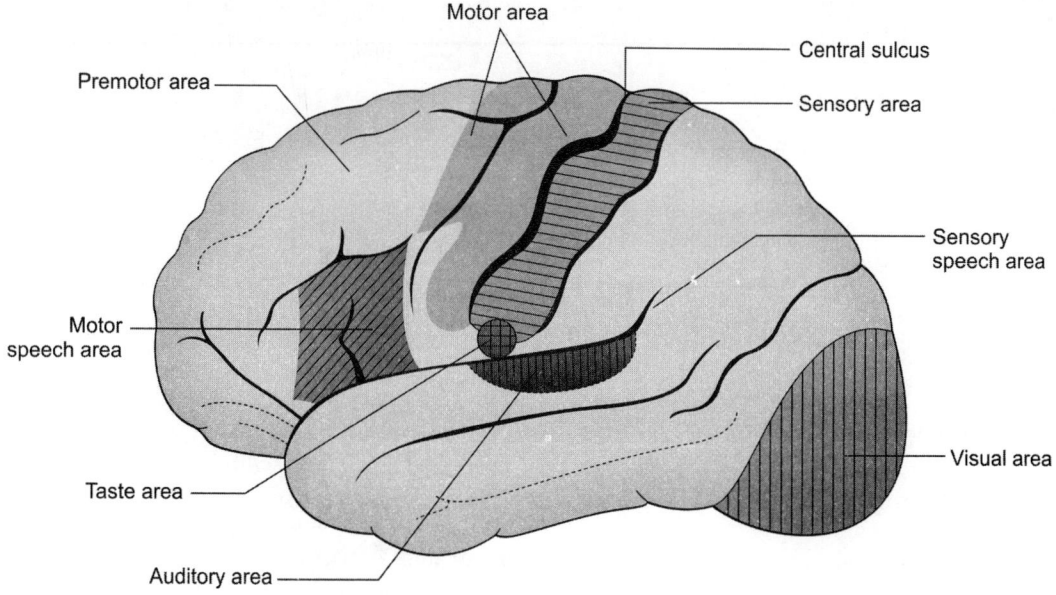

Fig. 14.9B: Superolateral surface of left cerebral hemisphere *(For colour Fig. see Plate 4)*

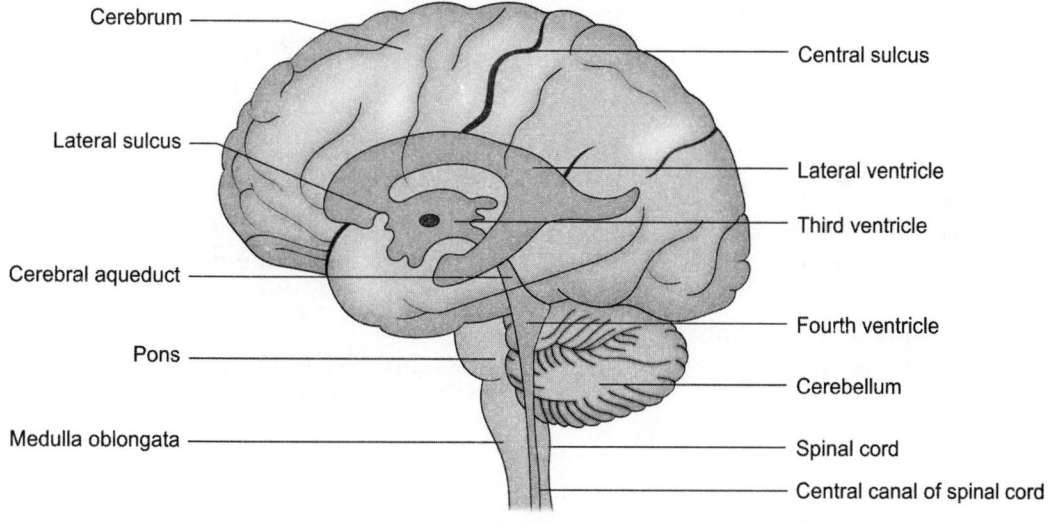

Fig. 14.9C: Ventricles of the brain with central canal of spinal cord *(For colour Fig. see Plate 4)*

Exercise

1. Identify the lobes of the hemisphere after reading the Chapter 8.
2. Learn the functional areas of brain.
3. Identify the ventricles of the brain.

Tissues

HISTOLOGY

There are four basic tissues in the body. These are:
1. Epithelial tissue
2. Muscular tissue
3. Connective tissue
4. Nervous tissue

Histolgoy of various subtypes of these tissues is given. The diagrams are accompanied by three points of identification as "Facts of Remember".

Epithelial Tissue

a. Squamous (Fig. 15.1)
b. Cuboidal (Fig. 15.2)
c. Columnar (Fig. 15.3)
d. Columnar with goblet cells (Fig. 15.4)
e. Stratified squamous non-keratinised (Fig. 15.5)
f. Stratified squamous keratinised (Fig. 15.6)
g. Transitional (Fig. 15.7)

Muscular Tissue

a. Striated (Fig. 15.8)
b. Smooth (Fig. 15.9)
c. Cardiac (Fig. 15.10)

Connective Tissue (Specialised)

a. Cartilage
  • Hyaline (Fig. 15.11)
  • Elastic (Fig. 15.12)
  • Fibrocartilage (Fig. 15.13)
b. Bone
  • Compact (Fig. 15.14)
  • Cancellous (Fig. 15.15)

Nervous Tissue

a. Neuron and neuroglia (Fig. 15.16)
b. Spinal cord (Fig. 15.17)
c. Nerve trunk (Haematoxylin and eosin stain) (Fig. 15.18)
d. Cerebellum (Fig. 15.19)
e. Cerebrum (Fig. 15.20)

SQUAMOUS EPITHELIUM

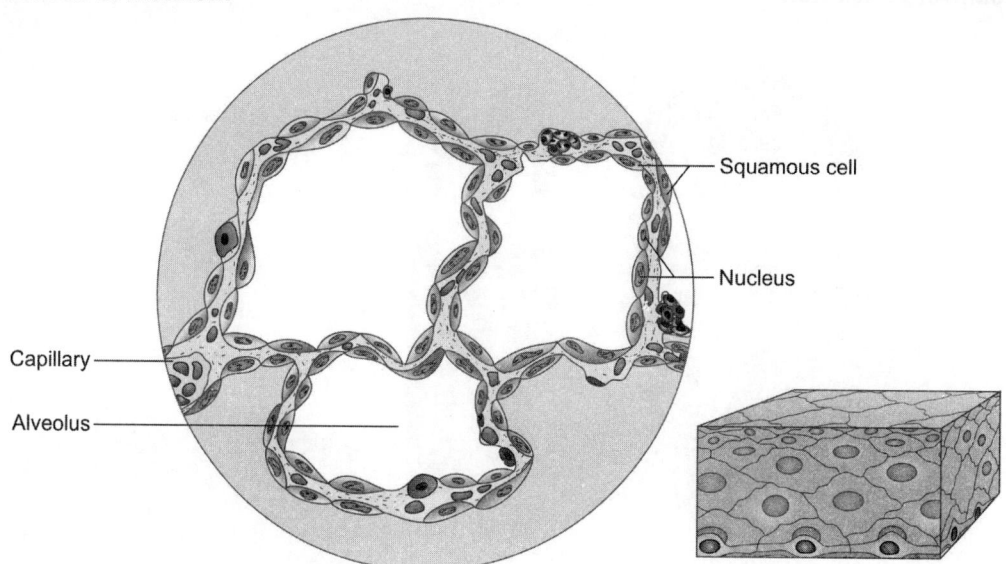

Squamous cell

Nucleus

Capillary

Alveolus

1. Flattened cells lining the lung alveoli
2. Capillaries in between the alveoli
3. Squamous cells permit exchange of gases

Fig. 15.1: Haematoxylin and eosin (H&E) stain

CUBOIDAL EPITHELIUM

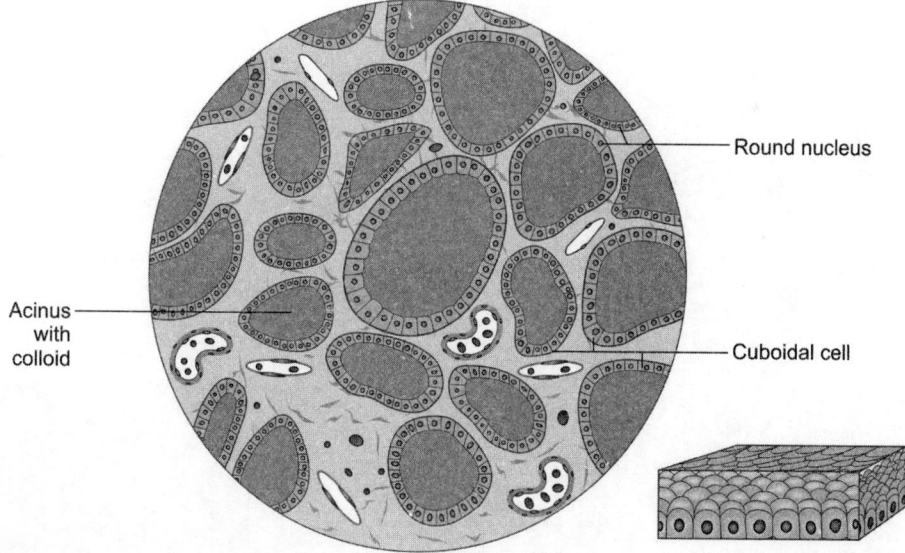

Round nucleus

Acinus with colloid

Cuboidal cell

1. The cells have same width and height
2. The cells contain a central nucleus
3. All the cells rest on the basement membrane

Fig. 15.2: Thyroid gland (H&E stain)

COLUMNAR EPITHELIUM

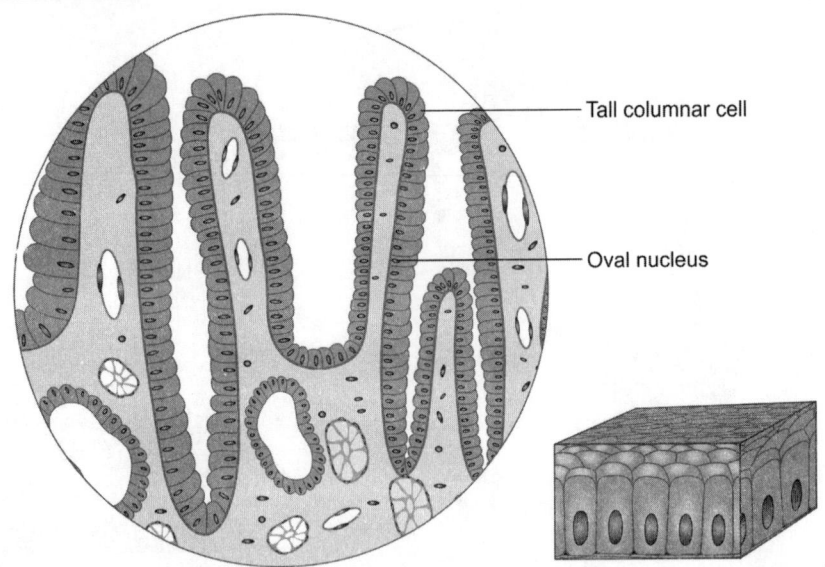

- Tall columnar cell
- Oval nucleus

Facts to Remember
1. The cells are three times taller than their width
2. Nucleus is basal and oval in shape
3. All the cells look alike

Fig. 15.3: Lining of stomach (H&E stain)

COLUMNAR EPITHELIUM WITH GOBLET CELLS

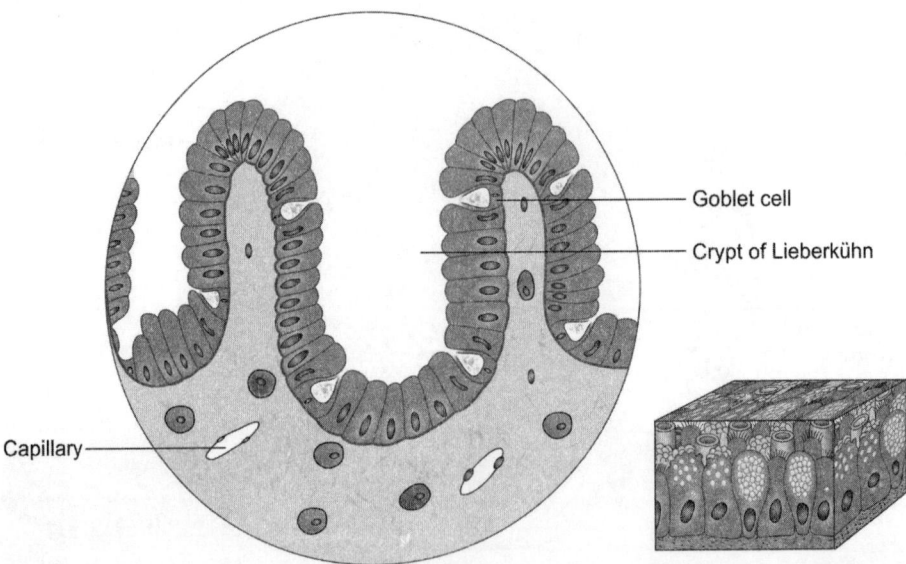

- Goblet cell
- Crypt of Lieberkühn
- Capillary

Facts to Remember
1. The columnar cells are interrupted due to presence of empty-looking goblet cells
2. The goblet cells contain basal peripheral nucleus
3. Goblet cells secrete mucus

Fig. 15.4: Small intestine (H&E stain)

STRATIFIED SQUAMOUS NON-KERATINISED EPITHELIUM

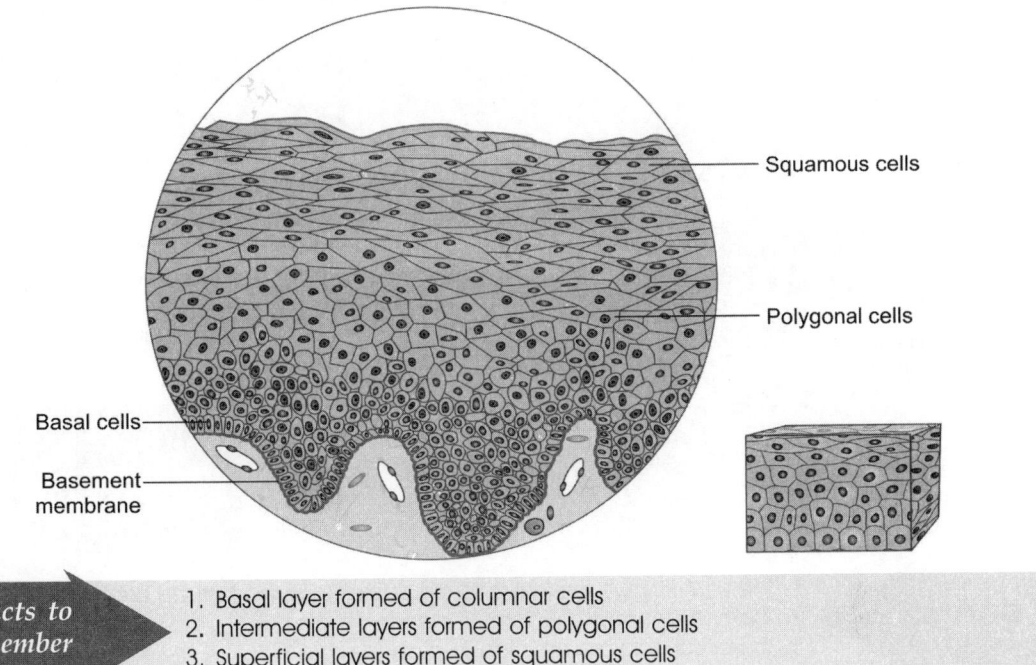

Squamous cells

Polygonal cells

Basal cells

Basement membrane

Facts to Remember

1. Basal layer formed of columnar cells
2. Intermediate layers formed of polygonal cells
3. Superficial layers formed of squamous cells

Fig. 15.5: Oesophagus

STRATIFIED SQUAMOUS KERATINISED EPITHELIUM

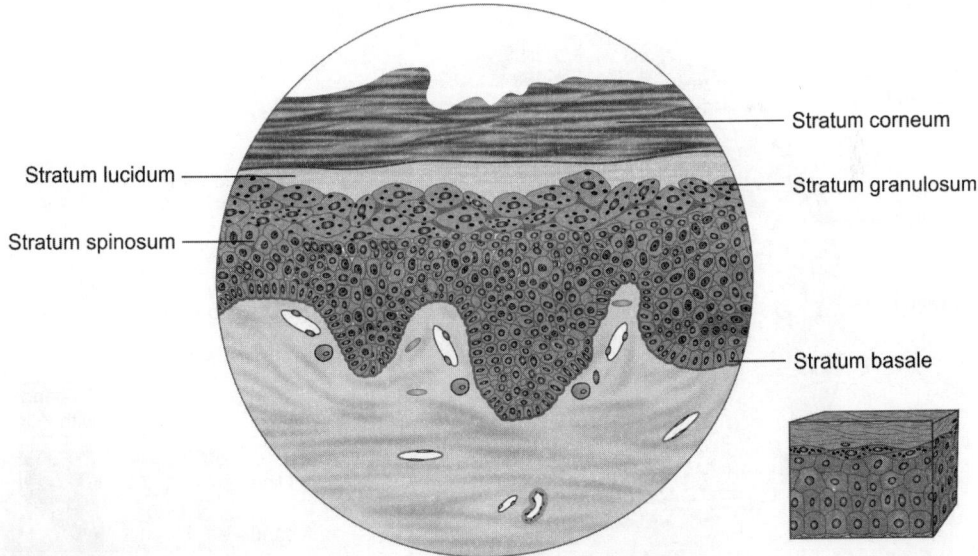

Stratum lucidum

Stratum spinosum

Stratum corneum

Stratum granulosum

Stratum basale

Facts to Remember

1. Columnar cells of stratum basale rest on the basement membrane
2. Stratum spinosum, stratum granulosum, stratum lucidum and stratum corneum form the succeeding layers
3. Stratum corneum is the waterproof layer

Fig. 15.6: Skin

TRANSITIONAL EPITHELIUM

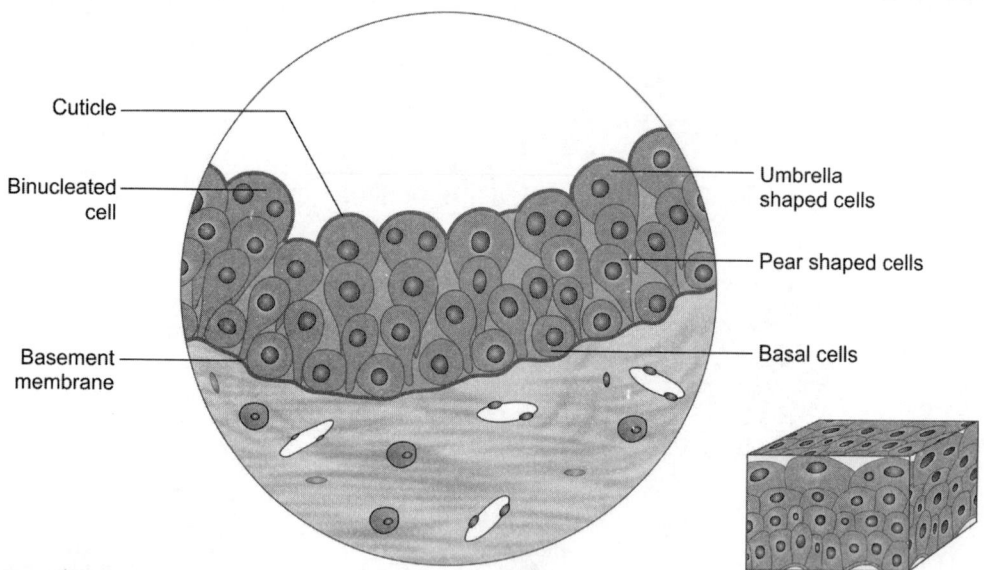

Cuticle

Binucleated cell

Basement membrane

Umbrella shaped cells

Pear shaped cells

Basal cells

Facts to Remember

1. The bright active luminal cells are umbrella-shaped, some are binucleated
2. The pear-shaped cells form intermediate layer
3. The basal cells are cuboidal in shape

Fig. 15.7: Urinary bladder

MUSCULAR TISSUE

Skeletal Muscle

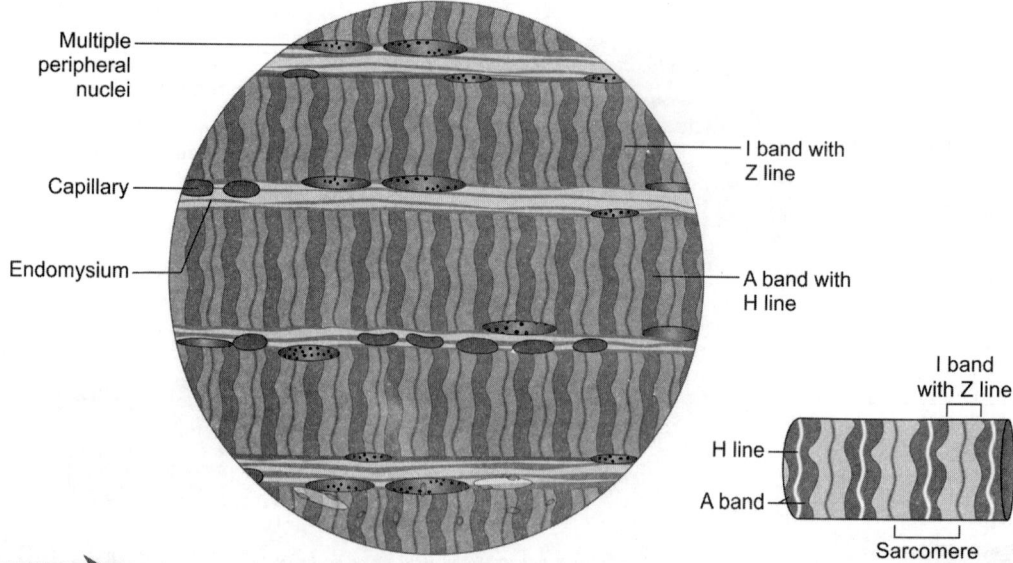

Multiple peripheral nuclei

Capillary

Endomysium

I band with Z line

A band with H line

I band with Z line

H line

A band

Sarcomere

Facts to Remember

1. Transverse and longitudinal striations
2. Dark and light bands
3. Multiple peripheral, flattened nuclei

Fig. 15.8: Biceps brachii muscle

Smooth Muscle

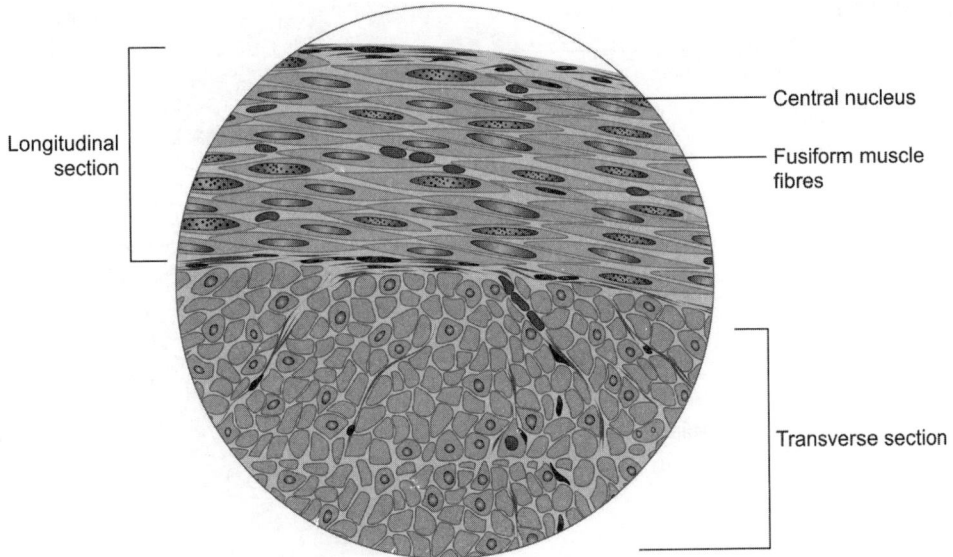

Longitudinal section

Central nucleus

Fusiform muscle fibres

Transverse section

Facts to Remember
1. Longitudinal striations
2. Single central nucleus
3. Transverse section shows round/oval fibres

Fig. 15.9: Stomach

Cardiac Muscle

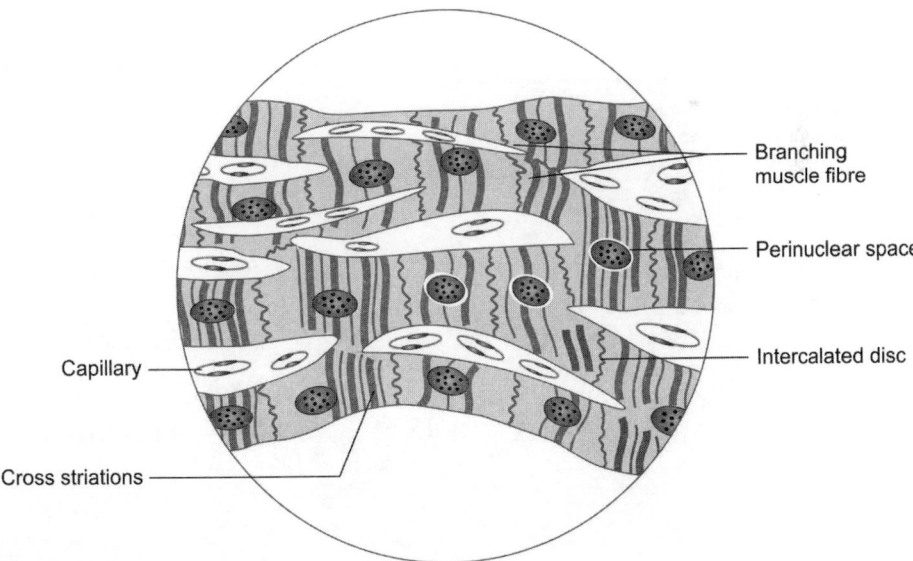

Branching muscle fibre

Perinuclear space

Intercalated disc

Capillary

Cross striations

Facts to Remember
1. Faint longitudinal and transverse striations
2. Branching muscle fibres
3. Presence of intercalated discs

Fig. 15.10: Heart

CONNECTIVE TISSUE (SPECIALISED)

Hyaline Cartilage

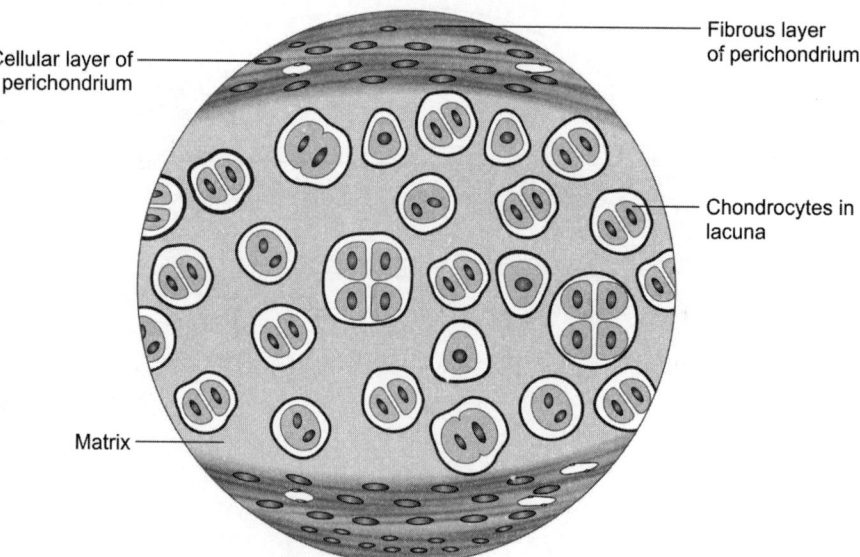

Cellular layer of perichondrium

Fibrous layer of perichondrium

Chondrocytes in lacuna

Matrix

Facts to Remember

1. Perichondrium seen all around
2. Ground substance appears homogeneous
3. Chondrocytes in lacuna lie in groups of 2–4 cells

Fig. 15.11: Trachea

Elastic Cartilage

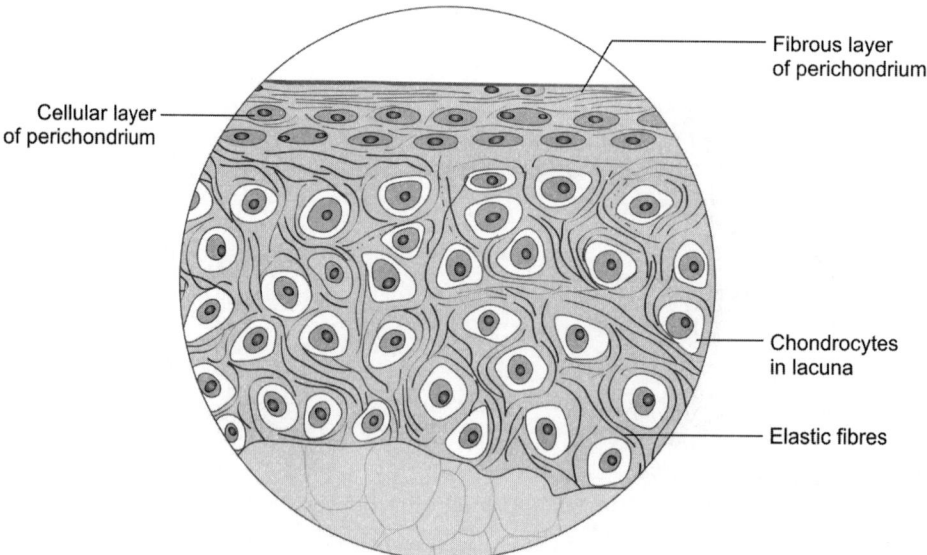

Cellular layer of perichondrium

Fibrous layer of perichondrium

Chondrocytes in lacuna

Elastic fibres

Facts to Remember

1. Perichondrium seen
2. Short yellow elastic fibres
3. Single chondrocytes seen in lacuna

Fig. 15.12: Epiglottis

Fibrocartilage

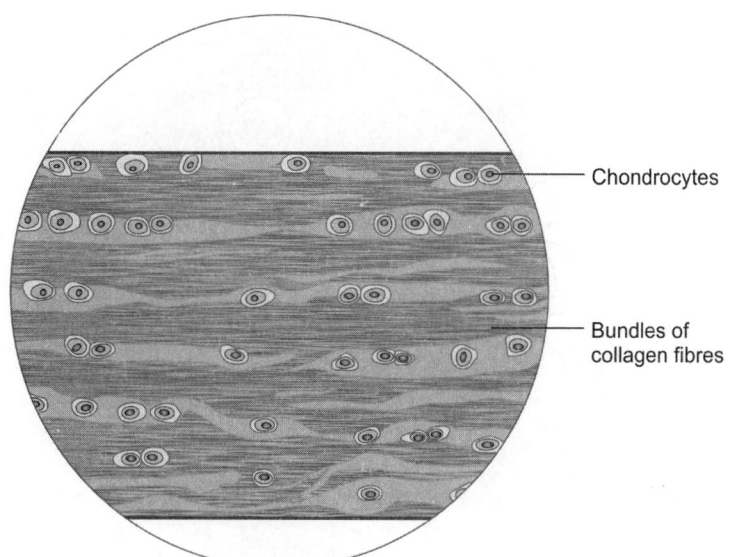

Chondrocytes

Bundles of
collagen fibres

Facts to Remember

1. Collagen fibres in bundles
2. A few chondrocytes in between
3. No perichondrium

Fig. 15.13: Fibrocartilage

BONE

Compact Bone

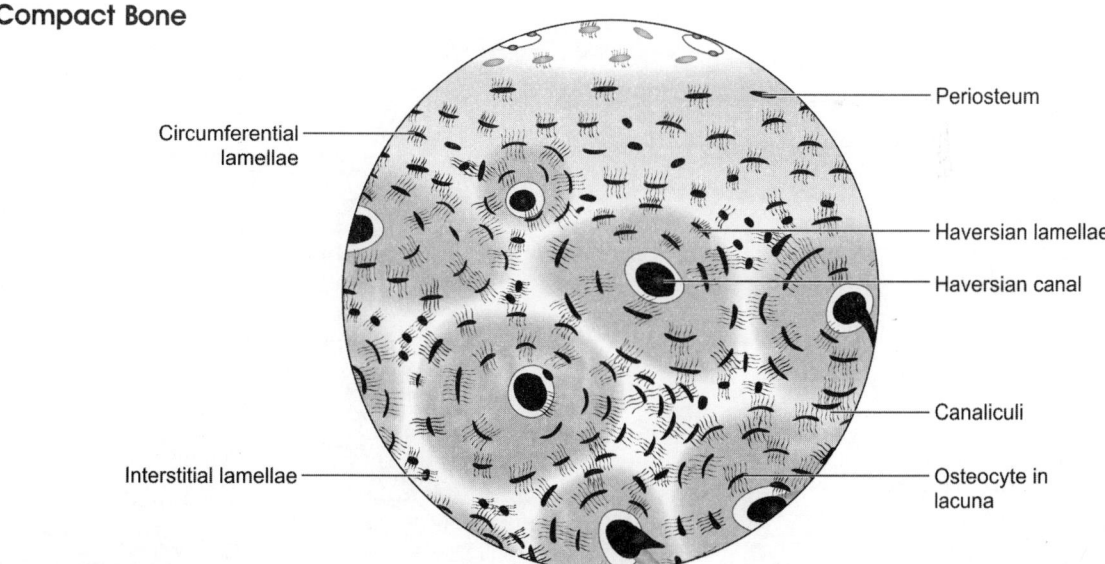

Periosteum

Circumferential
lamellae

Haversian lamellae

Haversian canal

Canaliculi

Interstitial lamellae

Osteocyte in
lacuna

Facts to Remember

1. Outer periosteum seen
2. Three types of lamellae seen: haversian, interstitial and circumferential
3. In between lamellae are osteocytes in the lacuna with canaliculi

Fig. 15.14: Compact bone

Cancellous Bone

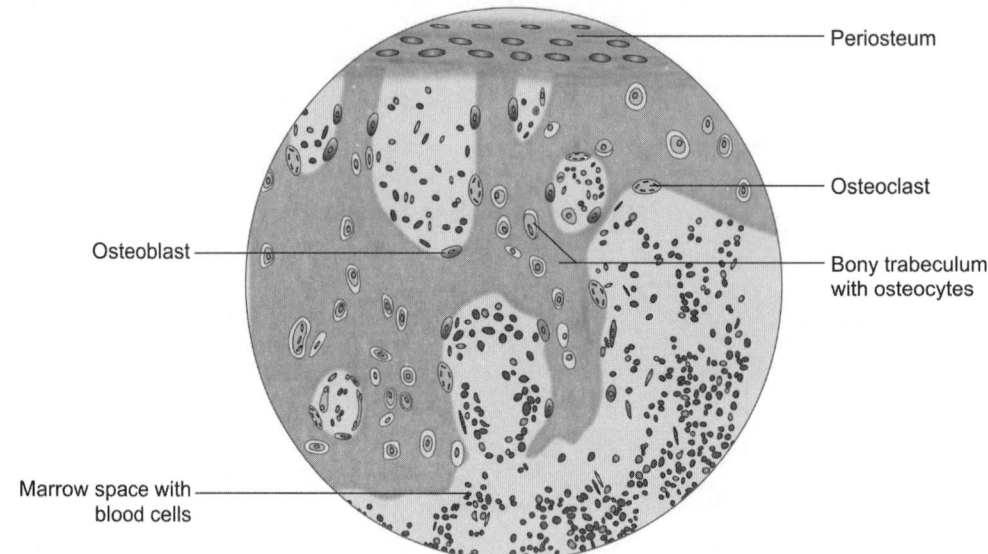

Facts to Remember
1. Periosteum on the outside
2. Bony trabeculae with osteocytes and a few osteoblast cells
3. Marrow space in between bony trabeculae

Fig. 15.15: Sternum

NERVOUS TISSUE

Neuron and Neuroglia

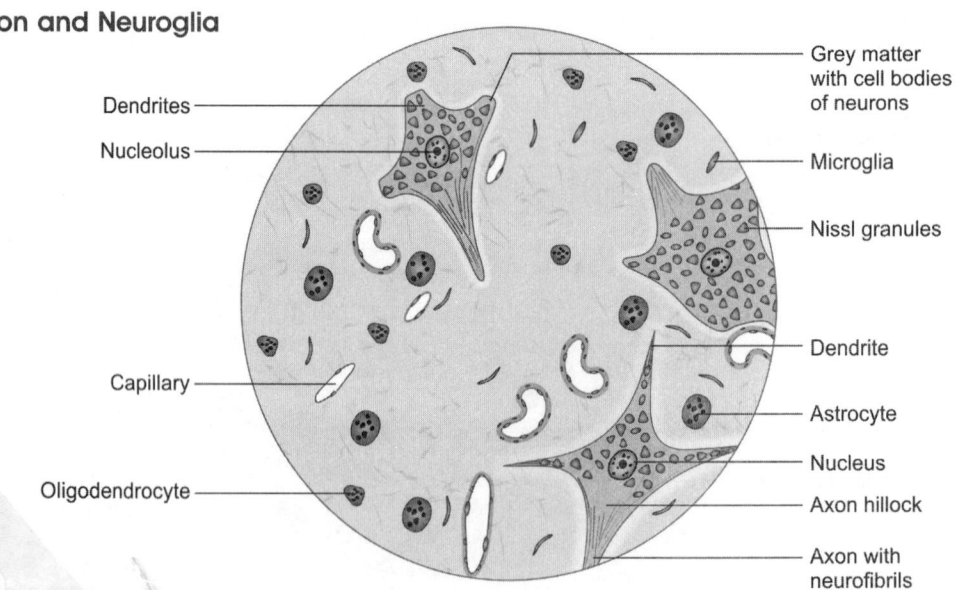

Facts to Remember
1. Multipolar neuron is large irregular cell with central nucleus
2. Has multiple dendrites, single axon
3. Also seen are the astrocyte, oligodendrocyte, microglia, capillaries

Fig. 15.16: Neuron and neuroglia

SPINAL CORD

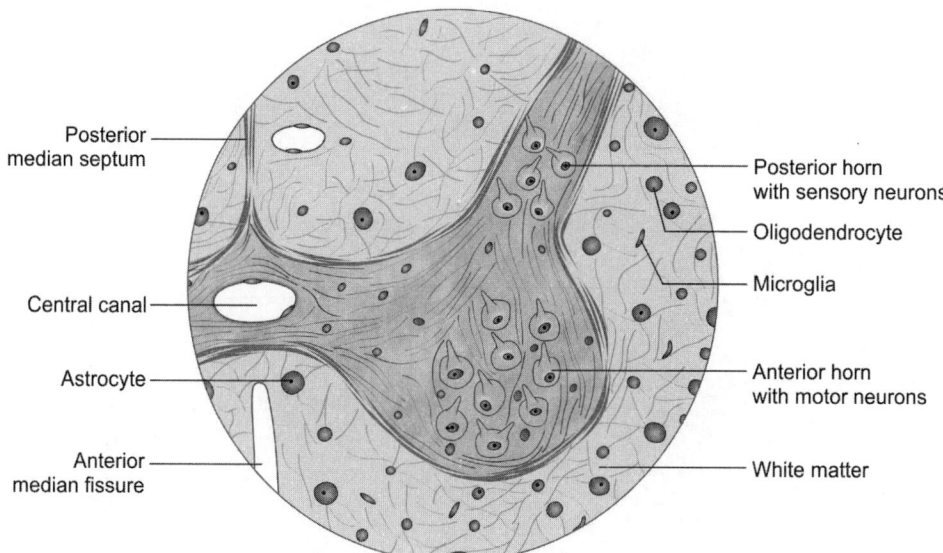

Posterior median septum

Central canal

Astrocyte

Anterior median fissure

Posterior horn with sensory neurons

Oligodendrocyte

Microglia

Anterior horn with motor neurons

White matter

Facts to Remember

1. Inner grey matter contains cell bodies of neurons
2. Outer white matter contains processes of neurons and neuroglial cells
3. Central canal lies in the grey commissure

Fig. 15.17: Spinal cord

NERVE TRUNK

Nerve Trunk Showing Axon

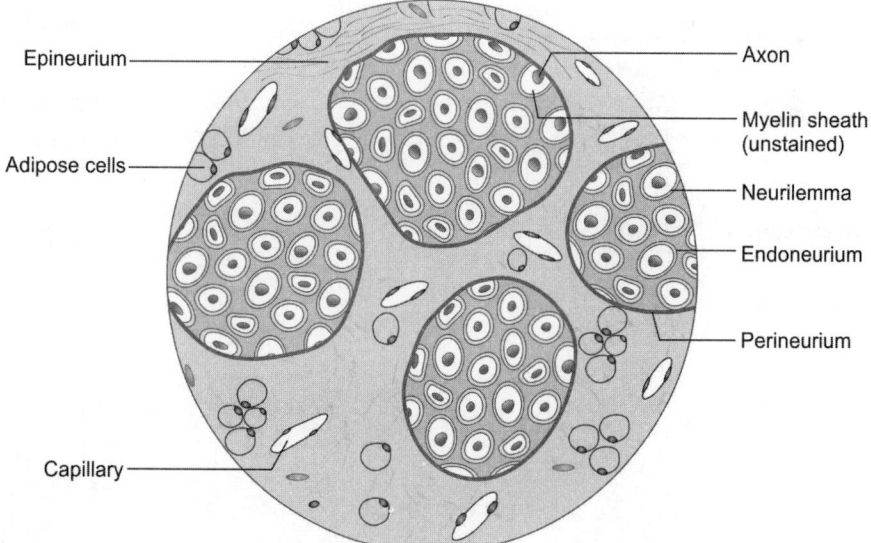

Epineurium

Adipose cells

Capillary

Axon

Myelin sheath (unstained)

Neurilemma

Endoneurium

Perineurium

Facts to Remember

1. The neurilemma is stained pink
2. The empty circle is the unstained myelin sheath
3. The inner structure is the stained axon

Fig. 15.18: Median nerve (H&E stain)

Cerebellum

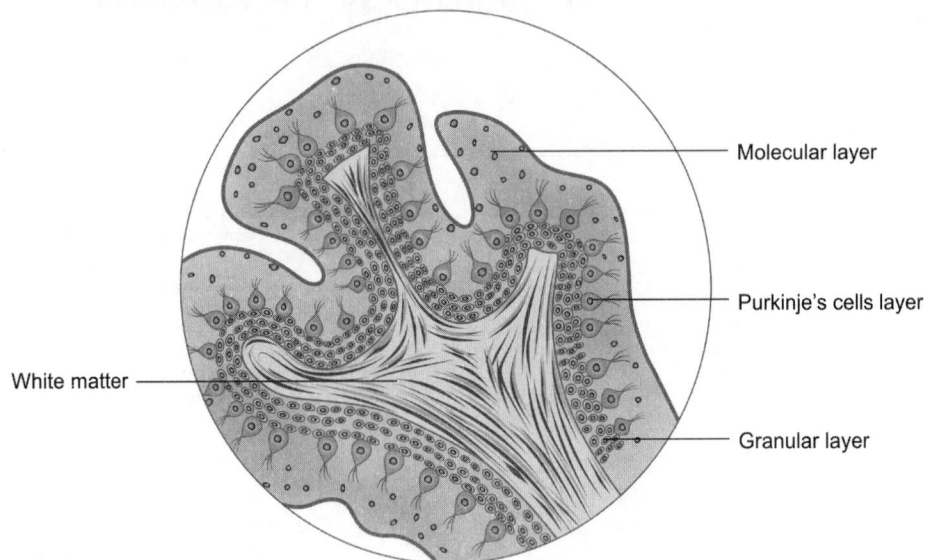

Molecular layer

Purkinje's cells layer

White matter

Granular layer

Facts to Remember

1. Outer molecular layer and inner granular layer
2. Purkinje's cells at the junction
3. Uniform structure

Fig. 15.19: Cerebellum

CEREBRUM

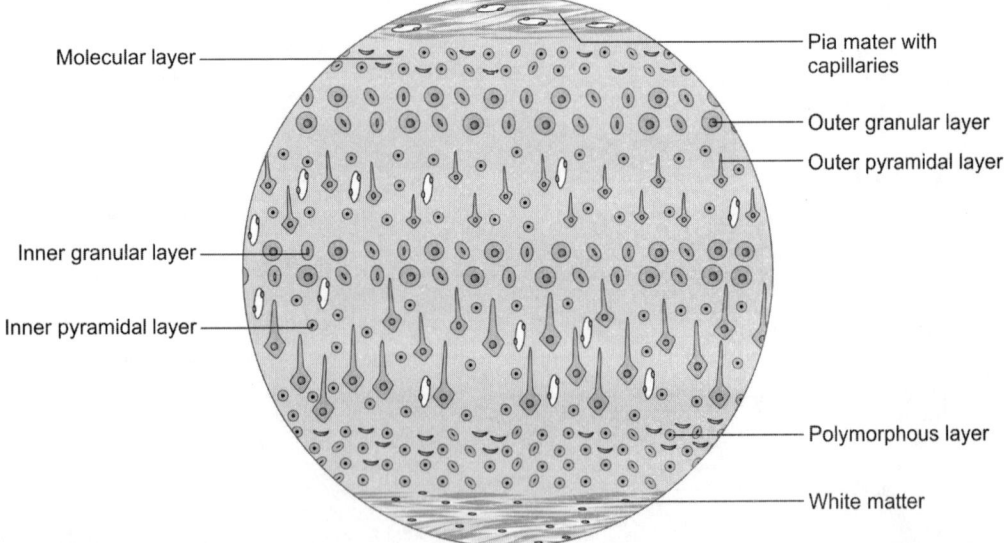

Molecular layer

Pia mater with capillaries

Outer granular layer

Outer pyramidal layer

Inner granular layer

Inner pyramidal layer

Polymorphous layer

White matter

Facts to Remember

1. Six layers of cells and fibres
2. Pyramidal cells more in motor cortex and granular cells more in sensory cortex
3. Numerous capillaries present

Fig. 15.20: Cerebrum

The Microscope

Study the different parts of a compound microscope and its use.

COMPOUND MICROSCOPE

The compound microscope is so called because it has two lenses system, i.e. the eyepiece and the objective lenses.

Broadly, the parts of compound microscope are divided into

a. Supporting parts (Fig. 16.1)
b. Focusing parts

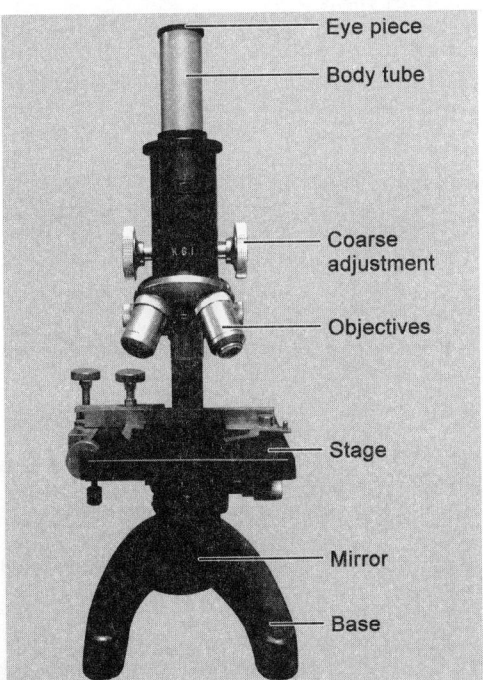

Fig. 16.1: Monocular compound microscope (front view)

c. Optical parts
d. Illumination parts

A. Supporting Parts

i. **Base:** It is horseshoe or U-shaped structure. It supports the microscope and provides stability.

ii. **Pillars:** There are two pillars between the base and handle. It is an upright structure. It is attached to the handle by a hinge joint.

iii. **Handle:** It is curved C shaped structure and it helps in tilting the microscope.

iv. **Body tube:** It is wide tube attached to the C shaped handle at the upper part. At the lower end it is attached to the nosepiece. Eyepiece is placed at the upper end.

v. **Stage:** Stage is comprised of two parts:

a. **Fixed stage:** It is a fixed square stage and has a round aperture at the centre. Object is placed at the centre for study. The light rays coming from below cross this aperture and strike the object which is to be focussed.

b. **Mechanical stage:** It is a calibrated stage (vernier scale) and is fitted on the fixed stage. There is a clip attached to it which holds the object. There are two screws attached to it which control sideways, forward and backward (to and fro) movements of the object. Movement of the object can be determined by engraved vernier scale on the mechanical stage.

B. Focusing Parts

Coarse and fine adjustment screw: If one side screw is moved then the other side screw also moves along with it automatically. These screws work in "Rack and Pinion" method. Circular movement (pinion) of these screws help in upward and downward movement (racking) of body tube.

a. **Coarse adjustment screw:** There are two coarse adjustment screws mounted at the top of the handle on either side. The focussing of an object is always done by using coarse adjustment screw first. The body tube is moved in upward and downward direction by the coarse adjustment screw.

b. **Fine adjustment screw:** There are two fine adjustment screws mounted at the top of the handle on either side. These are small sized screw or knob for fine and sharp focussing after coarse focussing has been made with the coarse adjustment screws.

C. Optical Parts

Optical parts of microscope help in image formation (Fig. 16.2).

i. **Body tube:** It is also consider as a part of optical system.

ii. **Eyepiece lens:** It is placed at the uppermost part of the body tube. The eyepiece lens has different magnifying power, i.e. 5X, 10X, etc. which can be changed according to the requirements. It is comprised of two lenses:

a. **Eye lens:** It is attached at top most part of eyepiece Lens

b. **Field lens:** It is present at the lower most part of eyepiece Lens

iii. **Nosepiece:** It has two parts fixed nosepiece and revolving nosepiece.

The fixed nosepiece is attached on the lower end of body tube.

Revolving nosepiece is fitted bellow the fixed nosepiece. Different objective lenses are attached to the revolving nosepiece.

iv. **Objective lenses:** There are four or three objective lenses with the different magnifying power attached to the revolving nosepiece. The magnifying power and the numerical aperture are engraved in each and every objective lens (Table 16.1).

D. Illumination Parts

i. **Light:** The source of light may be external or internal, i.e. light is attached with microscope itself (Fig. 16.3).

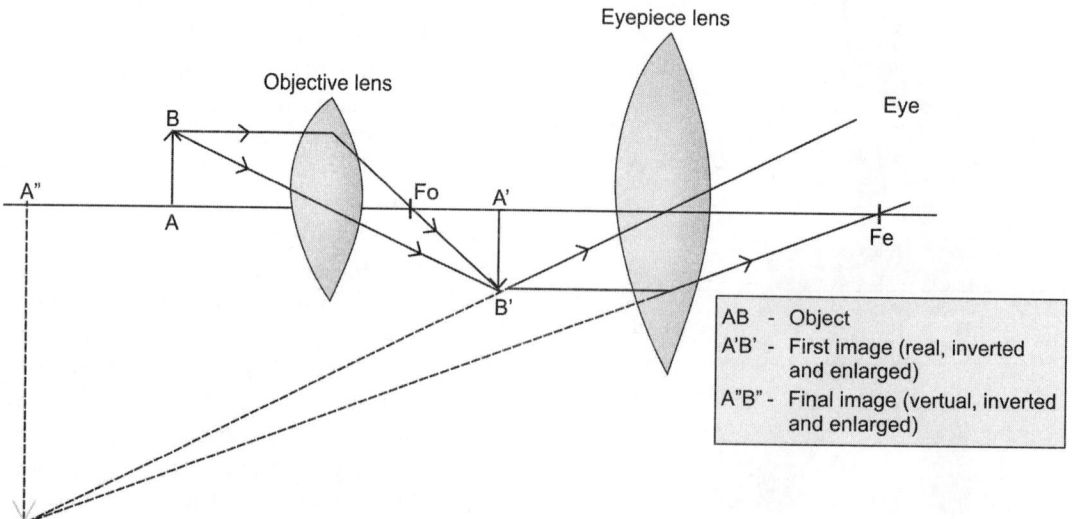

AB - Object
A'B' - First image (real, inverted and enlarged)
A"B" - Final image (vertual, inverted and enlarged)

Fig. 16.2: Optical ray diagram of image formation

Table 16.1: Magnification power, focal length, NA of objective lenses

Objective lenses	Magnification power	Focal length	Numerical aperture (NA)
Scanning objective lens	3X	40 mm	0.10
Low power objective lens	10X	16 mm	0.25
High power objective lens	40X or 45X	4 mm	0.65
Oil immersion objective lens	100X	Less than 2 mm	1.30

Total magnification power = Magnification power of eyepiece lens × Magnification power of objective lens

Sunlight or artificial light can be used as external source for microscope.

ii. **Planoconcave mirror:** It is double sided mirror. One side is plane and the other side is concave in nature. That's why it is known as planoconcave mirror. The plane mirror is used when sunlight is used as light source. Because sunlight rays are parallel in nature and reflected parallel to the condenser by plane mirror. The concave mirror is used in artificial light. Because artificial light rays are divergent in nature and reflected as parallel to the condenser by concave mirror.

iii. **Condenser:** It is just below the central aperture of fixed stage. It is a combination of two lenses fitted in a short cylinder. The function of condenser is to converge light

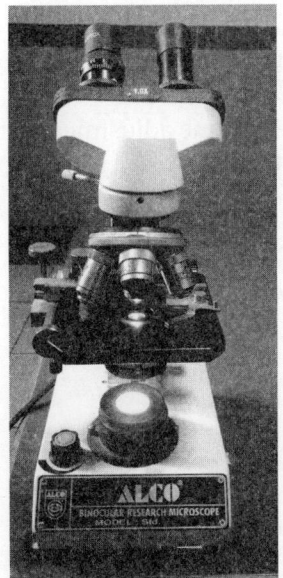

Fig. 16.3: Binocular compound microscope (front view)

at the central aperture of fixed stage. It also reduces the spherical and chromatic aberrations. By the help of a screw, fitted at one side, condenser can be moved in upward and downward direction. This screw also work in rack and pinion fashion.

While using scanning objective lens, the condenser should be at the lowermost position. During the use of low power objective lens, the condenser should be little bit upper from lowermost position. Position of condenser should be midway during the use of high power objective lens and at uppermost position while using oil immersion objective lens.

iv. **Iris diaphragm:** It is present just below the condenser. It controls the amount of light. Its size of aperture can be changed by moving a small lever fitted on the side.

It is opened least while using scanning objective lens. It is opened partially while using low power lens, almost open in high power and fully opened when oil immersion objective lens is used.

PROCEDURE: TO USE THE MICROSCOPE

Using of Low power Objective Lens

- Place the microscope in working table towards the light source.
- Select the mirror depending upon the source of light.
- Move the condenser at little bit upper from lower most position.
- Open iris diaphragm partially.
- Bring the low power objective lens in alignment by listening click sound (when low power objective lens is brought in the path

of light then a click sound is heard on its rotation).

- Adjust the light by looking through the eyepiece and by tilting the mirror towards light source.
- Now place the object at the centre of fixed stage.
- Lower the body tube (low power objective lens also move with body tube) gradually by coarse adjustment screw up to 3–4 cm away from the object.
- Then look through eye piece.
- The field should be equally and fully illuminated.
- Rotate coarse adjustment screw very slowly to move the body tube downward gradually until rough focus the object is done.
- Then use the fine adjustment screw to have animproved and clear focussing.

Using of High Power Objective Lens

- Bring the high power objective lens in alignment (in the path of light) by listening click sound.
- Bring the condenser at midway position.
- Open iris diaphragm almost fully.
- Lower the body tubegradually by coarse adjustment screw as far as possible without touching the object while looking from the side.
- Then look through eyepiece.
- The field should be equally and fully illuminated by little bit adjusting mirror if required.

- Now elevate the objective lens, i.e. body tube slowly with the help of coarse adjustment screw until the object is visible.
- Then use the fine adjustment screw to have an improved and clear focussing.

Using of Oil immersion Objective Lens

- Elevate the body tube at least 2 inch from the object.
- Bring the oil immersion objective lens in alignment (in the path of light) by listening click sound.
- Put one drop of cedar wood oil over the object (the part of the object which is just above the centre aperture). Cedar wood oil has approximately same refractive index as that of glass and it replaces the thin layer of air which is present in between the object and oil immersion objective lens. Hence, it prevents the refraction of light and object will be more clearly visible.
- Bring the condenser at highest position.
- Open iris diaphragm fully.
- Lower the body tube gradually by coarse adjustment screw until the tip of the oil immersion object touches the cedar wood oil drop while looking from the side.
- Then look through eyepiece.
- The field should be equally and fully illuminated by little bit adjusting mirror if required.
- Then use the fine adjustment screw to have an enhanced and clear focusing.

Determination of TLC*, DLC* and Blood Film for Malarial Parasite

DETERMINATION OF TOTAL LEUCOCYTE COUNT (TLC)

PRINCIPLE

Blood is diluted with Turk's fluid or WBC diluting fluid. Glacial acetic acid of WBC diluting fluid destroy the membrane of red blood cells and Gentian violet (another component of WBC diluting fluid) stain the nuclei of WBCs. After charging this mixture into counting chamber of improved version of Neubauer chamber, counting is done under low power objective lens of microscope. With the knowledge of the volume of the fluid examined and dilution of the blood obtained the number of leucocytes per cubic millimeter of undiluted whole blood is calculated.

APPARATUS REQUIRED

Microscope, Haemocytometer (Fig. 17.1) (only improved version of Neubauer chamber and

WBC pipette), watch glass, cover slip, WBC diluting fluid (Turks fluid), cotton swab dry, cotton swab soaked in alcohol, sterile lancet or pricking needle.

Composition of Turk's fluid or WBC diluting fluid: Glacial acetic acid, gentian violet and distilled water

Glacial acetic acid destroys the membrane of red blood cells.

Gentian violet stains the nuclei of WBCs.

Improved version of Neubauer chamber: This is a single, thick glass slide. At the centre H-shaped groove is present. H-shaped groove divide central part into two equal platforms. The central platform is 0.1 mm lower than the two pillars present laterally from the central platform. One cover slip is enough to cover

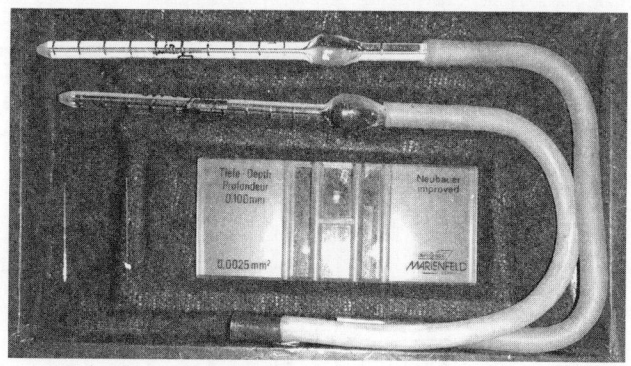

17.1: Hemocytometer

---

*TLC: Total leucocytic count; *DLC: Differential leucocytic count half of central platform and the depth under the cover is 0.1 mm (Fig. 17.2).

Two counting grids are engraved in central platform (one in each half). These counting grids are used for TLC and total RBC counts in blood. The area of each counting grid is a square measuring 3×3 mm^2. This area is divided into nine large squares, each having an area of 1 mm^2. The four large corner squares (1 mm^2 each) are used for total WBC count while the centre large square (1 mm^2) is used for total RBC count (Fig. 17.3).

Each large corner squares (WBC counting chambers) are further subdivided into 16 small squares, each measuring 1/16 mm^2. The central RBC counting chamber is divided into 25 medium sized squares each measuring 1/25 mm^2. Out of 25 medium sized squares only 5 medium sized squares are used for RBC counting. The four corner medium sized squares and the central medium sized squares are used.

Each medium sized square is further divided into 16 smallest squares. Total 400 smallest squares are present in the centre large square. The area of each smallest square is 1/400 mm^2. The red cells are counted in 80 smallest squares, i.e. 5 medium sized squares.

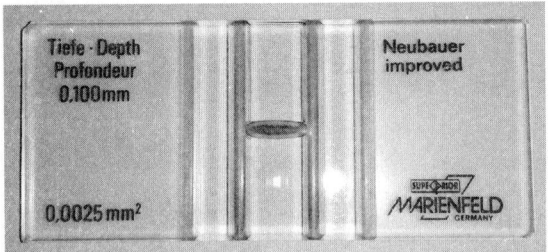

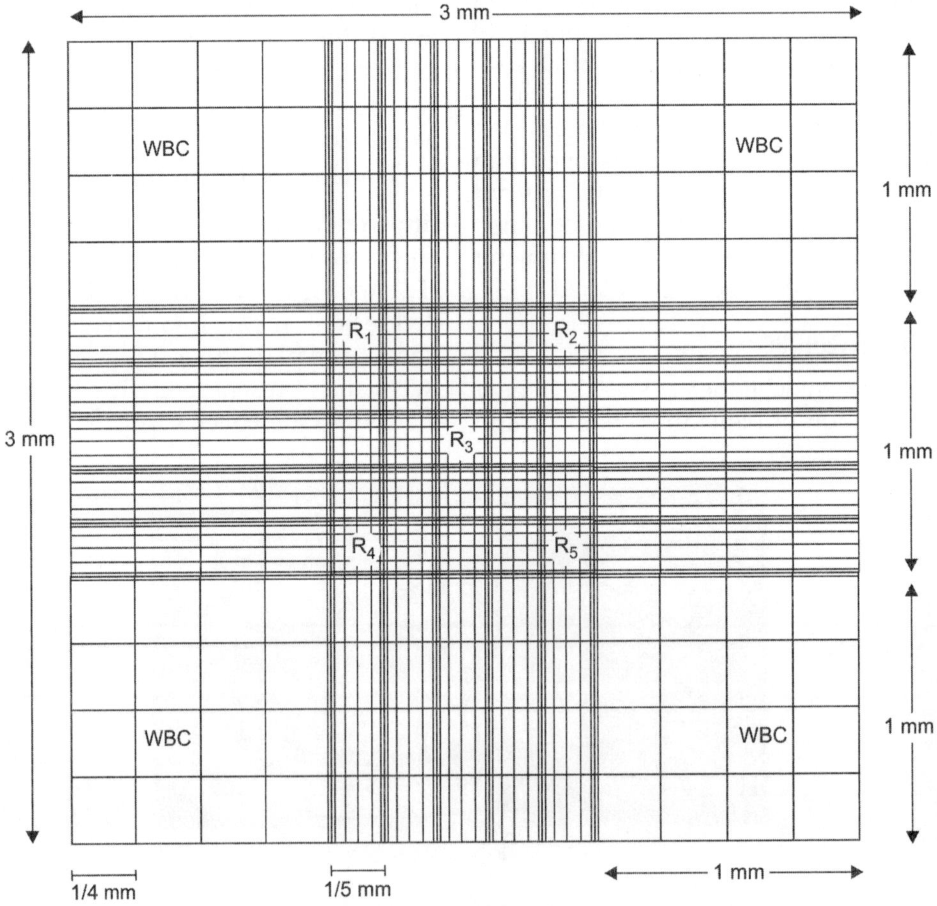

17.2: Improved version of Neubauer chamber

17.3: Counting grids

WBC pipette: Three markings are present in WBC pipette (Fig. 17.4). Two markings i.e. 0.5 and 1 are present in the stem part of pipette and third marking, i.e. 11 is present at neck region of pipette after the bulb.

Bulb size is smaller than RBC pipette.

One white bead is present inside the bulb for mixing of blood and WBC diluting fluid.

The mouth piece is white in colour.

RBC pipette: Three markings are present in RBC pipette. Two markings, i.e. 0.5 and 1 are present in the stem part of pipette and third marking, i.e. 101 is present at neck region of pipette after the bulb.

Bulb size is much larger than WBC pipette.

One red bead is present inside the bulb for mixing of blood and Hayme's fluid.

The mouthpiece is red in colour.

PROCEDURE

- Clean the improved Neubauer chamber, WBC pipette, cover slip and watch glass, thoroughly and then dry these completely.
- Take enough amount of Turk's fluid or WBC diluting fluid in watch glass.

Filling of the WBC Pipette

- Clean the tip of finger (never choose thumb and little finger for pricking) of non-dominant hand with cotton swab soaked in alcohol.
- Allow the finger to air dry completely.
- Squeeze that finger for few seconds just to accumulate blood at the tip of finger.

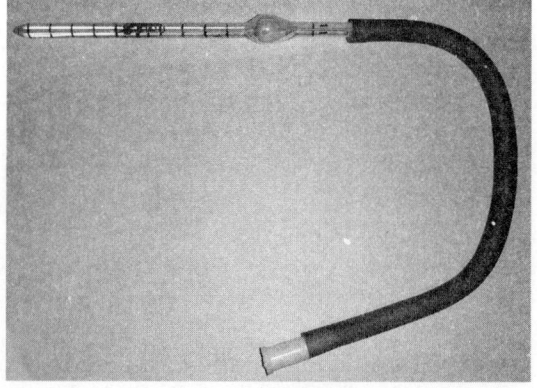

17.4: WBC pipette

- Prick the finger tip with a sterile lancet.
- Discard the first drop of blood with dry cotton swab.
- Make a large drop of blood on the finger tip.
- Dip the tip of the WBC pipette within the blood drop.
- Suck the blood exactly up to the 0.5 mark in the WBC pipette. No air bubble should be present in between the blood column.
- Wipe the outside part of the pipette tip.
- Suck Turk's fluid or WBC diluting fluid up to the '11' mark.
- Mix the blood and Turk's fluid by gently rotating the pipette after placing it horizontally in between the palms for at least 2 minutes.

Charging of the Improved Version of Neubauer Chamber

- Place a cover slip on the half part of central platform and the edge of the cover slip should be little bit outward from the end slit.
- Discard first 2–3 drops of content in a dry cotton because initially the stem part of WBC pipette only contains Turk's fluid not diluted blood.
- Hold the WBC pipette at 45° angle and allow to form a small drop of diluted blood at the tip of WBC pipette.
- Then touch the drop to the slit between counting chamber and cover slip and during the time of charging WBC pipette should be kept in 45° angle.
- The chamber is filled automatically by capillary action.
- When the diluted blood enter between the gap of counting chamber and cover slip then immediately WBC pipette should be removed.
- After charging the improved Neubauer chamber, allow it to stand for 3 to 4 minutes so that all the cells settle down otherwise one may get the faulty result (because of cell movement).

COUNTING OF LEUCOCYTES

- The Neubauer chamber placed in the stage of the microscope and focus under low power objective lens (Fig. 17.5).

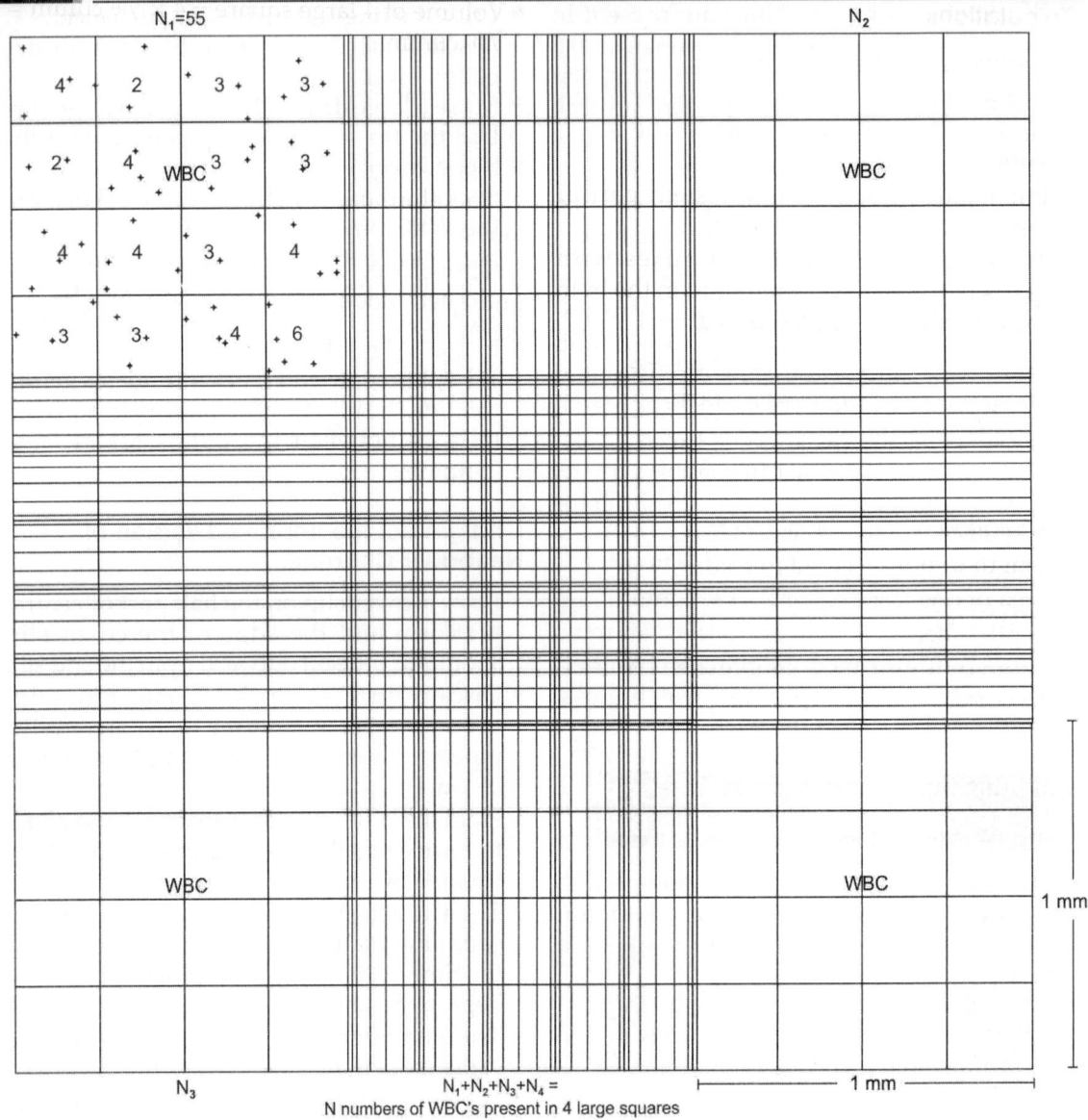

17.5: WBC counting chambers under low power objective lens

- Then recognise WBCs. They appear as round, dark blue dots and also try to differentiate foreign particles from WBCs (If air bubbles appears then clean the cover slip, improved Neubauer chamber and charge it again).
- Count in all four large corner squares (1 mm² each).
- Draw WBC squares in note book and enter the observation and calculate the final result.

Rules of Counting

- Never tilt the microscope during counting.
- WBCs which are present within the square are included in counting.
- If WBCs touching or laying on the upper horizontal line and left vertical line are included in that specific square then WBCs touching or laying on the lower horizontal line and right vertical line are omitted in that specific square.

Calculations

Calculation of Dilution Factor

Out of the 11 parts 0.5 parts is blood and 10.5 parts is WBCs diluting fluid in the WBC pipette.

But 1 part present in initial stem part of pipette is not mixed with blood.

Thus 0.5 part of the blood mixes with 9.5 parts of the WBC diluting fluid in the bulb to form 10 parts of diluted blood.

$$\text{Dilution factor} = \frac{\text{Final diluted blood volume achieved (10 parts)}}{\text{Original blood volume taken (0.5 parts)}} = 20$$

Calculation of Volume of Large Squares

- Length of one large square = 1 mm
- Area of one large square = 1×1 mm^2
- Depth when cover slip is placed = $1/10$ mm^2
- Volume of one large square $1 \times 1 \times 1/10 = 1/10$ cumm

- Volume of 4 large square = $4 \times 1/10$ cumm = $4/10$ cumm

Calculation of Total Leucocyte Count

WBCs present in $4/10$ mm^3 volume of diluted blood = N (say)

Therefore, cells in 1 mm^3 volume of diluted blood = N × $10/4$

Therefore, cells in 1 mm^3 volume of undiluted blood = N × $10/4$ × 20 = N × 50 = X (say)

So, Total Leucocyte Count is X/mm^3.

Normal Count of Total Leucocyte Count

Adults   : 4,000–11,000/mm^3 of the blood
Newborns : 10,000–25,000/mm^3 of the blood
Infants   : 6,000–18,000/mm^3 of the blood
Children   : 5,000–15,000/mm^3 of the blood

Note: TLC not differs with gender unlike RBC count.

PREPARATION OF PERIPHERAL BLOOD SMEAR AND PERFORMING DIFFERENTIAL LEUCOCYTE COUNT

PRINCIPLE

Apparatus Requirements

Glass slides, cotton swab dry, cotton swab soaked in alcohol, sterile lancet or pricking needle, Leishman's stain, distilled water or buffer solution, Pasteur pipette, compound microscope.

Leishmanís Stain

It is composed of methylene blue, eosin and methyl alcohol.

Methylene blue: It is basic dye and stains acidic parts of cells, e.g. nucleus of WBCs and cytoplasmic granules of basophils and cytoplasm of most of WBCs except eosinophil.

Eosin: It is an acidic dye and stains basic parts of cells, e.g. cytoplasm of RBCs and eosinophils and cytoplasmic granules of eosinophils.

Methyl alcohol: It helps in preservation and fixation of blood smear with slide.

PROCEDURE

Preparations of Peripheral Blood Smear

- Take two clean glass slides (Fi.g 17.6).
- Grease free glass slides by washing these with soap water and dry completely.
- Then select one slide as spreader. The narrow edge of spreader should be smooth.
- Clean the tip of finger (never choose thumb and little finger for pricking) of non dominant hand with cotton swab soaked in alcohol.
- Allow the finger to air dry completely.
- Squeeze that finger for few seconds just to accumulate blood at the tip of finger.
- Prick the finger tip with a sterile lancet.
- Discard the first drop of blood with dry cotton swab.
- Place a drop of blood on one end of a slide and it should be about 1 cm away from the narrow edge of one end (Fig. 17.6A).

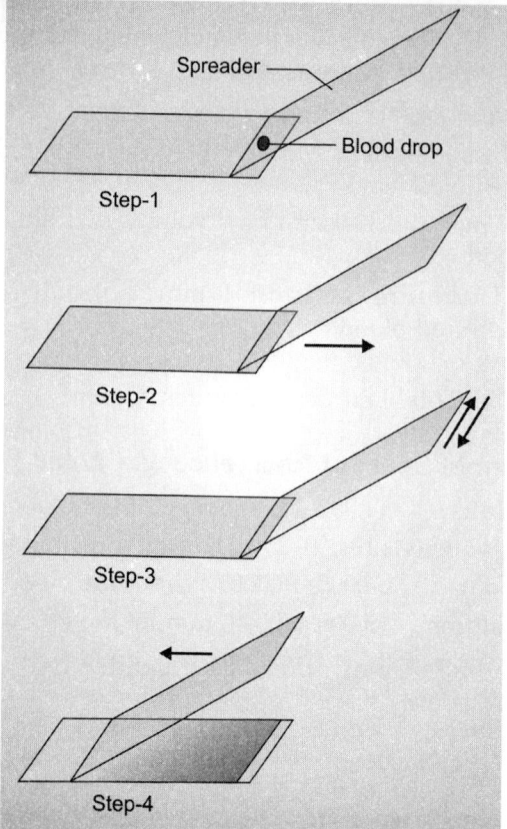

Step-1

Step-2

Step-3

Step-4

17.6: Steps of peripheral blood smear preparation *(For colour Fig. see Plate 5).*

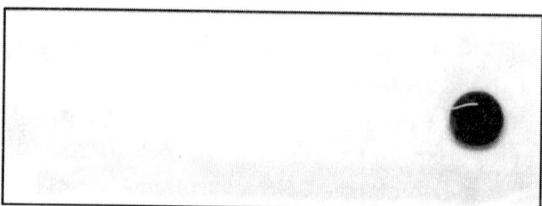

17.6A: Step 1

- The blood drop was placed by touching the blood drop to the slide.
- Keep the slide on working table and hold the slide firmly with the middle or index finger and thumb of the non dominant hand at the end part of the slide.
- Hold the spreader with dominant hand from its long edge by the help of middle or index finger and thumb.

- Place the spreader slide just in front of the blood drop at an approximate 45 degree angle (Fig. 17.6B).

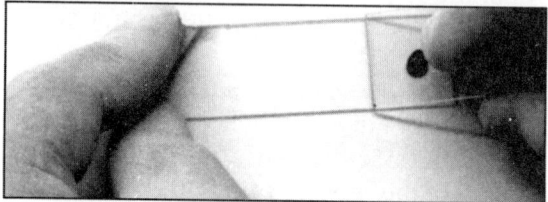

17.6B: Step 2

- Pull the spreader backward direction until it touches the blood drop and hold for few seconds at that place to spread the blood along the narrow edge of the spreader. The spreader can be slightly moved in side by side direction to accelerate the spreading of blood along the narrow edge (Fig. 17.6C).

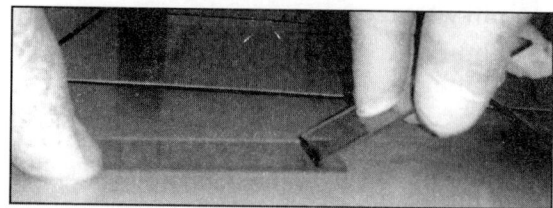

17.6C: Step 3

- Then pull the spreader to the forward direction (towards the other end of the slide) by maintaining approximate 45 degree angle till the end and pressure should be gentle and pulling should be uninterrupted and little bit quick (Fig. 17.6D).

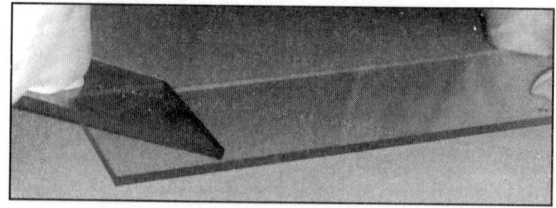

17.6D: Step 4

- Dry the peripheral blood smears completely (Fig. 17.7).

17.7: Step 5

Fixation and Staining of Peripheral Blood Smear

- Place the peripheral blood smear slide on the staining rack. The smear side should be facing upside.
- Pour few drops of Leishman's stain on the smear. The stain should be poured just to cover the smear and stain drops should be counted.
- Then wait for 2 minutes. The waiting time depends upon the stain concentration.
- Add distilled water or buffer solution with the help of Pasteur pipette on the smear. The number of drops of distilled water should be double as that of stain and if buffer solution is used then it should be same as that of stain. It should be taking care that the water or buffer solution does not spill out.
- Mix the stain and the water evenly by blowing air gently from mouth or by blowing air through a Pasteur pipette.
- Then wait for 10 minutes again that waiting time depends on stain concentration.
- Pour the stain and wash the slide gently under very slow speed tap water and place one finger at the upper part of the slide to prevent from direct flow of tap water on the smear and complete wash out.
- Dry it completely and then observe under microscope.

Examination of the Stained Blood Smear

Scanning the Whole Smear

- First scan the prepared stained blood smear under low power objective lens as quickly as possible.
- The extreme initial part (head part) and extreme end part (tail part) of the smear should not be included for counting. Because smear is very thick in the initial portion and blood cells are unevenly distributed in this part and there is clumping of RBCs. At the end part cells are also distributed unevenly and larger leucocytes, e.g. monocytes and eosinophils are high in number. So, both the places should be avoided for differential leucocyte count (DLC).
- The middle part should be always chosen for DLC as in this part smear is thin enough (one cell thickness) and blood cells are evenly distributed.

Selection of Site and Perform Differential Leucocyte Count

- Then switch the low power objective lens to oil immersion objective lens.
- Place one drop of cedar wood oil on the selected part of the smear.
- Make close contact the oil immersion objective lens with cedar wood oil.
- Use plane or concave mirror to get the light.
- Move the condenser at the upper most position.
- Iris diaphragm should be fully opened to get maximum intensity of illumination.
- After selection of the part, differential leucocytes count start from one end of the smear and proceed in a zigzag manner. No area should be repeated for counting.
- Place a drop of immersion oil on the slide (do not place on a cover slip) directly on the smear. Now switch to oil immersion objective lens. Move coarse adjusting screw, by seeing from the outside of microscope till the lens is immersed in the drop of cedar wood oil.
- Condenser should be at highest position and iris diaphragm should be opened completely.
- Then observe through eyepiece lens and focus the film by using fine adjustment screw.
- Identify different types of leucocytes by comparing with identifying character of leucocytes given in Table 17.1.
- Count at least 100 leucocytes by tally bar count or with help of manual cell counter.
- Determine the percentage of the various types of leucocytes. For counting the cells start from one end of the smear and proceed in a zigzag manner.

Table 17.1: Characteristics feature of erythrocytes and leucocytes

Types of cells	Cell size (μm)	Characteristics feature of nucleus	Characteristics feature of cytoplasm	Characteristics feature of cytoplasmic granules
RBC	7.2	• Mature RBC devoid of nucleus	• Pinkish in colour • Pale at the centre and peripheral part is little darker	Cytoplasmic granules absent
Neutrophil (Polymorph) (Fig. 17.8A)	10–14	• Deep violet or deep bluish in colour • Multi-lobed nucleus (2–6 lobes) and each lobes are connected by chromatin threads	Light bluish in colour *(For colour Fig. see Plate 5)*	• Fine cytoplasmic granules • Pink and blue both coloured granules are present (take both type of stain, almost 50% are eosinophilic and rest 50% are basophilic in nature) (Fig. 17.8B)
Eosinophil (Fig. 17.9A)	10–15	• Deep violet or deep bluish in colour • Bi-lobed nucleus (very few tri-lobed nucleus are visible) • It is headphone shaped	Light pinkish in colour *(For colour Fig. see Plate 5)*	• Coarse cytoplasmic granules • Pinkish in colour (eosinophilic in nature) (Fig. 17.9B)
Basophil (Fig. 17.10A)	10–14	• Deep violet or deep bluish in colour • "S" shaped • Nucleus not visible because of high concentration of cytoplasmic granules	Light bluish in colour *(For colour Fig. see Plate 5)*	• Coarse cytoplasmic granules • Blue in colour (basophilic in nature) • These cytoplasmic granules crowded all over the cell that's why nucleus not visible (Fig. 17.10B)
Small Lymphocyte (Fig. 17.11A)	7–10	• Deep violet or deep bluish in colour • Large and single • Almost cover the whole cell	• Light bluish in colour • Amount of cytoplasm is very scanty and hardly visible	Cytoplasmic granules are absent (Fig. 17.11B) *(For colour Fig. see Plate 5)*
Large Lymphocyte (Fig. 17.12A)	10–14	• Deep violet or deep bluish in colour • Large and single • Present at the centre • Almost circular or oval	• Light bluish in colour • Amount of cytoplasm is larger than small lymphocytes	Cytoplasmic granules are absent (Fig. 17.12B) *(For colour Fig. see Plate 5)*
Monocyte (Fig. 17.13A)	15–18	• Deep violet or deep bluish in colour • Large and single • Kidney or bean shaped • Eccentric or placed at the periphery	• Light bluish in colour • Abundant amount	Cytoplasmic granules are absent (Fig. 17.13B) 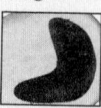 *(For colour Fig. see Plate 5)*

Normal Values of Different Leucocytes:

Neutrophils	:	50–70%
Eosinophils	:	1–4%

Basophils	:	0–1%
Lymphocytes	:	20–40%
Monocytes	:	3–8%

EXAMINATION OF BLOOD FILM FOR MALARIA PARASITE

Principle

The direct microscopic visualization of the parasite in the thick and thin blood smears has been the accepted method for the diagnosis of malaria.

Methods of Examination of Malaria Parasite from Blood Film

Two methods are used to examine of malaria parasite:
1. Thin smear
2. Thick smear

THIN SMEAR METHOD

Apparatus required: Glass slides, cotton swab dry, cotton swab soaked in alcohol, sterile lancet or pricking needle, methanol, Leishman's stain or Gimsa stain or Field's Stain, distilled water or buffer solution, Pasteur pipette, compound microscope.

Preparations of Thin Peripheral Blood Smear

- Take two grease free clean glass slides.
- Then select one slide as spreader. The narrow edge of spreader should be smooth.
- Clean the tip of finger (never choose thumb and little finger for pricking) of non-dominant hand with cotton swab soaked in alcohol.
- Allow the finger to air dry completely.
- Squeeze that finger for few seconds just to accumulate blood at the tip of finger.
- Prick the finger tip with a sterile lancet.
- Discard the first drop of blood with dry cotton swab.
- Place a drop of blood on one narrow edge end of a slide it should be about 1 cm away from the narrow edge of one end.
- Make thin blood smear with the help of a spreader at 45° angle (method similar to the

peripheral smear preparation which is described earlier).
- Dry the thin blood smears completely (Fig. 17.14).

Fixations of Thin Blood Smear

- After complete drying, the thin smear should be fixed in methanol.
- This can be done by either dipping the thin smear into methanol for 30 seconds or by touching lightly the thin smear with a methanol-soaked cotton ball.

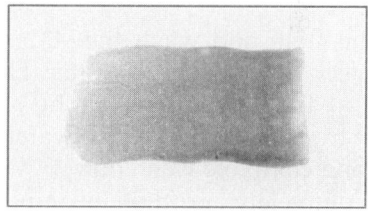

17.14: Thin peripheral blood smear

Staining of Thin Blood Smear

A number of Romanowsky stains like Field's, Giemsa's and Leishman's stain are suitable for staining the thin smears:
a. Staining with Giemsa stain
b. Staining with Leishman's stain
c. Staining with Field's stain.

a. Staining with Giemsa Stain

- Prepare a 10% Giemsa in buffered water of pH 7.2.
- Pour few drops of the prepared 10% Giemsa stain on the smear. The stain should be poured just to cover the smear.
- Wait for 30–45 minutes.
- Rinse the slide gently in tap water for a few seconds till the excess stain is removed.
- Drain the excess water.
- Then dry the smear completely and examine under microscope.

b. Staining with Leishman's Stain

- Pour few drops of Leishman's stain on the smear. The stain should be poured just to cover the smear and stain drops should be counted.
- Then wait for 1–2 minutes. The waiting time depends upon the stain concentration.
- Add distilled water or buffer solution with the help of Pasteur pipette on the smear. The number of drops of distilled water should be double as that of stain and if buffer solution is used then it should be same as that of stain. It should be taking care that the water or buffer solution does not spill out.
- Mix the stain and the water evenly by blowing air gently from mouth or by blowing air through a Pasteur pipette.
- Then wait for 8–10 minutes again that waiting time depends on stain concentration.
- Pour the stain and wash the slide gently under very slow speed tap water. Finger is placed at the upper part of the slide to prevent from direct flow of tap water on the smear and complete wash out.
- Dry it completely and then examine under microscope.

c. Staining with Field's Stain

- Prepare a dilute Field's B stain by diluting it in buffered water of pH 7.2 in 1:4 ratio (1 part Field's B stain and 4 part buffer water of pH 7.2).
- Pour few drops of the prepared dilute Field's B stain on the smear. The stain should be poured just to cover the smear.
- Add immediately equal amount of Field's A stain.
- Wait for one minute.
- Rinse the slide gently in tap water for a few seconds till the excess stain is removed.
- Drain the excess water.
- Then dry the smear completely and examine under microscope.

THICK SMEAR METHOD

Thick smear method is 30 times more sensitive than thin smear method.

Apparatus required: Glass slides, cotton swab dry, cotton swab soaked in alcohol, sterile lancet or pricking needle, Giemsa stain or Field stain, buffer solution of pH 7.2, Pasteur pipette, compound microscope.

Preparations of Thick Blood Smear

- Take two grease free clean glass slides.
- Then select one slide's corner as spreader.
- Clean the tip of finger (never choose thumb and little finger for pricking) of non-dominant hand with cotton swab soaked in alcohol.
- Allow the finger to air dry completely.
- Squeeze that finger for few seconds just to accumulate blood at the tip of finger.
- Prick the finger tip with a sterile lancet.
- Discard the first drop of blood.
- Place a large drop of blood at the centre of a slide.
- Spread the drop of blood in a circle. The diameter of the circle should be around 1–2 cm and not more than that. Thickness of the smear should allow newsprint to be just visible through it.
- Wait until the thick film is completely dry before staining (Fig. 17.15).

17.15: Thick blood smear

Staining of Thick Blood Smear

There are three methods by which thick smear can be stained:

a. Rapid staining with Giemsa stain
b. Rapid staining with Field's stain
c. Standard staining with Giemsa stain

a. Rapid Staining with Giemsa Stain

- Do not fixed with methanol.
- First prepare a 10% Giemsa in buffered water of pH 7.2.
- Dip the slide in the prepared 10% Giemsa stain for 5 minutes.

- Rinse gently for 1 or 2 seconds in a jar of tap water.
- Drain the excess water.
- Then dry the smear completely and examine under microscope.

b. Rapid Staining with Field's Stain

Field's stain has two components. Field's A is a buffered solution of azure dye and Field's B is a buffered solution of eosin.

- Do not fixed with methanol.
- Dip the slide in into coplin jar containing Field's A stain for 3 seconds.
- Then remove it from coplin jar containing Field's A stain.
- Dip the slide in into coplin jar containing Field's B stain for another 3 seconds.
- Then remove it from coplin jar containing Field's B stain.

- Rinse the slide gently in tap water for a few seconds till the excess stain is removed.
- Drain the excess water.
- Then dry the smear completely and examine under microscope.

c. Standard Staining with Giemsa Stain

- Do not fixed with methanol.
- First prepare a 4% Giemsa in buffered water of pH 7.2.
- Dip the slide (after drying for several hours) in the prepared 4% Giemsa stain.
- Wait for 30–45 minutes.
- Rinse the slide gently in tap water for a few seconds till the excess stain is removed.
- Drain the excess water.
- Then dry the smear completely and examine under microscope.

Determination of RBC*, BT&CT*, ESR* and Haemoglobin

PRINCIPLE

Blood is diluted 200 times with Hayem's fluid or RBC diluting fluid. After charging this mixture into counting chamber of improved version of Neubauer chamber, counting is done under high power objective lens of microscope. With the knowledge of the volume of the fluid examined and dilution of the blood obtained the number of erythrocytes per cubic millimeter of undiluted blood is calculated.

APPARATUS REQUIRED

Microscope, haemocytometer (only improved version of Neubauer chamber and RBC pipette), watch glass, cover slip, RBC diluting fluid (Hayem's fluid), cotton swab dry, cotton swab soaked in alcohol, sterile lancet or pricking needle.

Composition of Hayem's fluid or RBC diluting fluid: Sodium sulphate 2.5 gm, sodium chloride 0.5 gm, mercuric chloride 0.25 gm (corrosive sublimate), distilled water to make up to 100 ml.

Improved version of Neubauer chamber: This is a single, thick glass slide. At the centre H-shaped groove is present. H-shaped groove divide central part into two equal platforms. The central platform is 0.1 mm lower than the

two pillars present laterally from the central platform. One cover slip is enough to cover half of central platform and the depth under the cover is 0.1 mm.

Two counting grids are engraved in central platform (one in each half). These counting grids are used for TLC and total RBC counts in blood. The area of each counting grid is a square measuring 3×3 mm^2. This area is divided into nine large squares, each having an area of 1 mm^2. The four large corner squares (1 mm^2 each) are used for WBC count while the centre large square (1 mm^2) is used for RBC count.

The central RBC counting chamber is divided into 25 medium sized squares each measuring 1/25 mm^2. Out of 25 medium sized squares only 5 medium sized squares are used for RBC counting. The four corner medium sized squares and the central medium sized squares are used (Fig. 18.1).

Each medium sized square is further divided into 16 smallest squares. Each central large square has 400 smallest squares. The area of each smallest square is 1/400 mm^2. The red cells are counted in 80 smallest squares, i.e. 5 medium sized squares.

RBC pipette: Three markings are present in RBC pipette (Fig. 18.2). Two, i.e. 0.5 and 1 are present in the stem part of pipette and third

---

*RBC: Red blood cell, BT&CT: Bleeding time and clotting time, ESR: Erythrocyte sedimentation rate

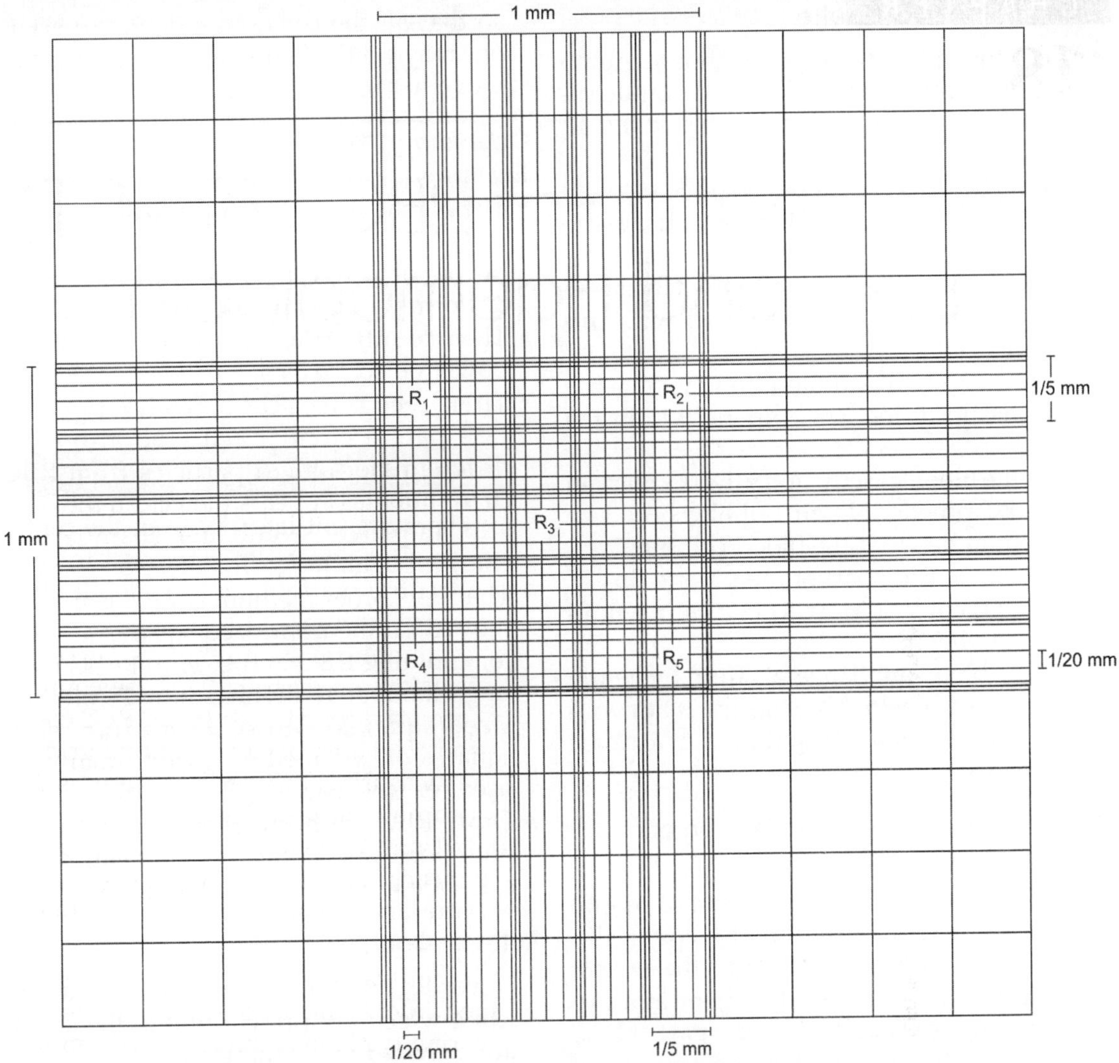

Fig. 18.1: RBC counting chambers in improved version of Neubauer chamber

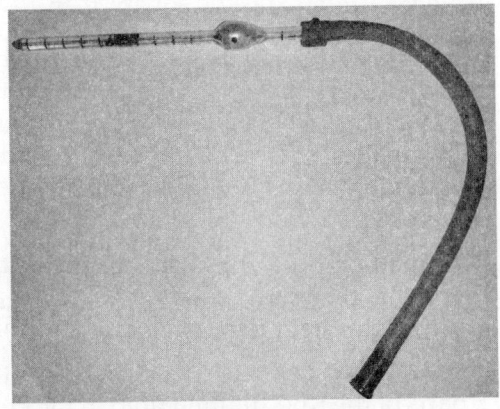

Fig. 18.2: RBC pipette

marking, i.e. 101 is present at neck region of pipette after the bulb.

Bulb size is much larger than WBC pipette One red bead is present inside the bulb for mixing of blood and Hayem's fluid.

The mouth piece is red in colour.

PROCEDURE

- Clean the improved Neubauer chamber, RBC pipette, cover slip and watch glass, thoroughly and then dry these completely.
- Take enough amount of Hayem's fluid or RBC diluting fluid in watch glass.

Filling of the RBC Pipette

- Clean the tip of finger (never choose thumb and little finger for pricking) of non-dominant hand with cotton swab soaked in alcohol.
- Allow the finger to air dry completely.
- Squeeze that finger for few seconds just to accumulate blood at the tip of finger.
- Prick the finger tip with a sterile lancet.
- Discard the first drop of blood with dry cotton swab.
- Make a large drop of blood on the finger.
- Dip the tip of the RBC pipette within the blood drop.
- Suck the blood exactly up to the 0.5 mark in the RBC pipette. No air bubble should be present in between the blood column.
- Wipe the outside part of the pipette tip.
- Suck Hayem's fluid or RBC diluting fluid up to the 101 mark.
- Mix the blood and Hayem's fluid by gently rotating the pipette after placing it horizontally in between the palms for at least 2 minutes.

Charging of the Improved Version of Neubauer Chamber

- Place a cover slip on the half part of central platform and the edge of the cover slip should be little bit outward from the end slit
- Discard first 2–3 drops of content in a dry cotton because initially the stem part of RBC pipette only contains Hayem's fluid not diluted blood.
- Hold the RBC pipette at 45° angle and allow to form a small drop of diluted blood at the tip of RBC pipette.
- Then touch the drop to the slit between counting chamber and cover slip and during the time of charging RBC pipette should be kept in 45° angle.
- The chamber is filled automatically by capillary action.
- When the diluted blood enter between the gap of counting chamber and cover slip then immediately RBC pipette should be removed.
- After charging the improved Neubauer chamber, allow it to stand for 3 to 4 minutes

so that all the cells settle down otherwise one may get the faulty result (because of cell movement).

Counting of RBC
Examine

- The Neubauer chamber placed in the stage of the microscope and focus under low power objective lens to confirm whether uniformly RBCs are distributed or not.
- Then counting of RBCs done under high power objective lens.
- Then recognise RBCs. They appear as transparent circular cell and also try to differentiate foreign particles from RBCs (If air bubbles appears then clean the cover slip, improved Neubauer chamber and charge it again).
- The four corner medium sized squares and the central medium sized squares are used for counting RBCs. (The central RBC counting chamber is divided into 25 medium sized squares. Out of 25 medium sized squares only 5 medium sized squares are used for RBC counting.)
- Draw RBC counting chamber squares in note book and enter the observation and calculate the final result (Fig. 18.3).

Rules of Counting

- Never tilt the microscope during counting.
- RBCs which are present within the square are included in counting.
- If RBCs touching or laying on the upper horizontal line and left vertical line are included in that specific square then RBCs touching or laying on the lower horizontal line and right vertical line are omitted in that specific square.

CALCULATIONS
Calculation of Dilution Factor

Out of the 101 parts 0.5 parts is blood and 100.5 parts is RBCs diluting fluid in the RBC pipette.

But 1 part present in initial stem of pipette is not mixed with blood.

Thus 0.5 part of the blood mixes with 99.5 parts of the RBC diluting fluid in the bulb to form 100 parts of diluted blood.

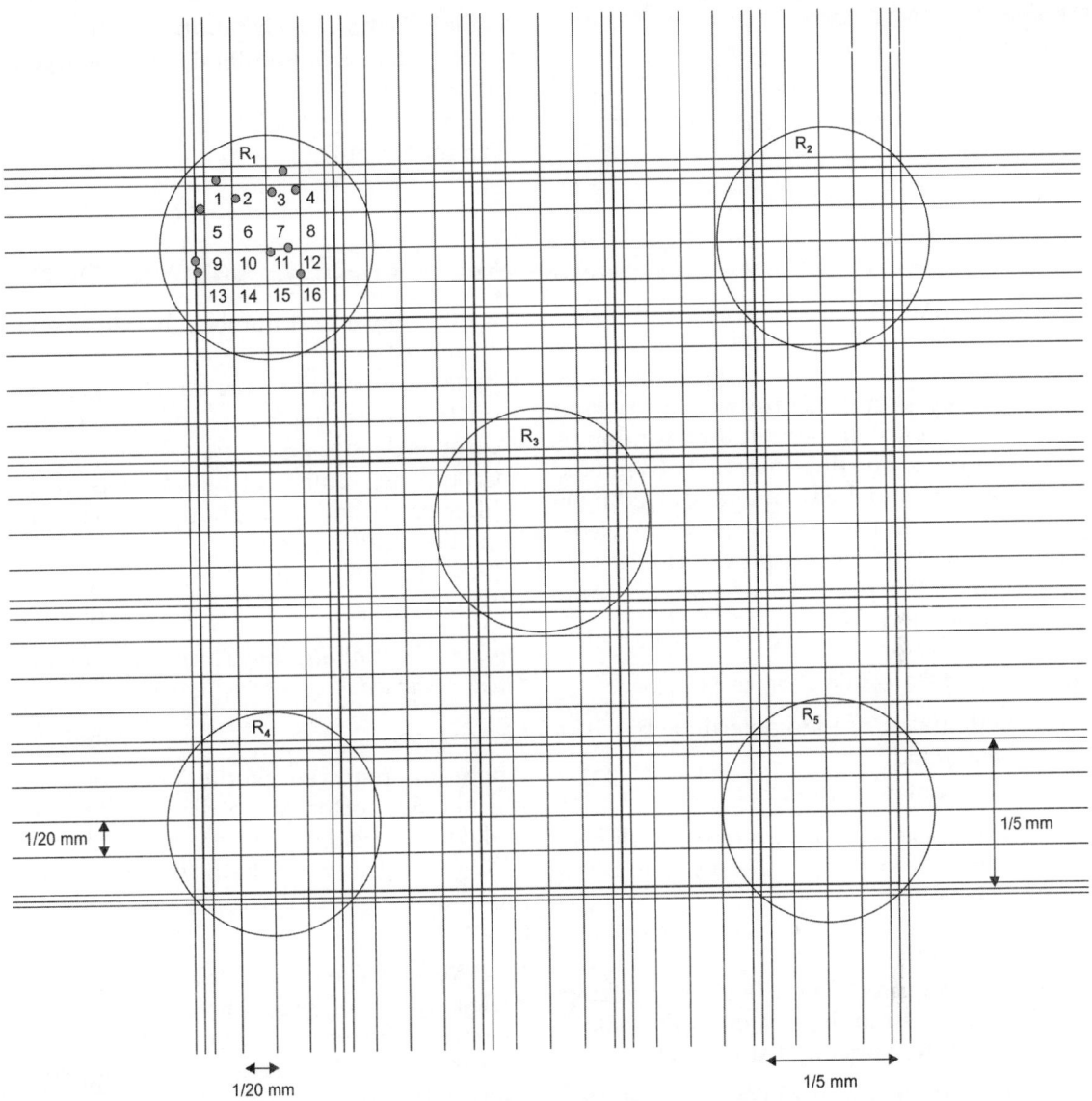

Fig. 18.3: RBC counting chambers under high power objective lens

Dilution factor = $\dfrac{\text{Final diluted blood volume}}{\text{Original blood volume}} = 200$
$\phantom{\text{Dilution factor}} \dfrac{\text{achieved (100 parts)}}{\text{taken (0.5 parts)}}$

- Volume of one medium square $\frac{1}{5} \times \frac{1}{5} \times \frac{1}{10}$
  = $\frac{1}{250}$ mm^3
- Volume of 5 medium square = $5 \times \frac{1}{250}$ mm^3
  = $\frac{1}{50}$ cumm.

Calculation of Volume of Large Squares

- Length of one medium square = $\frac{1}{5}$ mm
- Area of one medium square = $\frac{1}{5} \times \frac{1}{5}$ mm = $\frac{1}{25}$ mm^2
- Depth when cover slip is placed = $\frac{1}{10}$ mm^2

Calculation of Total Erythrocyte Count

- RBCs present in $\frac{1}{50}$ mm^3 volume of diluted blood = N (say)
- Therefore, RBCs present in 1 mm^3 volume of diluted blood = N × 50

- Therefore, RBCs present in 1 mm^3 volume of undiluted blood $= N \times 50 \times 200$
$$= N \times 10000 = X \text{ (say)}$$
So, total erythrocyte count is X/mm^3

Normal Total Erythrocyte Count

- Adult males: 5–6 million/µl (average 5.5 million/µl).
- Adult females: 4.5–5.5 million/µl (average 5.5 million/µl).

DETERMINATION OF BLEEDING TIME AND CLOTTING TIME

BLEEDING TIME (BT)

Principle

After a deep skin puncture with a pricking needle, bleeding will continue for few minutes and then stops. The time interval between the skin puncture and the stoppage of bleeding is bleeding time. The BT depends on vaso-constriction and platelet plug formation. It determines the function of platelets and integrity of the capillaries.

Methods of Determination of BT

Two methods are used to determine BT:
1. Duke method
2. Copley-Lalitch method

Duke method is usually preferred in clinical laboratories even though the Ivy method is more reliable one.

Duke's Method

Apparatus required: Sterile lancet or pricking needle, cotton swab dry, cotton swab soaked in alcohol, filter paper and stopwatch.

Procedure of Duke's method
- Clean the tip of finger (never choose thumb and little finger for pricking) of non-dominant hand with cotton swab soaked in alcohol.
- Allow the finger to air dry completely.
- Squeeze that finger for few seconds just to accumulate blood at the tip of finger.
- Prick the finger tip with a sterile lancet and puncture should be deep enough (at least 3 mm deep).
- Immediately start stopwatch.
- Remove the drops of blood after every 15 seconds by touching the skin gently with

a filter paper and number the blood spots 1 onwards.
- Note the time when there is no trace of blood on the filter paper, i.e. when bleeding completely stopped.
- Count the number of blood spots on the filter paper and multiply by 15 seconds to get the bleeding time.
- Enter the observation in note book (Fig. 18.4A).

Normal Value of Bleeding Time: 1–5 minutes in Duke's Method.

Ivy Method

Apparatus required: Sterile lancet or pricking needle, cotton swab dry, cotton swab soaked in alcohol, beaker containing water at 37°C (placed in water bath to maintain this particular temperature), water bath and stopwatch.

Procedure of Copley-Lalitch method
- Clean the tip of finger (never choose thumb and little finger for pricking) of non-dominant hand with cotton swab soaked in alcohol.
- Allow the finger to air dry completely.
- Squeeze that finger for few seconds just to accumulate blood at the tip of finger.
- Prick the fingertip with a sterile lancet and puncture should be deep enough (at least 3 mm deep).
- Immediately start stopwatch.
- Dip the pricked finger in a beaker containing water at 37°C and placed in water bath to maintain the temperature at this particular point.
- The blood flows to the bottom of the beaker in a continuous slow stream.

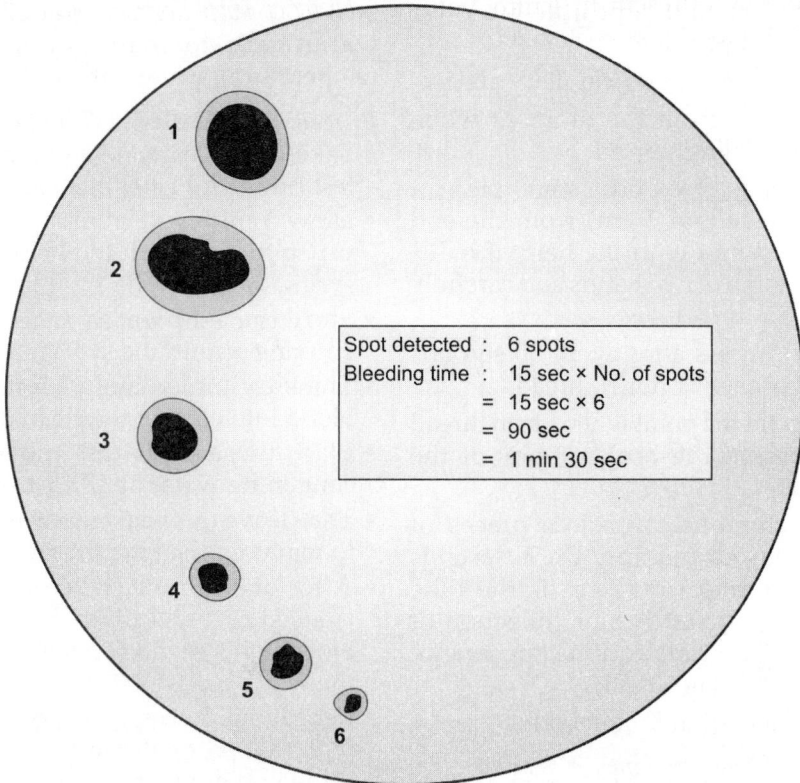

Spot detected : 6 spots
Bleeding time : 15 sec × No. of spots
                = 15 sec × 6
                = 90 sec
                = 1 min 30 sec

Fig. 18.4A: Determination of bleeding time *(For colour Fig. see Plate 6)*

- Note the time when the bleeding stops spontaneously.
- The time interval between the skin puncture and the stoppage of bleeding is bleeding time.
- Enter the observation in note book.

Normal Value of Bleeding Time: 2–6 minutes in Ivy's method.

CLOTTING TIME (CT)

Principle

If blood is kept in a glass capillary or a test tube then blood coagulates into a jelly-like mass. The time interval between the collection of blood within the capillary tube and clot formation is clotting time. The CT depends on coagulation mechanism.

Methods of Determination of CT

Two methods are used to determine CT:
1. Capillary tube method
2. Lee-White method.

The capillary tube method is most commonly used in determination of CT.

Wright's Capillary Tube Method

Apparatus required: Sterile lancet or pricking needle, cotton swab dry, cotton swab soaked in alcohol, capillary tube and stopwatch.

Procedure of Wright's capillary tube method
- Clean the tip of finger (never choose thumb and little finger for pricking) of non-dominant hand with cotton swab soaked in alcohol.
- Allow the finger to air dry completely.
- Squeeze that finger for few seconds just to accumulate blood at the tip of finger.
- Prick the finger tip with a sterile lancet.
- Discard the first drop of blood.
- Make a large drop of blood on the finger.
- Dip one end of a clean and dry capillary tube within the blood drop and other end of

capillary tube should kept little bit lower from horizontal position.

- Blood will fill the tube by capillary action.
- Start stopwatch from the moment when capillary tube filling started.
- After 30 seconds break off a small piece of capillary tube (about 1 cm) from the end which is filled first with the help of index finger and thumb of two hands and carefully look for fibrin thread.
- Repeat this process after every 30 seconds till the appearance of fibrin thread.
- Note the time of the point when fibrin thread is seen between the broken ends of the capillary tube.
- Count the number of broken pieces of capillary tube and multiply by 30 seconds to get the clotting time (this is the time interval between starting of collection of blood in capillary tube and the appearance of fibrin thread) (Fig. 18.4B).
- Enter the observation in notebook.

Normal Value of Clotting Time: 3–9 minutes by Wright's capillary tube method.

Lee and White Test Tube Method

Apparatus required: Sterile 5 ml syringe with needle, cotton swab dry, cotton swab soaked in alcohol, three clean and dry small test tubes,

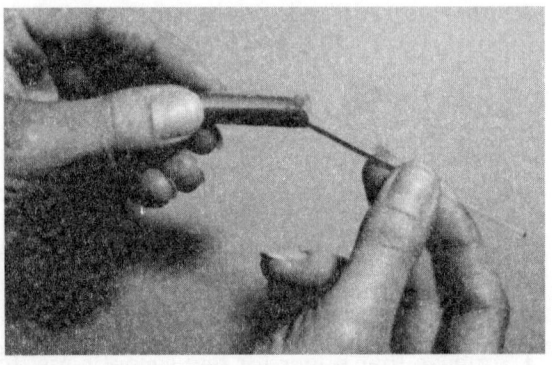

Fig. 18.4B: Determination of clotting time *(For colour Fig. see Plate 6)*

beaker containing water at 37°C (placed in water bath to maintain this particular temperature), water bath and stopwatch.

Procedure of Lee and White test tube method

- Take three clean and completely dry small test tubes and label them as 1, 2 and 3.
- Draw 5 ml blood from anticubital vein by venepuncture with the help of 5 ml sterile syringe with needle.
- Start the stopwatch when blood stars entering within the syringe.
- Transfer immediately 1.5 ml of collected blood into each of the clean dry test tubes.
- Place these three test tubes in a beaker containing water at 37°C.
- Then leave this beaker in water bath at 37°C to maintain the temperature of the beaker.
- After one minute, take out the test tube labelled as 1 and tilt that at 45° of angle. If blood spills then keep the test tube back in the water bath.
- Repeat the process in every 30 seconds gap with that particular test tube (labelled as 1) till the point when tilting of the test tube is possible without spilling of blood.
- Note the time gap and this is the clotting time for first (1) test tube.
- Then take the test tube labelled as 2 and tilt it as before till the blood clots.
- Note the time gap and this is the clotting time for second (2) test tube.
- Then same method should be followed with the third test tube, i.e. labelled as 3.
- Note the time gap and this is the clotting time for third (3) test tubes.
- Clotting time of third test tube should be considered as the final result. Because coagulation process is accelerated by repeated tilting and the third test tube tilted lesser time.
- Enter the observation in notebook.

Normal Value of Clotting Time: 5–10 minutes by Lee and White test tube method.

DETERMINATION OF ESR

PRINCIPLE

When mixture of blood and anticoagulant is allowed to stand in a very slender tube then the erythrocytes gradually settled down at the bottom part of the tube and at the upper part clear straw colored plasma appears. The "Rouleaux" formation, i.e. stacking of RBC on one another is the reason of sedimentation of erythrocytes in anti-coagulated blood kept in undisturbed condition. After "Rouleaux" formation density of stacked erythrocytes are increased and promotes sedimentation. The rate at which erythrocytes are sedimented or settled down is known as erythrocyte sedimentation rate (ESR). ESR depends upon the rate at which "Rouleaux" formation is occurring.

The ESR, expressed as mm/hr.

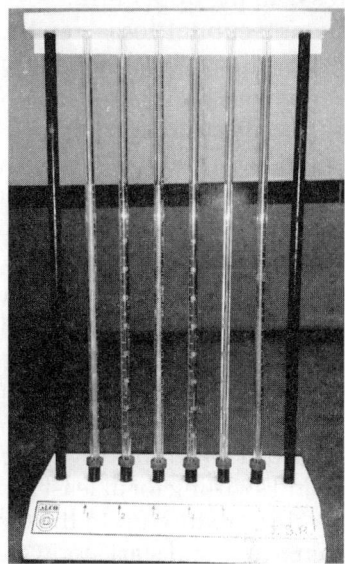

Fig. 18.5: Westergren tubes and stand *(For colour Fig. see Plate 6)*

METHODS OF DETERMINATION OF ESR

Two methods are used to determine ESR:
1. Westergren's method
2. Wintrobe's method.

Westergren's Method

The Westergren's method is more sensitive than Wintrobe's method because the Westergren's tube is much longer than Wintrobe's tube.

Apparatus Required

Syringe (5 ml) with needle, Westergren's pipette and stand (Fig. 18.5), pasteur pipette, i.e. dropper with long nose pointed tip, anticoagulant-sodium citrate (3.8 gm%), tourniquet, cotton swab dry, cotton swab soaked in alcohol.

Westergren's Pipette

It is a 30 cm long graduated tube and opened at both side.

The inner width of the tube is 2.5 mm.

Graduation is present in lower 2/3rds part of the tube.

0 to 200 markings are there (Fig. 18.6).

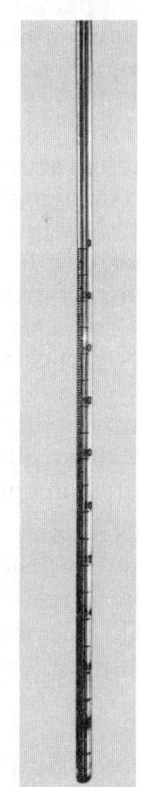

Fig. 18.6: Westergren pipette marking *(For colour Fig. see Plate 7)*

Procedure
- Wrap the tourniquet 2 inch above the antecubital fossa in the upper arm.
- Clean the antecubital fossa region (particularly the median cubital vein region) with alcohol soaked swab.
- Then dry that place completely.
- Locate the median cubital vein.
- Insert the needle of the syringe in median cubital vein (preferably) swiftly at an angel of 20 to 30°.
- Collect 5 ml of blood by venipuncture.
- Mix the 4 ml blood of the syringe with 1 ml 3.8% sodium citrate (anticoagulant) in a container. The blood and anticoagulant ratio should be 4:1.
- Mixing should be done thoroughly by inversion and swirling for at least 2 minutes.
- Then suck this mixture up to the 0 mark of Westergren's tube and start stopwatch from the moment when Westergren's tube filling started.
- Block tightly the upper open end with the help of thumb immediately to prevent the leaking of blood mixture from the bottom open end.
- Place the lower end of Westergren's tube in the rubber pad present at the bottom section of the Westergren stand and fix it vertically. The upper end of Westergren's tube should be fixed by the metal clip or screw provided on the upper section of that stand.
- Allow the tube to stand for hour and gradually at the upper part clear straw colored plasma appears.
- Note the level up to which the red cell column has fallen down after 1 hour.
- Enter the observation in note book.

Normal value of ESR by Westergren's method:
In male normal value of ESR is 3–10 mm at the end of one hour.

In female normal value of ESR is 5–12 mm at the end of one hour.

Wintrobe's Method

In Wintrobe's method two experiments can be done simultaneously from the same sample, i.e. ESR and Haematocrit Value.

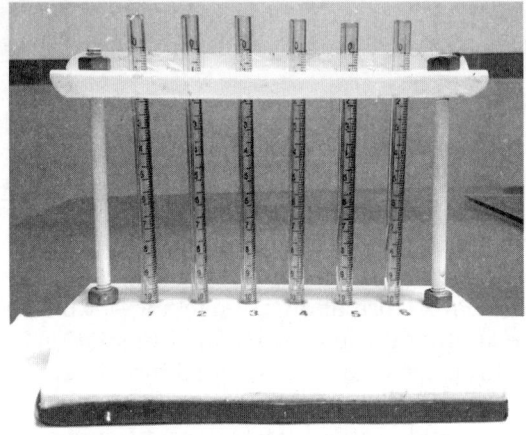

Fig. 18.7: Wintrobe tubes and stand

Apparatus Required
Syringe (5 ml) with needle, Wintrobe's tube and stand (Fig. 18.7), pasteur pipette, i.e. dropper with long nose pointed tip, anticoagulant-double oxalate (ammonium oxalate + potassium oxalate: 6 mg + 4 mg), tourniquet, cotton swab dry, cotton swab soaked in alcohol.

Wintrobe's Pipette
It is a short 11 cm graduated tube and opened only at one side.

The inner width of the tube is 2.5 mm.

Two similar types of graduations are present but direction is different.

In one type of graduation 0 to 10 marking in upside down direction and in another type 0 to 10 marking in downside up direction (Fig. 18.8).

Each small marking denotes 0.1 mm.

Procedure
- Wrap the tourniquet 2 inch above the antecubital fossa in the upper arm.
- Clean the antecubital fossa region (particularly the median cubital vein region) with alcohol soaked swab.
- Then dry that place completely.
- Locate the median cubital vein.
- Insert the needle of the syringe in median cubital vein (preferably) swiftly at an angel of 20 to 30°.
- Collect 5 ml of blood by venipuncture.

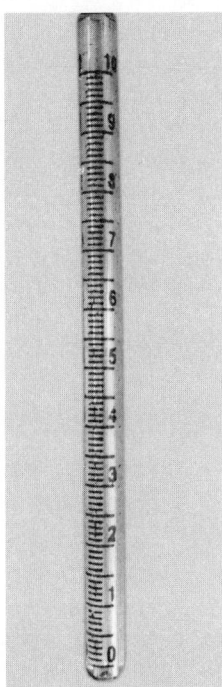

Fig. 18.8: Wintrobe tube marking 10 to 0 *(For colour Fig. see Plate 7)*

• Mix the 2 ml blood of the syringe with double oxalate anticoagulant (ammonium oxalate + potassium oxalate: 6 mg + 4 mg) in a container.

• Mixing should be done thoroughly by inversion and swirling for at least 2 minutes.

• With a long-necked pasteur pipette or transfer pipette fill the Wintrobe's tube with this mixture up to the 0 mark of Wintrobe's tube (Out of two graduation scale, the scale where 0 is the uppermost mark and 10 is the lowermost mark is chosen).

• Start stopwatch from the moment when Wintrobe's tube filling started.

• Place the Wintrobe's tube vertically in the Wintrobe's stand.

• Allow the tube to stand for hour and gradually at the upper part clear straw coloured plasma appears.

• Note the level up to which the red cell column has fallen down after 1 hour.

• Enter the observation in notebook.

Normal value of ESR by Westergren's method

• In male normal value of ESR is 2–8 mm at the end of one hour.

• In female normal value of ESR is 4–10 mm at the end of one hour.

ESTIMATION OF HAEMOGLOBIN CONCENTRATION IN BLOOD BY SAHLI'S METHOD

PRINCIPLE

N/10 HCl breaks the membrane of erythrocytes. Then haemoglobin present within the erythrocytes converted into acid haematin by reaction with N/10 HCl. The acid haematin is brown in colour. It is necessary to allow stand for 10 minutes before dilution, so that all the haemoglobin present in 20 µl blood is converted into acid haematin. This solution is further diluted until its colour is matched visually with the standard coloured glass rods of Sahli's comparator. The haemoglobin concentration is measured directly from the Sahli's graduated tube.

Apparatus Required

Sahli's haemoglobinometer or haemometer, N/10 HCl, distilled water, cotton swab dry, cotton swab soaked in alcohol, sterile lancet or pricking needle.

Sahli's haemoglobinometer or haemometer: It contains a Sahli's comparator, graduated tube, haemoglobin pipette, stirrer and dropper (Fig. 18.9).

Comparator: It has three columns of slots. Two lateral columns are covered and fitted with non-fading brown-tinted glass rods standardised against acid haematin. At the middle portion of three columns there is a vacant slot which accommodates the Sahli's graduated tube. At the back side of this comparator an opaque white glass is attached (Fig. 18.10).

Graduated tube: Two types of marking or graduations are there. At one side gram

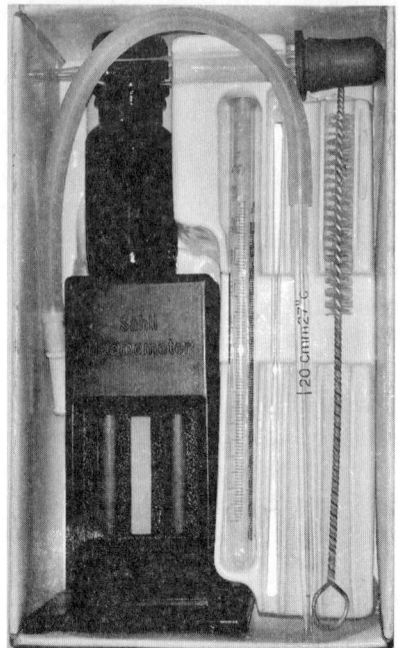

Fig. 18.9: Sahli's haemometer

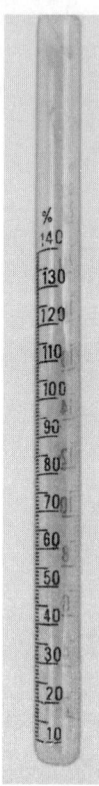

Fig. 18.11: Sahli's graduated tube percentage marking *(For colour Fig. see Plate 7)*

and in % scale denotes 1%. Out of the two scales gram% is always preferred over % scale (Fig. 18.11).

Haemoglobin pipette: This pipette has only one marking of 20 µl (20 cu mm) and no bulb is present in this pipette (Fig. 18.12).

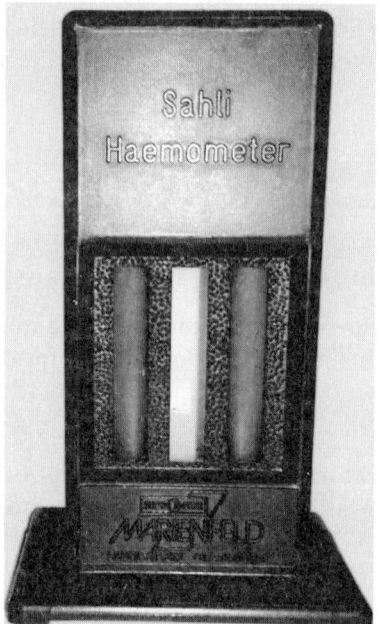

Fig. 18.10: Sahli's comparator

percent (gm%) markings (2 to 22 gm%) are present, and on the other side percentage (%) markings (10 to 140%) are present. Each small marking in gram% scale denotes 0.2 gram%

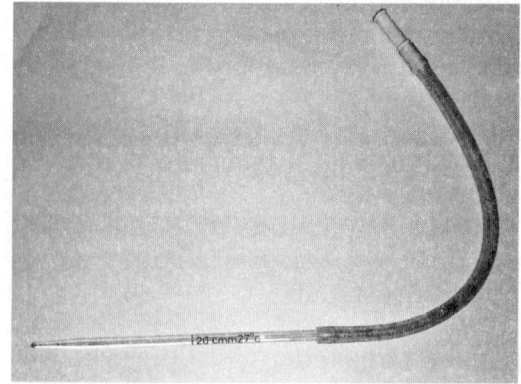

Fig. 18.12: Haemoglobin pipette *(For colour Fig. see Plate 7)*

Stirrer: It is a thin glass rod for mixing the solution during dilution with distilled water.

Procedure

- Sahli's graduated tube and haemoglobin pipette should be completely dry before starting the work.
- Take N/10 HCl up to 2 gram% mark or 20% mark with help of a dropper.
- Clean the tip of finger (never choose thumb and little finger for pricking) of non-dominant hand with cotton swab soaked in alcohol.
- Allow the finger to air dry completely.
- Squeeze that finger for few seconds just to accumulate blood at the tip of finger.
- Prick the finger tip with a sterile lancet.
- Discard the first drop of blood with dry cotton swab.
- Make a large drop of blood on the finger.
- Dip the tip of the pipette within the blood drop.
- Suck the blood exactly up to the mark of 20 cumm or 20 µl in the haemoglobin pipette. No air bubble should be present in between the blood column of haemoglobin pipette.
- Wipe the outside part of the pipette tip.
- Then gently blow the blood of haemoglobin pipette into the graduated tube containing N/10 HCl.
- Rinse the pipette with the N/10 HCl of the graduated tube at least for two times and take out the pipette from graduated tube.
- Rotate the graduated tube for few seconds keeping it in between the palms to mix the blood properly with N/10 HCl.
- Allow the graduated tube to stand for about 10 minutes so that all haemoglobin present

in 20 µl blood is converted into acid haematin.

- After 10 minutes dilute the acid haematin solution by adding distilled water drop by drop with help of a dropper.
- Mix it with the help of stirrer and match the colour of the solution in the tube with the standards brown-tinted glass rods of the comparator.
- Add distilled water till the colour is not matched with standards brown-tinted glass rods of the comparator and the stirrer should be kept above the solution while matching the colour with comparator. Do not take it out from the graduated tube until the final reading is taken.
- When colour matched, remove the stirrer from graduated tube.
- Hold the graduated tube at your eye level and the graduated tube should be hold in such a way that the graduation on it do not face directly in front side and interfere in the matching of colour.
- Note the reading by looking at the gram% marking where lower meniscus of this transparent colour solution touched the graduated tube (If % scale is taken then 14.8 gm/dl should be consider as 100% irrespective of gender and % value should be taken in similar way).

Normal Haemoglobin Concentration

In gram% scale:

Adult males   :   14–18 gm/dl
                   (average 15.5 gm/dl)
Adult females :   12.5–15.5 gm/dl
                   (average 13.5 gm/dl)

In % scale:

14.8 gm/dl considered as 100% irrespective of gender.

Recording of Body Temperature, Pulse/Heart Rate, BP and ECG

RECORDING OF BODY TEMPERATURE

INTRODUCTION

Body temperature represents the balance between heat production and heat loss. If the rate of heat generated equates to the rate of heat lost, the core body temperature will be at stable condition. All metabolising body cells manufacture heat in varying amounts. Therefore, body temperature is not evenly distributed across all the body.

Body temperature is one of the four main vital signs that must be monitored to ensure safe and effective care.

Location of Body for Temperature Measurement

a. Oral
b. Axilla (armpit)
c. Rectal
d. Ear canal
e. Forehead

Oral Temperature Measurement

Oral temperature measurement is the most common method to measure body temperature in adult subject. If subject is contentiously sneezing, coughing, shivering or in unconscious stage then this method should be avoided.

Apparatus Required

Clinical glass thermometer and stopwatch.

Clinical Glass Thermometer

One bulb (mercury reservoir) is present at the tip of the thermometer. Clinical glass thermometer has a loop or constriction in the inner tube so that once the mercury column cross the loop or constriction it cannot go down again until it is shaken. If you do not shake the thermometer before use, otherwise it will result in an inaccurate reading.

Two types of graduation scales are present on the outer glass wall of thermometer. One scale is in Fahrenheit and other one is in Celsius (Fig. 19.1).

Procedure of Oral Temperature Measurement

- Clean the clinical glass thermometer and dry it properly.
- Hold the thermometer at the upper end.
- Shake the thermometer to direct mercury column at the lower end (bulb part at the tip).
- Place the bulb part of thermometer in oral cavity just below the tongue.
- Instruct the subject to hold the thermometer firmly by using the lips (not with the help of teeth).

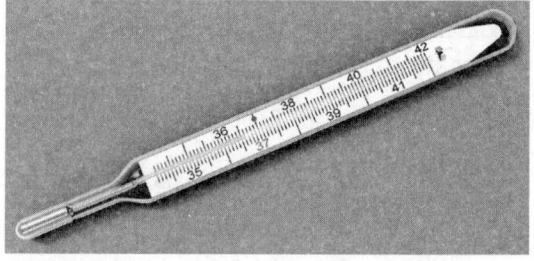

Fig. 19.1: Clinical glass thermometer for oral and axillary temperature measurement *(For colour Fig. see Plate 7)*

- Wait for at least two minutes.
- Then hold the thermometer and instruct the subject to open the mouth.
- Remove the thermometer from the oral cavity.
- Hold the thermometer at eye level and read the mark up to which mercury column reach.
- Enter the observation in notebook.

Axillary Temperature Measurement

This is the safest place to measure body temperature. But in this method we get little bit lower temperature in comparison to the core body temperature.

Apparatus Required

Clinical glass thermometer and stopwatch.

Procedure of Oral Temperature Measurement

- Clean the clinical glass thermometer and dry it properly.
- Hold the thermometer at the upper end.
- Shake the thermometer to direct mercury column at the lower end (bulb part at the tip).
- Place the bulb part of clinical glass thermometer in the centre of axilla (armpit).
- Instruct subject to hold the thermometer firmly by adducting the upper arm close to the midaxillary line and by placing the forearm across the chest.
- Leave the thermometer on that place for 3–4 minutes.
- Then hold the thermometer and remove the thermometer from axillary region of subject.
- Hold the thermometer at eye level and read the mark up to which mercury column reach.
- Enter the observation in notebook.

Rectal Temperature Measurement

This is the most accurate method to measure core body temperature. This method takes more time to achieve core body temperature. This method mainly used in infants and children. In this method privacy should be maintained properly.

Apparatus Required

Rectal thermometer and stopwatch.

Rectal Thermometer

One bulb (mercury reservoir) or probe is present at the tip of the thermometer. This bulb is smaller and rounded than clinical glass thermometer.

Two types of graduation scales are present on the outer glass wall of thermometer. One scale is in Fahrenheit and other one is in Celsius.

Procedure of Rectal Thermometer Measurement

- Clean the rectal thermometer and dry it properly.
- Hold the thermometer at the upper end.
- Apply lubricant jelly (water based) on the probe or bulb part at the tip.
- Gently insert the rectal thermometer 5 to 7 cm in the rectum.
- Leave the thermometer on that place for 4–5 minutes.
- Then hold the thermometer at the end part and remove the thermometer gently from rectal region of subject.
- Hold the thermometer at eye level and read the mark up to which mercury column reach.
- Enter the observation in notebook.

Auditory Canal or Tympanic Temperature Measurement

This method gives an accurate picture of internal body temperature.

Apparatus Required

Tympanic thermometer and stopwatch.

Tympanic Thermometer

It has a projection at the upper part which has an infrared probe or prod (can sense the infrared energy). This probe is covered by a disposable envelop. This particular part is inserted into the ear canal. Tympanic thermometer can sense the infrared energy which is emitted from internal auditory canal and then display the temperature digitally on the display area.

Procedure of Auditory Canal or Tympanic Temperature Measurement

- Clean the probe of tympanic thermometer and dry it properly.
- Insert the tympanic thermometer into the external auditory canal.
- Press and hold the button present in body part of the tympanic thermometer to record the temperature.
- After few seconds recorded temperature displayed in LCD display part of thermometer.
- Enter the observation in notebook.

Forehead Temperature Measurement

This method does not give an accurate picture of body temperature.

Apparatus Required

Band thermometer and stopwatch.

Band Thermometer

It is a typical band like structure. It is a plastic strip thermometer. Temperature sensitive marking are present on the band. It is mercury free and flexible.

Procedure of Forehead Temperature Measurement

- Dry the subject's forehead completely before sticking or placing band thermometer.
- Stick the band thermometer if it is sticky or hold the band thermometer at both ends and press flat against the forehead (half inch above the eyebrows).
- Hold or stick for at least 20–30 seconds.

- Observe the colour change while it is in the forehead to get the body temperature.
- Green colour indicates the body temperature of the subject (colour changing option as indicator of body temperature may vary with different manufacturer are present in details within the band thermometer packet).
- Enter the observation in notebook.

Temporal Artery Temperature Measurement

This method does not give an accurate picture of body temperature. But in this method temperature can be measured in infants during sleep also.

Apparatus Required

Temporal artery thermometer and stopwatch.

Temporal Artery Thermometer

It has a small projection at the upper part which has an infrared probe or prod. This probe can sense the infrared energy which is emitted from the skin over temporal artery. This probe has no cover.

Procedure of Temporal Artery Temperature Measurement

- Place the temporal artery thermometer at the centre of forehead of subject.
- Press and hold the button present in body part of the temporal artery thermometer.
- Slide the probe horizontally on the forehead towards the hairline.
- After few seconds recorded temperature displayed in LCD display part of thermometer.
- Enter the observation in notebook.

EXAMINATION OF PULSE/HEART RATE

INTRODUCTION

Arterial pulse is the pressure wave produced by alternate expansion and relaxation of arteries. Ejection of blood to the aorta during ventricular systole is the reason of expansion of arterial wall (Windkessel effect) and relaxation of arterial wall is occurred during ventricular diastole. Arterial pulse is transmitted along the column of flowing blood in arteries. It is not transmitted by the wall of arteries. That is why arterial pulse is absent at the distal part of obstruction point in the lumen of the artery even when the arterial walls are intact.

Arterial pulse rate is equal to the heart rate except in pulse deficit.

Sites for Pulse Rate Measurement

a. Radial artery
b. Carotid artery

Other sites for pulse rate measurement
a. Brachial artery
b. Femoral artery
c. Pedal pulse
d. Temporal pulse
e. Popliteal pulse

Pulse Rate Measurement from Radial Artery

This is the most common site to measure pulse rate.

Apparatus required: Stopwatch.

Procedure of Pulse Rate Measurement from Radial Artery

- Ask subject to sit comfortably and relax for at least 5 minutes (5–10 minutes) for recording resting pulse rate.
- Ask the subject for permission to assess the pulse.
- Ask the subject to keep his or her hand on the working table.
- Keep the wrist of the subject's hand in semi-flexed and semi-pronated position.
- Palpate the pulse by placing the pad (flat part) of index finger, middle finger and ring finger on the radial artery against the lower

end of radius bone (around 2 cm below the base of the thumb or proximal to the wrist joint) (Fig. 19.2).
- Place all the three fingers in same line and apply very gentle pressure on the radial artery to palpate the pulse (Fig. 19.3).
- Count the pulse for 30 seconds and then multiply with 2 to get the pulse rate in one minute.

Note the following characters of pulse
  i. **Rhythm:** Pulse rate reflects the cardiac rhythm. Normally pulse is regular.

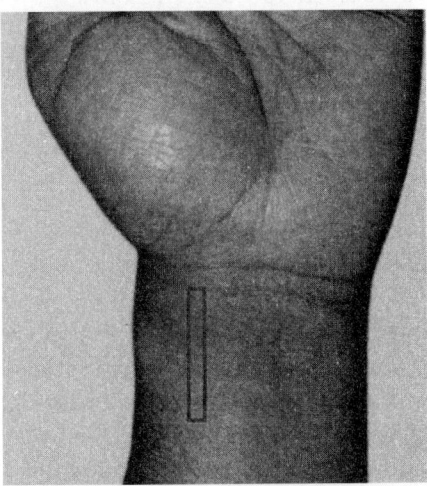

Fig. 19.2: Location of radial artery *(For colour Fig. see Plate 8)*

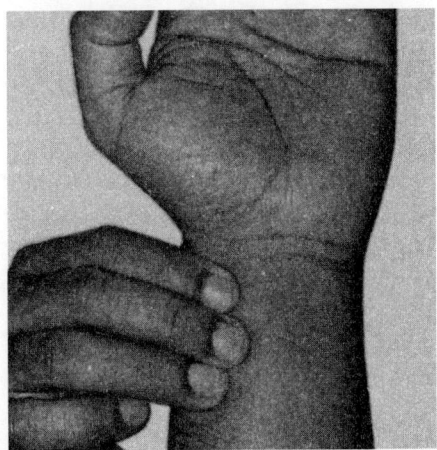

Fig. 19.3: Pulse rate measurement from radial artery *(For colour Fig. see Plate 8)*

When the pulse waves are repeated at regular interval in the consecutive beats then the rhythm is regular, if not, then it is irregular.

Check carefully whether pulse is regular or irregular.

If pulse is irregular then very carefully examine whether it is regularly irregular or irregularly irregular.

Pulse is regularly irregular in respiratory sinus arrhythmia.

Pulse is irregularly irregular in atrial fibrillation.

ii. **Volume of the pulse:** Volume of the pulse is a measure of pulse pressure.

It is assessed by the amplitude of lifting of the fingers felt during palpation. The amplitude of movement of expansion felt by the fingers at the time of palpation is due to passage of pulse wave.

High pulse volume pulse is found in aortic insufficiency, thyrotoxicosis, hypervolemia, etc.

Low volume pulse is found in hypovolemia, aortic stenosis, etc.

iii. **Condition of the arterial wall:** Apply extra pressure on the radial artery by the thumb.

Roll the radial artery against the radial bone by the examining fingers.

Normally, it cannot be felt or is just palpable.

If the artery is hardened, it will feel like a cord.

Pulse Rate Measurement from Carotid Artery

There are two (right and left) carotid arteries. The right carotid artery is located in a groove on the right side of the larynx and the left carotid artery is located in a groove on the left side of the larynx. Either artery can be used to take the carotid pulse.

Apparatus Required

Stopwatch.

Procedure of Pulse Rate Measurement from Carotid Artery

- Ask subject to sit comfortably and relax for at least 5 minutes (5–10 minutes) for recording resting pulse rate.
- Ask the subject for permission to assess the pulse.
- Palpate the carotid pulse by placing the pad (flat part) of index and middle fingers between the larynx and anterior border of sternocleidomastoid muscle of subject's neck.
- Apply very gentle pressure on the carotid artery to palpate the pulse and never assess both carotid arterial pulse simultaneously.
- Count the pulse for 30 seconds and then multiply with 2 to get the pulse rate in one minute.

Examination of Pulse Rate Other than Radial Artery and Carotid Artery

- The temporal pulse is felt at the temple near the ear.
- The brachial pulse is felt on the inside of the elbow.
- The femoral pulse is felt in the groin area (between the anterior portion of the iliac crest and the pubic tubercle).
- The popliteal pulse is felt behind the knee.
- The pedal pulse is felt on top of the foot in the middle of the dorsum of the foot just lateral to the tendon of extensor hallucis longus.

RECORDING OF BLOOD PRESSURE

Blood pressure: The lateral pressure exerted on the wall of blood vessels by the flowing blood is known as blood pressure.

Systolic blood pressure: The maximum lateral pressure exerted on the wall of blood vessels by the flowing blood during the time of systole is known as systolic blood pressure. It denotes the force of contraction of ventricle. Normal value is 110–130 mm Hg.

Diastolic blood pressure: The minimum lateral pressure exerted on the wall of blood vessels by the flowing blood during the time of diastole is known as diastolic blood pressure. It denotes the peripheral resistance. Normal value is 74 to 84 mm Hg.

Pulse pressure: It is the difference between systolic blood pressure and diastolic blood pressures. Normal pulse pressure is around 40 mm Hg.

Mean pressure: It is the average pressure present throughout the cardiac cycle. It is calculated by adding 1/3 pulse pressure to the diastolic pressure.

Methods of Measurement of Blood Pressure

A. Direct method

B. Indirect method

A. Direct Method of Measurement of Blood Pressure

It is an invasive technology. In this method a cannula tube or catheter is directly inserted into the subject's blood vessel. The catheter is then connected to a blood pressure transducer which generates an electrical signal. Nowadays, this method is used in research based experiment.

B. The Indirect Method of Measurement of Blood Pressure

It is a noninvasive technology. In this method, blood flow through the brachial artery of arm (or femoral artery in leg) is occluded by inflating Riva Rocci cuff which is tied on the upper arm (or thigh). After that the pressure is gradually released to start the blood flow through the constricted artery and the changes are studied by palpatory method or oscillatory method or auscultatory method to record the blood pressure.

There are three methods by which indirect blood pressure can be measured:

 i. Palpatory method

 ii. Oscillatory method

iii. Auscultatory method.

Apparatus Required for Measurement of Blood Pressure by Indirect Method

Sphygmomanometer, stethoscope (only required for auscultatory method).

Stethoscope

It has three parts (Fig. 19.4)

a. **Chest Piece:** This part is comprised of two portions—one is bell-shaped part and other is the diaphragm. The bell-shaped part of chest piece is used for listening low pitched sound and the diaphragm part of chest piece is used for listening high pitched sound.

b. **Stem Part:** It is present in between the chest piece and rubber tube. A "click" sound can be heard if the stem part is rotated. By this

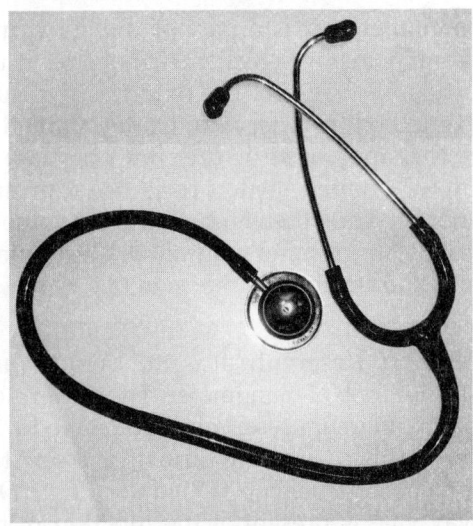

Fig. 19.4: Stethoscope

rotation it can be locked or unlocked and sound transmit from the diaphragm can be blocked or unblocked.

c. **Rubber Tube:** This is a flexible single rubber tube. At the lower end it is connected to the chest piece and at the upper end connected to the ear tube. The function of this rubber tube is to transmit the sound from chest piece to the ear tube.

Few stethoscopes have double lumen tube, i.e. two sound paths inside a single-outer tube which helps to get more clear sound especially used during cardiac examination.

d. **Ear Tubes:** It is made up of metal. It is present in between the rubber tube and ear tips. It transmits sounds from the rubber tube to the ear. This ear tubes are little bit angular in structure just to fit properly in ear canal.

e. **Ear Tips:** Two separate ear tips or ear pieces are attached at tip of metal ear tubes. These are made up of plastic. These ear tips are designed in such a way that can easily and tightly fit in the external auditory canal. The ear tips provide an excellent auditory seal and comfortable fit.

Sphygmomanometer

It is an apparatus for determining arterial blood pressure and consists of following parts (Fig. 19.5):

a. **Manometer:** It is a part of the sphygmo-manometer by which the pressure in the inflatable bag, i.e. the external pressure exerted on the artery can be determined. It is U-shaped in structure. But one limb of this U-shaped structure is broader and shorter. The other limb of the manometer is long, narrow and graduated. The broader and shorter limb is the mercury reservoir (Fig. 19.6).

b. **Mercury Reservoir:** It is the broader and shorter limb of manometer. The uppermost part of mercury reservoir is connected with the rubber tube originating from the inflatable rubber bag of Riva Rocci cuff. One way vale is present at the junction of the rubber tube and uppermost part mercury

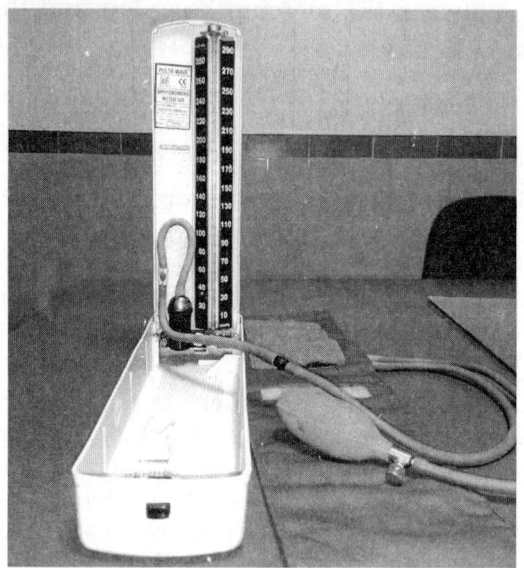

Fig. 19.5: Sphygmomanometer

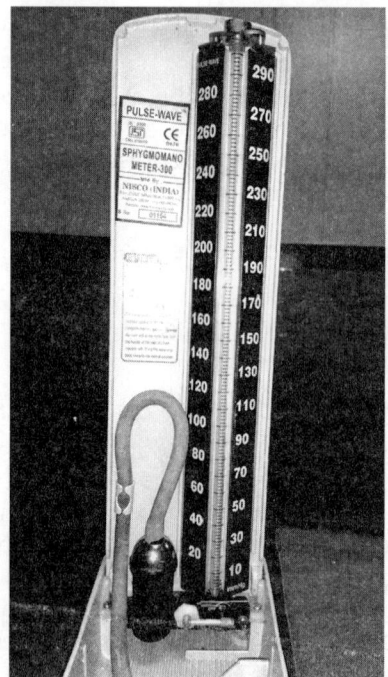

Fig. 19.6: Sphygmomanometer marking

reservoir. This one way valve allow air pressure to transmit from the rubber tube of inflatable bag to the mercury column in the reservoir and also prevent the spilling of mercury when lid of sphygmomano-meter is closed. One stopcock is present in between the mercury reservoir and the long-graduated tube. This stopcock prevents the movement of mercury in between the two limbs of manometer when in closed or switch off condition. But free flow of mercury is possible when it is open or switch on condition.

c. **Graduated Tube:** This is the long and narrow limb of manometer. The tube is graduated into 0 to 300 mm Hg. Each smallest division denotes 2 mm Hg.

d. **Riva Rocci Cuff:** It is comprised of a inner inflatable bag which is enclosed in non-distensible cotton fabric. Normally, the inner inflatable bag is 12–13 cm wide and 24 cm long for arm and 15–18 cm wide and 30 cm long for leg.

Two rubber tubes are attached with the inflatable bag of Riva Rocci cuff. The other end of one rubber tube is attached with the air pump through leak valve screw.

The other end of second tube is connected with the uppermost part of mercury reservoir.

e. **Air Pump:** It is designed in such way that it can easily fit in the fist of normal adult. This air pump is oval in shape. At the lower end one way valve is present. When this one valve opens, air from the external environment can enter in the air pump. It also has a leak valve screw at the upper stem part. The Riva Rocci cuff can be inflated by tightly closing the leak valve screw along with alternate squeezing and relaxation of air pump.

Procedure of Indirect Method of Measurement of Blood Pressure

i. Palpatory Method

Only systolic blood pressure can be measured in this method. Diastolic pressure cannot be determined by this method.

Procedure:
• Ask the subject to sit comfortably or lie down in the couch and relax (mentally and physically) for at least 5 minutes for recording resting blood pressure.

• Ask the subject to keep his or her hand on the working table if the subject is in sitting posture or arm should be kept on the bed if subject is in lie down or supine posture.
• Keep the sphygmomanometer at the heart level. If subject is in sitting posture then sphygmomanometer should be kept at the heart level and if subject is in lie down or supine posture then it should be kept in bed.
• Fully open the lid of sphygmomanometer.
• Switch on the stopcock of mercury reservoir.
• Tie the Riva Rocci cuff around the upper arm just 2–3 cm above the antecubital fossa. The Riva Rocci cuff should not be very tight or very loose.
• Palpate the pulse by placing the pad (flat part) of index finger, middle finger and ring finger on the radial artery against the lower end of radius bone (around 2 cm below the base of the thumb or proximal to the wrist joint).
• Tightly close the leak valve screw.
• Alternately squeeze and relax the air pump to inflate the cuff.
• Raise the mercury column slowly up to 150 to 160 mm Hg (at least 40 mm Hg above the point when pulse disappeared).
• Then, open the leak valve screw in such a way that mercury column will fall in a rate of 2–3 mm Hg at each time.
• Record the pressure at which point pulse again reappeared for the first time.
• The height of the mercury in graduated manometer at this moment denotes the systolic blood pressure.
• Enter the observation in notebook.

ii. Auscultatory Method

This is the most convenient and reliable method out of three method. Systolic and diastolic pressure both can be measured in this method and is generally used in daily practice.

Procedure
• Ask the subject to sit comfortably or lie down in the couch and relax (mentally and physically) for at least 5 minutes for recording resting blood pressure.

- Ask the subject to keep his or her hand on the working table if the subject is in sitting posture or arm should be kept on the bed if subject is in lie down or supine posture.
- Keep the sphygmomanometer at the heart level. If subject is in sitting posture then sphygmomanometer should be kept at the heart level and if subject is in lie down or supine posture then it should be kept in bed.
- Fully open the lid of sphygmomanometer.
- Switch on the stopcock of mercury reservoir
- Tie the Riva Rocci cuff around the upper arm just 2–3 cm above the antecubital fossa. The Riva Roccicuff should not be very tight or very loose.
- Locate the place at antecubital fossa where brachial artery bifurcated into radial and ulnar artery. This place is just medial to the tendon of the bicep at antecubital fossa.
- Hold the chest piece of the stethoscope with the help of index, middle and ring finger of your dominant hand.
- Place the chest piece of the stethoscope with three fingers at that particular area and place the thumb at posterior part of the cubital fossa.
- Tightly close the leak valve screw.
- Alternately squeeze and relax the air pump to inflate the cuff.
- Raise the mercury column slowly up to 150 to 160 mm Hg (at least 40 mm Hg above the point of systolic blood pressure determined by palpatory method).
- Then, open the leak valve screw in such a way that mercury column will fall in a rate of 2–3 mm Hg at each time.
- Record the mercury column or pressure at which point the first sharp, clear, tapping sound appeared. This pressure denotes the systolic blood pressure.

  At a point where pressure in the cuff just balances the arterial pressure (or arterial pressure just overcomes pressure in cuff) an intermittent flow of blood begins in the narrow artery distal to the cuff producing a sharp light and tapping sound which is audible by stethoscope. This pressure is the systolic blood pressure.

- As the mercury column reduced this sound changes its intensity and quality and can be divided into 5 phases (Korotokoff sounds), i.e.
  1. **Clear tapping sound or Phase I:** It is first heard at systolic blood pressure point and it is continued for 10–12 mm Hg when the pressure gradually lowered.
  2. **Murmurish sound or Phase II:** For next 10–15 mm Hg the sound becomes changed into murmurish sound.
  3. **Loud banging sound or Phase III:** In the next phase sound is much louder, clear and knocking or banging like sounds auscualtated. It is continued for next 10–14 mm Hg.
  4. **Muffled sound or Phase IV:** Suddenly the sound becomes muffled and it is continued for next 5–6 mm Hg.
  5. **Disappearance of sound or Phase V:** After phase IV sound finally disappears.
- Record the mercury column or pressure at which point sound completely disappears. This pressure indicates diastolic pressure.
- Some people prefer to note the diastolic pressure at the point where sudden muffling of sound appears (stage IV) rather than when it completely disappears.
- Enter the observation in notebook.

iii. Oscillatory Method

Procedure

- Ask the subject to sit comfortably or lie down in the couch and relax (mentally and physically) for at least 5 minutes for recording resting blood pressure.
- Ask the subject to keep his or her hand on the working table if the subject is in sitting posture or arm should be kept on the bed if subject is in lie down or supine posture.
- Keep the sphygmomanometer at the heart level. If subject is in sitting posture then sphygmomanometer should be kept at the heart level and if subject is in lie down or supine posture then it should be kept in bed.
- Fully open the lid of sphygmomanometer.
- Switch on the stopcock of mercury reservoir.

- Tie the Riva Rocci cuff around the upper arm just 2–3 cm above the antecubital fossa. The Riva Roccicuff should not be very tight or very loose.
- Tightly close the leak valve screw.
- Alternately squeeze and relax the air pump to inflate the cuff .
- Raise the mercury column slowly up to 150 to 160 mm Hg (at least 40 mm Hg above the point of systolic blood pressure determined by palpatory method).
- Then, open the leak valve screw in such a way that mercury column will fall in a rate of 2–3 mm Hg at each time.

- Record the mercury column or pressure at which point the first oscillation in the mercury column is observed. This pressure denotes the systolic blood pressure.
- Record the mercury column or pressure at which point oscillation in the mercury column is completely disappears. This pressure denotes the diastolic blood pressure.
- Enter the observations in notebook.

Normal Value of Blood Pressure

- Average systolic blood pressure 120 mm Hg
- Average diastolic blood pressure 80 mm Hg

RECORDING OF ELECTROCARDIOGRAM (ECG)

INTRODUCTION

Electrocardiography refers to the recording of summed up electrical events of all cardiac muscle fibers generated during each heart beat. Willem Einthoven developed the technique of electrocardiography.

Apparatus Required

ECG machine (electrocardiograph), electrodes (leads), ECG graph paper and electrode gel.

A. ECG Machine

ECG machine record the electrical events from the entire heart muscle (i.e. the atria and the ventricles). It consists of very sensitive Galvanometer provided with a stylus or pen, which gets electrically heated up and inscribes on a thermosensitive graph paper. The machine operates on battery or electricity.

There are various controlling switch in ECG machine.

Power on/off switch: This switch controls the power supply in ECG machine (Fig. 19.7).

Calibration controlling switch: This switch controls calibration. Amplitude is represented vertically in millvolts in ECG graph paper, which is adjusted with calibration switch.

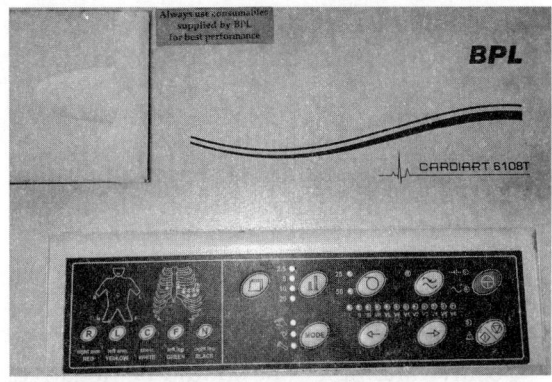

Fig. 19.7: ECG machine (For colour Fig. see Plate 8)

Before recording ECG, the machine should be calibrated to show a displacement of 10 mm for 1 mV.

Centring switch: By pressing this switch the base line of the stylus or pen can be adjusted at the centre of the paper.

Speeds control switch: ECG paper can be moved in two speeds. Speed can be selected either in 25 mm/second or 50 mm/second. Normally, a speed of 25 mm/second is used.

Various leads selector switch: By the help of these switches one can record the specific lead's result.

B. Electrodes and Electrode Gel

Electrodes are made up of metal. These are either plate like structure (electrode of limb leads) or cup like structure (electrode of chest leads). Electrodes are connected with the ECG machine by cables.

Electrode gel is thick and highly conductive in nature. Before placing the leads at particular part of body, electrode gel is applied at that part.

C. Electrocardiographic Leads

Two types of electrocardiographic leads are there:

a. Bipolar leads

b. Uniploar leads

a. **Bipolar leads:** Both the electrodes are active in bipolar leads.

The bipolar leads are of two types: The standard bipolar limb leads and bipolar chest leads.

The standard bipolar limb leads: The original electrocardiographic leads system was developed by Willem Einthoven (1860–1927).

The standard bipolar limb leads record the potential difference between two active electrodes out of which one should be positive and other one should be negative.

The standard limb leads are designated by Roman numerals. These are:

- Lead I = Left arm LA (+) and right arm RA (–), i.e. [LA–RA]

- Lead II = Left leg LL (+) and right arm RA (–), i.e. [LL–RA]

- Lead III = Left leg LL (+) and left arm LA (–), i.e. [LL–LA]

In 12 leads electrocardiography, Lead I, Lead II and Lead III records are included.

The bipolar chest leads: The bipolar chest leads are not normally used in recording of ECG.

b. **Unipolar leads:** In unipolar lead has only one active electrode (exploring electrode).

This leads record the potential difference between an exploring electrode (active electrode) and an indifferent electrode (reference electrode with zero potential).

The "exploring" electrode is placed on an area of the body surface.

The "indifferent" electrode is kept at approximately zero potential by connecting all the electrodes placed on the right arm, left arm and left leg to a central terminal (V_T) through a 5000 ohm resistance. Because of this high voltage resistance, indifferent electrode keeps on at constant voltage.

The unipolar leads are of two types:

i. Unipolar limb leads

ii. Unipolar precordial leads or Unipolar chest leads.

i. **Unipolar limb leads:** These are designated by letter V

There are VR, VL and VF

VR: Potential difference between right arm (exploring electrode) and an indifferent electrode

VL: Potential difference between left arm (exploring electrode) and an indifferent electrode

VF: Potential difference between left leg (exploring electrode) and an indifferent electrode.

- VF reflects the electrical activity of inferior surface of the heart.

- VL that of the left upper side of heart.

- VR the cavity of the ventricles.

- But the amplitude of deflection is very small and sometimes difficult to interpret.

- So, unipolar limb leads are not much used in practice.

- Augmented limb leads are generally used in recent practice.

Augmented limb leads

There are three augmented limb leads: **aVR, aVL and aVF** ("a" denotes augmented).

This augmentation is done by removing the contribution of the respective limb to the V_T. In augmented limb leads the amplitude of wave increased by around 50% in comparison to the unaugmented lead.

This augmented limb leads record potential difference between one limb and the other two limbs.

In aVR exploring electrode connected to the right arm

In aVL exploring electrode connected to the left arm

In aVF exploring electrode connected to the left leg

1. aVR: Potential difference between Right Arm (RA) and Left Arm (LA) + Left Leg (LL), i.e. RA – (LA+LL)

2. aVL: Potential difference between Left Arm (LA) and Right Arm (RA) + Left Leg (LL), i.e. LA – (RA+LL)

3. aVF: Potential difference between Left Leg (LL) and Right Arm (RA) + Left Arm (LA), i.e. LL – (RA+LA)

ii. Unipolar chest leads or precordial leads: Chest lead is a small metal cup electrode with a rubber bulb at the back side. The electrode is kept in position by vacuum created by squeezing the rubber bulb.

These leads record the potentials from the anterior surface of the heart from the right side towards the left side.

The positions of the leads are as follows:

- V_1: 4th intercostal space at the right border of sternum.
- V_2: 4th intercostal space at the left border of sternum.
- V_3: In between V_2 and V_4
- V_4: 5th left intercostal space at the midclavicular line
- V_5: 5th left intercostal space at left anterior axillary line
- V_6: 5th left intercostal space at the mid-axillary line.

D. ECG Graph Paper

The ECG graph paper is a thermosensitive graph paper. It is chemically treated for proper writing by ECG machine stylus or pen. It is divided into one millimetre squares by thin lines. Every fifth line is thickened both horizontally and vertically.

ECG is recorded on standard speed (25 mm/sec.). Therefore, horizontally, one square represents 0.04 sec.

Procedure of Recording ECG

- Ask the subject to lie down on a couch or bed, comfortably and fully relaxed condition.
- Ask subject to remove any short of metal if present in contact of subject's body.
- Apply electrode gel on the following places of the body and connect the appropriate electrode.

  a. Just below the two wrists and connect the electrode clip RA at right arm and LA at left arm.

  b. Just above the two ankles and connect the electrode clip RL at right leg and LL at left leg.

  c. V_1 marked electrode with rubber bulb in 4th intercostals space at the right border of sternum.

  d. V_2 marked electrode with rubber bulb in 4th intercostal space at the left border of sternum.

  e. V_3 marked electrode with rubber bulb in between V_2 and V_4.

  f. V_4 marked electrode with rubber bulb in 5th left intercostal space at the mid-clavicular line.

  g. V_5 marked electrode with rubber bulb in 5th left intercostal space at left anterior axillary line.

h. V_6 marked electrode with rubber bulb in 5th left intercostals space at the mid axillary line.

- Connect the connector cable of electrode to the ECG machine.
- Check whether sufficient amount ECG graph paper roll is present or not.
- Switch on the ECG machine and centre the stylus.
- Adjust calibration control switch to check deflection at 10 mm for 1 mV.
- Adjust the speed at 25 mm/second by speeds control switch.
- Then press the automatic mode switch in ECG machine to record twelve leads, i.e. I, II, III, aVR, aVL, aVF and V_1, V_2, V_3, V_4, V_5 and V_6 or selective lead ECG can be taken in manual mode.
- Paste the ECG paper in the note book and enter the observation in notebook.
- The ECG record shows. P, Q, R, S, T waves.
- Recording and analysis of ECG gives information about:

a. The anatomical orientation of the heart.

b. The relative size of its chambers.

c. Variety of disturbances of rhythm and conduction.

d. The extent, location and progress of ischaemic damage to the myocardium.

e. The effect of altered electrolyte concentrations.

f. Heart rate can also be calculated from ECG.

1

Measurements

INTERNATIONAL SYSTEM (SI)

Base Units

Unit	Quantity	Symbol
metre	length	M
kilogram	mass	Kg
second	time	S
litre	volume	L
mole	amount of matter	Mol
pascal	pressure	Pa
joule	energy	J

Temperature Conversion

- Celsius (C) to Fahrenheit (F)
  $$°F = (°C × 1.8) + 32$$
- Fahrenheit (F) to Celsius (C)
  $$°C = (°F − 32) ÷ 1.8$$

Prefixes

Prefix	Multiplier	Symbol
tera-	10^{12}	T
giga-	10^9	G
mega-	10^6	M
kilo-	10^3	k
hecto-	10^2	h
deca-	10^1	da
deci-	10^{-1}	d
centi-	10^{-2}	c
milli-	10^{-3}	m
micro-	10^{-6}	μ
nano-	10^{-9}	n
pico-	10^{-12}	p
femto-	10^{-15}	f

2 Normal Value for Selected Blood Tests

Test (specimen)		SI units (traditional units)
Aminotransferases (serum)		
Alanine aminotransferase (ALT)		0–35 U/L (same)
Aspartate aminotransferase (ALT)		0–35 U/L (same)
Ammonia (plasma)		12–55 mmol/L (20–120 μg/dL)
Bilirubin (serum)	Conjugated	< 5.0 pmol/L (< 0.5 mg/dL)
	Unconjugated	18–20 pmol/L (0.2-1.0 mg/dL)
Blood urea nitrogen (BUN) (serum)		2.9–9.3 mmol/L (8–26 mg/dL)
Cholesterol, total (plasma)		< 5.2 mmol/L (< 200 mg/dL)
HDL cholesterol (plasma)		> 1.0 mmol/L (> 40 mg/dL)
LDL cholesterol (plasma)		< 3.2 mmol/L (< 130 mg/dL)
Creatinine (serum)	Males	10–40 pmol/L (0.15–0.5 mg/dL)
	Female	30–70 pmol/L (0.35–0.9 mg/dL)
Creatine phosphokinase (CPK) (serum)		0–130 U/L
Creatinine (serum)		45–105 μmol/L (0.5–1.2 mg/dL)
Electrolytes (plasma)	Calcium (total)	2.1–2.6 mmol/L (9–10.5 mg/dL)
	Chloride	95–105 mmol/L (95–105 mEq/L)
	Magnesium	0.7–1.2 mmol/L (1.3–2.1 mEq/L)
	Potassium	3.5–5.0 mmol/L (3.5–5.0 mEq/L)
	Sodium	136–148 mmol/L (136–148 mEq/L)

Contd...

Test (specimen)		SI units (traditional units)
Glucose (plasma)		3.9–6.1 mmol/L (70–110 mg/dL)
Haemoglobin (whole blood)	Males	140–180 g/L (14–18 g/100 mL)
	Females	120–160 g/L (12–16 g/100 mL)
Iron, total (serum)	Males	14–32 μmol/L (80–180 μg/dL)
	Females	11–29 μ mol/L (60–160 μg/dL)
Lactic dehydrogenase (LDH) (serum)		71–207 U/L (same)
Lipids (serum)	Total	4.0–8.5 g/L (400–850 mg/dL)
	Triglycerides	0.1–1.9 g/L (100–190 mg/dL)
pH (blood)		7.35–7.45
Platelet count (whole blood)		150,000–400,000/μL
Protein (serum)	Total	60–80 g/L (6–8 g/dL)
	Albumin	40–60 g/L (4–6 g/dL)
	Globulin	23–35 g/L (2.3–3.5 g/dL)
Red blood cell count	Males	4.5–6.5 millon/μL
(whole blood)	Females	3.9–5.6 millon/μL
Uric acid (serum)		120–420 μmol/L (2.0–7.0 mg/dL)
White blood cell count (whole blood)		5,000–10,000/μL
Neutrophils		60–70% of all WBCs
Basophils		0.5–1% of all WBCs
Eosinophils		2–4% of all WBCs
Lymphocytes		20–25% of all WBCs
Monocytes		3–8% of all WBCs

Key to symbols

g: gram; mg: milligram; μg: microgram; U: units; L: litre; dL: decilitre; mL: millilitre; μ: microlitre; mEq/L: Milliequivalents per litre; mmol/L: millimoles per litre; μmol/L: micromoles per litre; >: greater than; <: less than.

Index